Losch, Henry

German-English medical thesaurus

Inktank publishing

Losch, Henry

German-English medical thesaurus

Inktank publishing, 2018

www.inktank-publishing.com

ISBN/EAN: 9783747745359

A GERMAN-ENGLISH Medical Thesaurus,

OR

Treasure of Single and Compound Medical Words and Terms, With Dialogues, Idiomatic Phrases and Proverbs, Etc., Etc.

AND

GERMAN AND ENGLISH INDEXES

FOR

PHYSICIANS AND MEDICAL STUDENTS.

BY

REV. HENRY LOSCH, M. D.,

AUTHOR OF "IMPROVED METHOD AND COMPLETE MANUAL FOR THE SYSTEMATIC AND PRACTICAL STUDY OF THE GERMAN LANGUAGE;" AUTHOR OF "PSALTER, HARP AND SONG;" TRANSLATOR OF GOETHE'S POETICAL WORKS, INCLUDING BOTH PARTS OF "FAUST," IN THE ORIGINAL METRES, ETC., ETC., ETC.

PHILADELPHIA, PA.:
PUBLISHED BY THE AUTHOR.
1895.

PREFACE.

From the frequent inquiries coming to me concerning the nature of a convenient manual like the following, I could not mistake the suggestion, that a book of this kind was a great desideratum. By the advice of a few friends, whom I consulted regarding this subject, and from the increasing conviction that the book was positively needed, I felt encouraged to undertake the work, although the task of writing such a book seemed to me not altogether without difficulty. The success of my "Improved Method and Complete Manual for the Systematic and Practical Study of the German Language," however, filled me with confidence, giving me also the sure and true basis for the practical construction of this work. In regard to the various parts of the book, much labor was necessary for the information I desired to present, and to what extent this had to be done, can be judged from the manifold contents of the book, demonstrating also that the parts and subjects treated, were what the scope of such a work seemed to demand. The German and English indexes alone contain over twenty thousand words. For accurate and convenient reference I have added, at the close of the book, the complete schedule of declensions and list of irregular verbs of my German Grammar. The reason for making this addition arose from the conviction that if persons studying or having studied the German Language, on the one hand, can classify a noun at sight by looking at the schedule of the terminations of each declension, in as much as there are four different classes of declensions in German, after which the nouns must be declined, wherefore every representative noun in this work has attached the number of the respective class of declension, to which it belongs; and on the other hand such persons also know the irregular verbs and can readily refer by looking at the schedules of conjugations of these verbs, to the various changes they undergo in the process of conjugation in the various tenses, etc., they certainly have overcome two of the foremost difficulties in the study of this language. To study a language effectively and successfully is to study its various parts of speech. Though these are nominally the same in German as in English, there is still a vast difference in the extent of the study these various parts require in order to become familiar with them for ready comprehension in reading and in speaking the language. The study of the German articles, for instance, the first of the ten parts of speech, requires infinitely more study in German than in English, because in English there is but one article for the three genders, masculine, feminine and neuter, but in German every gender has a special article which is declined differently in each of the four cases, Nominative, Genitive, Dative and Accusative in the singular. There are besides many definite words standing often in the place of the definite articles, declined like these, and many indefinite words standing often in place of the indefinite articles, declined like these in the singular, but like the definite articles in the plural. To study thoroughly and successfully these and other complicated and difficult parts of speech in the German Language cannot be accomplished by so-called easy-phrase-object-picture-methods. There must be faithful and persistent study with the aid of a thorough grammar, I am frank to say, like mine, not only the latest, but also the most complete in the market. And the pronunciation of the words of the German Language can only be acquired from the lips of a competent teacher, a native German. It cannot be taught by parrot-method or burlesque sound-imitation in letters and words having no real existence and hanging merely like spiderwebs in the mind, etc.

Hoping and trusting that the book will fulfill the purpose for which it is designed, I solicit the favorable consideration of every physician and student desiring to familiarize themselves with the vast treasures of the German Medical Terminology, through the unusually numerous compounds, the special basis of this work in the German Medical Literature.

PHILADELPHIA. HENRY LOSCH.

CONTENTS.

Part First.

Medical Terms Considered Systematically.

A. Man Considered Generically.

Part Second.

Gesundheitliche, Medizinische, Chirurgische and Häusliche Angelegenheiten, Maszregeln und Mittel, Hygienic, Medical, Chirurgical and Domestic Affairs, Measures and Means.

Part Third

PART FIRST.

SIMPLE AND COMPOUND MEDICAL TERMS SYSTEMATIZED.

A. MAN CONSIDERED GENERICALLY.

§ 1. *Construction of Compounds* (*Komposita, zusammengesetzte Wörter*).

Though a simple word or term is easily understood, it needs to be said that a compound consists, either in several nominatives put together, or the first word of the compound, generally appearing in the genitive form (singular or plural), to which one or several words in the nominative form adhere, is joined to the *root* of the last word of the compound which contains the *rootsyllable* from which it is derived, e. g.

1* **Brust-schlüsselbein-zitzenfortsatz-muskel-schwund,** m. 1.,† (literally: breast-clavicle-mastoid process-muscle atrophy) i. e. atrophy of the sterno-cleido-mastoid muscle.—The rootword is Schwund, m. 1. atrophy (from v. ir. schwinden, to diminish, shrink).

2 **Augen-muskel-lähmung,** f. paralysis of the muscle of the eye; Lähmung, f. (from lähmen, to paralyze) is the rootword.

3 **Bacillen-Lehre,** f. (from Bacillen, bacilli, and Lehre, f. doctrine) means: Bacteriology.

4 **Lebens-anfang,** m. 1. (from Leben, n. 1. life, in the genitive form, and Anfang, m. 1. beginning (from v. ir. anfangen, to begin) means: beginning of life, etc.

In compound words formed of nouns, adjectives, adverbs, etc., the entire word becomes an adjective, e. g.:

5 **bacillen-haltend,** adj. (from Bacillen, in the nominative form, plural, and haltend, adj. (from v. ir. halten, to hold) means: bacilli-containing.

6 **lebens-voll,** adj. (from Leben, life, gen. sing. and voll, adj. full) means: full of life.

Familiarity, therefore, with the rootword or the last word in compounds, is absolutely necessary for the full understanding of German Medical literature, since so unusually many compound words are used.

§ 2. *Generic Term Man.*

The *generic* name (Gattungsname, m. 2.) regarding the

7 **Art,** f. kind, sort, race, sex, species of a man, as a human being (menschliches Wesen, n. 2.) is:

8 **Mensch,** m. 3. man, and applies to *any* man, e. g.:

---

* These numbers correspond with the numbers of the respective words in the dictionaries for easy reference.

† *m.* for *masculine* is attached to *masculine* nouns, *f.* for *feminine* and *n.* for *neuter* nouns. The number attached to a noun indicates the form or class of declension, to which it belongs. Feminine nouns are not numbered, because all belong to the fourth class of declensions. See schedule of declensions at the close.

9 **Arzt**, m. 1. doctor, physician.
10 **Ärztin**, f. female physician.
11 **Doktor**, m. 2. doctor.
12 **Chirurg**, m. 3. } surgeon, etc.
13 **Wundarzt**, m. 1. }
(For a full list in compounds see § 33, 4.)

§ 3. *A Man's General Condition.*

The following *adjectives* may be applied to a man, who may be:

14 **abnorm**, abnormal, irregular.
15 **abwesend**, absent.
16 **achtbar**, honorable, respectable.
17 **achtlos**, inattentive.
18 **achtsam**, attentive.
19 **acclimatisiert**, acclimatized.
20 **accomodiert**, accommodated.
21 **accreditiert**, accredited.
22 **aktiv**, active, effective.
23 **albern**, silly, simple, dull.
24 **alemanisch**, } Allemannic,
allemannisch, } German.
25 **allein** (e), alone, single.
26 **alt**, old.
27 **altersschwach**, weak by old age.
28 **amerikanisch**, American.
29 **ängstlich**, } anxious, fearful.
30 **angstvoll**, }
31 **anwesend**, present.
32 **arbeitsam**, industrious, laborious.
33 **arg**, bad, malicious.
34 **ärgerlich**, angry, fretful.
35 **argwöhnisch**, suspicious.
36 **arm**, } poor, needy.
37 **ärmlich**, } miserable.
38 **armselig**, } wretched.
39 **artig**, } courteous.
40 **höflich**, } polite.
41 **aufgelegt**, disposed (either ill or well).
42 **aufgeregt**, excited.
43 **aufgeweckt**, awake, awakened.
44 **aufmerksam**, attentive.
45 **barsch**, harsh, sharp.
46 **bayerisch**, Bavarian.
47 **bedächtig**, } careful, heedful.
48 **bedachtsam**, }
49 **bedauerlich**, deplorable.
50 **bedürftig**, needy.
51 **begünstigt**, favored, encouraged.
52 **behaftet** (with), afflicted, infected with.
53 **behaglich**, easy, comfortable.
54 **beherzt**, bold, courageous.
55 **bejammert**, pitied, lamented.
56–7 **beklagenswert or -würdig**, commiserable, deplorable, miserable.
58 **beklommen** (fr. v. ir. beklemmen, to press, oppress), burdened.
59 **bekümmert**, afflicted.
60–1 **beneidenswert or -würdig**, enviable.
62 **benötigt**, needy of, to be in need of.
63 **beraubt**, deprived of.
64 **berauscht**, } inebriated or in-
65 **betrunken**, } toxicated.
66 **besinnungslos**, senseless.
67 **besorgt**, afraid, apprehensive.
68 **bestürzt**, perplexed.
69 **betrübt**, grieved, troubled, vexed.
65 **betrunken** (see berauscht).
70 **beunruhigt**, alarmed, uneasy.
71 **bevollmächtigt**, empowered.
72 **bewuszt**,* conscious of.
73 **bewusztlos**, unconscious.
74 **blöde**, timid, bashful.
75 **bös or böse**, } angry, irritable,
76 **bösartig**, } passionate.
77 **mürrisch**, }
78 **brav or** } gentle, brave, stal-
79 **(gut)**, } wart, valiant.
80 **comatös**, comatose or (comatous), morbidly drowsy.
81 **dankbar**, grateful, thankful.
82 **deutsch**, German.
83 **ehelich**, married.
84 **ehelos**, unmarried.

---

* Whenever the German *sz* (which as a compound consonant cannot be divided) as here in bewuszt, occurs, I prefer to give it by *sz* and not by *ss*, the common rendering of it. In words, therefore, like Fusz (foot), Grösze (greatness), etc., not *ss*, so *incorrectly* universally used (though some represent it now in German in Roman type by the character *fz*, unknown in English), but *sz* must stand. For otherwise writing the plural of Fusz, e. g., Füsse, it would be divided Füs-se, whilst its plural, given correctly, is Füsze, and, therefore, must be divided Fü-sze, etc., etc.

85 **ehrbar or ehrlich**, honest.
86 **elend or elendig**, miserable, distressed.
87 **eitel**, vain.
88 **epileptisch or** } epileptical,
89 **fallsüchtig**, }
90 **erschlafft**, relaxed, enervated.
91 **europäisch**, European.
92 **fett**, } fat, obese, corpulent.
93 **fettleibig**, }
94 **fieberfrei**, } not feverish.
fieberlos, }
95 **fieberhaft**, } aguish.
96 **fieberisch**, }
97 **französisch**, French.
98 **freisinnig**, free-thinking.
99 **freudig**, joyful.
100 **friedlich**, } peaceful.
101 **friedsam**, }
102 **froh**, } cheerful.
fröhlich, } mirthful.
103 **frugal**, saving, economical.
104 **gefühllos**, apathetic, insensible.
105 **gefühlvoll**, sensitive.
106 **gegenwärtig**, present.
107 **geisteskrank**, } imbecile.
108 **geistesschwach**, }
109 **geistesstumpf**, torpid.
110 **geistreich**, genial, ingenious.
111 **geistvoll**, spirited, full of spirit.
112 **gekränkt**, grieved, mortified, vexed.
113 **gelassen**, } calm, quiet, cool,
geduldig, } patient.
114 **gemütlich**, tender, kind-hearted, good-natured.
115 **gemütskrank**, melancholy.
116 **genügsam**, contented, satisfied.
117 **germanisch**, German.
118 **geschäftig**, busy, occupied.
119 **geschickt**, skilful.
120 **gesellschaftlich**, social, sociable.
121 **gesund**, healthy, well, sound.
122 **gewissenhaft**, conscientious.
123 **gewissenlos**, not conscientious.
124 **gichtbrüchig**, }
125 **gichtig**, } gouty.
gichtisch, }
126 **gierig**, avaricious.
127 **gleichartig**, congenial, homogeneous.
128 **gleichgültig**, indifferent.
129 **glücklich**, } happy, blessed.
130 **glückselig**, }
131 **gräszlich**, ugly.
132 **grausam**, cruel, inhuman.
133 **grindig**, scabby, scurfy.
134 **grosz**, big, great, large.
135 **groszsprecherisch**, boastful.
136 **grübelnd**, } worrying,
137 **grübelkrank**, } splenetic.
138 **gutmütig**, good-hearted.
139 **gynäkomorphisch**, shaped like a woman.
140 **gynäkophonisch**, having a womanly voice.
141 **habsüchtig**, grasping.
142 **hadersüchtig**, quarrelsome.
143 **halbtot**, half dead.
144 **halsstarrig**, obstinate.
145 **händelsüchtig**, quarrelsome.
146 **harsch**, blunt, unpolished.
147 **harthörig**, hard of hearing.
148 **hartköpfig**, obstinate.
149 **hartleibig**, costive.
150 **hartnäckig**, obstinate, stubborn.
151 **hassenswert**, } hateful.
hassenswürdig, }
152 **häszlich**, ugly, detestable.
153 **hastig**, } hasty.
eilig, }
154 **häuslich**, domestic.
155 **heftig**, vehement.
156 **heidnisch**, heathenish, barbarous.
157 **heil**, healed, whole, sound.
158 **heilbar**, curable.
159 **heimtückisch**, obstinate.
160 **heiszblütig**, hot-blooded.
161 **heiter**, cheerful.
162 **hektisch**, hectic.
163 **heldenmütig**, heroic.
164 **helvetisch**, Helvetic.
165 **heroisch**, heroical.
166 **herzhaft**, hearty, heartily.
167 **herzlos**, coolly, heartless.
168 **hessisch**, Hessian.
169 **heuchlerisch**, hypocritical.
170 **hilf or hülfreich**, helpful.
171 **hitzig**, quick, acute, inflammatory.
172 **hochmütig**, proud, haughty, arrogant.
173 **hochtönig**, high-toned.
174 **hoffärtig**, vain.
175 **höflich**, polite.
176 **holländisch**, Dutch.
177 **human**, humane.
178 **humoristisch**, humorous.
179 **hypochondrisch**, hypochondriacal.
180 **hypogastrisch**, hypogastric.

181 **idealistisch,** idealistic.
182 **idiopathisch,** idiopathic.
183 **idiotisch,** idiotic.
184 **imaginär,** imaginative.
185 **impertinent,** impertinent.
186 **intellectuel,** intellectual.
187 **italienisch,** Italian.
188 **jung,** young.
189 **kahl,** bald.
190 **kahlköpfig,** bald-headed.
191 **kalt,** cold.
192 **kaltblütig,** cold-blooded.
193 **keusch,** chaste.
194 **kindisch,** childish.
195 **kindlich,** child-like.
196 **klagend,** lamenting.
197 **klein,** little, short, small.
198 **kleindenkend,** narrow-minded.
199 **klug,** prudent.
200 **knirschend,** (Zähne, teeth), grinding.
201 **kräftig,** mighty, strong, powerful.
202 **krank,** ill, sick, indisposed.
203 **krätzig,** itchy.
204 **kritisch,** critical.
205 **kühn,** audacious, bold.
206 **kurzatmig,** short-breathed.
207 **kurzsichtig,** near-sighted.
208 **lahm,** lame.
209 **langmütig,** long-suffering, patient.
210 **langsam,** slow.
211 **lästig,** troublesome.
212 **launenhaft,** capricious.
213 **launich,** } peevish, whimsical.
launisch, }
214 **lebendig,** } alive, gay,
215 **lebhaft,** } lively, brisk,
216 **lebenskräftig,** } energetic, vigorous.
217 **ledig,** } single,
218 **unverheiratet,** } unmarried.
219 **leichtfertig,** frivolous.
220 **leichtherzig,** light-minded.
221 **leidend,** suffering.
222 **leidenschaftlich,** passionate, eager.
223 **lungensüchtig,** consumptive, phthisical.
224 **lustig,** jolly, merry.
225 **mager,** thin, lean.
226 **mondsüchtig,** lunatic.
227 **müde,** fatigued, tired.
228 **munter,** mirthful, awake.
229 **mürrisch,** peevish, angry looking.
230 **nachläszig,** negligent, neglectful.
231 **naiv,** ingenious, natural.
232 **nüchtern,** sober, quiet.
233 **ohnmächtig,** powerless, fainting, swooning.
234 **ordentlich,** orderly.
235 **östreichisch,** Austrian.
236 **pachämisch,** pachemic, thick-blooded.
237 **pfälzisch,** from the Palatinate or Bavaria on the Rhine.
238 **passiv,** passive.
239 **permanent,** permanent, continuing, lasting.
240 **phantastisch,** phantastical.
241 **phlegmatisch,** phlegmatic, indifferent.
242 **polnisch,** Polish.
243 **rasend,** raging, raving.
244 **rastlos,** restless.
245 **reizbar,** irritable.
246 **röchelnd,** wheezing.
247 **ruhelos,** restless, unquiet.
248 **ruhig,** quiet, tranquil.
249 **rüstig,** vigorous.
250 **schmächtig,** feeble.
251 **schmutzig,** dirty, unclean.
252 **schnarchend,** rattling with noise in the throat, wheezing.
253 **schwach,** } weak,
254 **schwächlich,** } feeble.
255 **schwermütig,** } melancholy, hypochon-
256 **melancholisch,** } driacal.
257 **sinnlich,** sensitive, sensual.
258 **sinnlos,** senseless.
259 **sorgfältig,** careful.
260 **sorglos,** careless.
261 **spanisch,** Spanish.
262 **stark,** strong, mighty.
263 **starrsüchtig,** cataleptic.
264 **stockblind,** totally blind.
265 **stocktaub,** totally deaf.
266 **sympathetisch,** sympathetic
267 **sympathisch,** sympathic.
268 **syphilitisch,** syphilitic.
269 **taubstumm,** deaf and dumb.
270 **thätig,** active, busy.
271 **thöricht,** foolish, unwise.
272 **toll,** frantic, insane.
273 **tot,** dead.
274 **träge,** indolent, lazy.
275 **treu,** faithful, watchful.
276 **trübsinnig,** dejected, melancholy.
277 **tüchtig,** valiant, stalwart.
278 **unbekümmert,** careless, listless.
279 **unfreundlich,** not friendly.
280 **ungesund,** unhealthy.
281 **ungetreu,** unfaithful, treacherous.

282 **ungleichartig**, dissimilar, heterogeneous.
283 **ungarisch,** / **ungrisch,** } Hungarian.
284 **unheilbar**, incurable.
285 **unmäszig**, intemperate.
286 **unordentlich**, disorderly.
287 **unpäszlich**, indisposed, unwell.
288 **unregelmäszig**, disorderly, unregular.
289 **unverheiratet**, unmarried.
290 **unwohl**, unwell.
291 **väterlich**, fatherly.
292 **vaterlos**, fatherless.
293 **venerisch**, venereal.
294 **verdächtig**, suspicious.
295 **verheiratet**, married.
296 **vernünftig**, prudent.
297 **verständig**, intelligent, wise.
298 **verrückt**, crazy, insane.
299 **verwirrt**, confused.
300 **verzagt**, timid, bashful.
301 **vollblütig**, fullblooded, sanguine.
302 **vorsichtig**, careful, cautious.
303 **wachsam**, vigilant, watchful.
304 **wackelig**, loose, shaky, rickety, tottering.
305 **wacker**, vigorous, gallant.
306 **wahnsinnig**, mad, insane.
307 **wehmütig**, sad, melancholy.
308 **weise**, wise, sagacious.
309 **wunderlich**, rare, peculiar.
310 **würdig**, worthy, deserving.
311 **zerrüttet**, disordered in mind.
312 **zerstreut**, dissipated, absent-minded, etc.

§ 4. **MENSCH**, in compounds:

313 **Menschenadel**, m. 2. dignity, nobility of man or of human nature.
314 **menschenähnlich**, adj. like a human being.
315 **Menschenalter**, n. 2. age, generation.
316 **Menschenantlitz**, n. 1. human face.
317 **menschenfeindlich**, adj. misanthropic.
318 **Menschenfleisch**, n. 1. man's flesh.
319 **menschenfreundlich**, adj. philanthropic.
320 **Menschengattung**, f. race of men.
321 **Menschengebeine**, pl. n. 1. human bones.
322 **Menschengefühl**, n. 1. human feeling.
323 **Menschengeschlecht**, n. 1. mankind, human species.
324 **Menschengesicht**, n. 1. human countenance.
325 **Menschengestalt**, f. human shape.
326 **Menschengewalt**, f. power of man.
327 **menschengleich**, adj. like man, human.
328 **Menschenhaar**, n. 1. man's hair.
329 **Menschenhand**, f. man's hand. hand of art (considered or contrasted with nature).
330 **Menschenherz**, n. 1. (fig.) feeling of man.
331 **Menschenklasse**, f. class of men.
332 **Menschenknochen**, m. 2. human bone.
333 **menschenkundig**, adj. knowing the nature of man.
334 **menschenleer**, adj. deserted, not visited or frequented by men.
335 **Menschenleben**, n. 1. life of man, or human life.
336 **Menschenliebe**, f. human love, philanthropy, charity.
337 **Menschenmörder**, m. 2. manslayer.
338 **Menschennatur**, f. human nature.
339 **Menschenopfer**, n. 2. human sacrifice.
340 **Menschenpocken**, f. pl. variolae
341 **Menschenquäler**, m. 2. tormentor of man.
342 **menschenreich**, adj. well-peopled or populated.
343 **Menschenschädel**, m. 2. human skull.
344 **Menschenscheu**, f. shunning of (from scheuen, to shun) mankind.
345 **menschenscheu**, adj. shunning mankind, unsociable.
346 **Menschenschlag**, m. 1. race of men.
347 **Menschensohn**, m. 1. son of man (as applied to Jesus Christ).
348 **Menschenstimme**, f. human voice.
349 **Menschensinn**, m. 1. sense of man (common sense).
350 **Menschentritt**, m. 1. human footstep.

351 **menschentümlich**, adj. according to human nature.

352 **Menschenverstand**, m. 1. common sense.

353 **Menschenweisheit**, f. human wisdom.

354 **Menschenwelt**, f. mankind, human world.

355 **Menschenwerk**, n. 1. work of man.

356 **Menschenwohl**, n. 1. weal, welfare of mankind.

357 **Menschenwürde**, f. dignity of man.

358 **Menschlichkeit**, f. humanity (from :

359 **menschlich**) adj. human, humane.

360, 361 §5. *Geist, Körper, Leben, Leib, Seele, applied as Bestandteile* (fr. v. ir. bestehen, to consist of). *components of Man, in compounds :*

362 **GEIST**, m. 1. spirit, soul, mind, in compounds :

363 **geistesabwesend**, adj. absent-minded.

364 **Geistesabwesenheit**, f. absence of mind.

365 **Geistesanbau**, m. 1. cultivation of the mind.

366 **Geistesanmut**, f. grace of mind.

367 **geistesanstrengend**, adj. trying to the mind.

368 **Geistesanstrengung**, f. exertion of the mind.

369 **Geistesarbeit**, f. work of thought or meditation.

370 **geistesarm**, adj. spiritless.

371 **Geistesarmut**, f. poverty of the mind.

372 **geistesbegabt**, adj. possessing talents.

373 **Geistesbildung**, f. cultivation of the mind.

374 **Geistesdrang**, m. 1. ardor, impulse of the mind.

375 **Geistesentwickelung**, f. development of the mind.

376 **geisteserquickend**, adj. refreshing the mind.

377 **Geisteserquickung**, f. refreshment of the mind.

378 **Geistesgabe**, f. (fr. v. ir. geben, to give), mental gift.

379 **Geistesgegenwart**, f. presence of mind.

380 **Geistesgrösze**, f. magnanimity.

381 **Geisteskraft**, f. faculty of the soul, mental power.

382 **geisteskrank**, adj. diseased in mind.

383 **Geisteskrankheit**, disorder of the mind, mental debility.

384 **Geisteskultur**, f. cultivation of the mind.

385 **geisteslähmend**, adj. laming the spirit.

386 **Geistesleere**, f. vacancy of the mind.

387 **Geistesnahrung**, f. nourishment of the mind.

388 **Geistesrichtung**, f. tendency of the mind.

389 **Geistesruhe**, f. tranquility of mind.

390 **geistesschwach**, adj. feeble or narrow-minded.

391 **Geistesschwäche**, f. impotence or weakness of the mind, imbecility.

392 **Geistesschwächung**, f. weakening of the mind.

393 **Geistesschwung**, m. 1. (from v. ir. schwingen, to swing). enthusiasm of mind.

394 **Geistesspannung**, f. exertion, stretch of mind.

395 **Geistesstärke**, f. vigor, fortitude of the mind.

396 **Geistesstörung**, f. disturbance of the mind.

397 **geistesstumpf**, adj. torpid.

398 **geistestötend**, adj. killing the spirit.

399 **geistesträge**, adj. heavy, dull.

400 **Geistesträgheit**, f. dulness of the mind, imbecility.

401 **geistesverwandt**, adj. congenial of mind.

402 **Geistesverwandtschaft**, f. congeniality of the mind.

403 **Geistesverstörung**, f. delirium.

404 **Geistesverwirrung**, f. wildness of mind.

405 **geistesverwirrt**, adj. distracted.

406 **Geisteszerrüttung**, f. disorder or derangement of the mind.

407 **geistig**, adj. mental, spirituous, alcoholic.

408 **geistlähmend**, adj. paralyzing the mind.

409 **geistleer**, adj. spiritless, stupid.

410 **geistlich**, adj. clerical, spiritual.

411 **geistlos**, adj. dull, heavy, vacant.
412 **Geistlosigkeit**, f. dulness, heaviness of mind.
413 **geistreich**, adj. ingenious, genial, etc.
414 **KÖRPER**, m. 2. body, in compounds.
415 **Körperanlage**, f. character, temperament.
416 **Körperanstrengung**, f. physical exertion.
417 **Körperbau**, m. 1. (fr. v. bauen. to build), structure of body, constitution.
418 **Körperbeben**, n. 2. tremor.
419 **Körperbeschaffenheit**, f. diathesis, condition of the body, constitution.
420 **Körperbewegung**, f. movements of the body, physical exercise.
421 **Körperbildung**, f. figure, form or shape of the body.
422 **Körperflüssigkeit**, f. fluid of the body (mostly used in the plural).
423 **Körperfülle**, f. corpulence.
424 **Körpergestalt**, f. figure, frame or structure of the body.
425 **Körpergewicht**, n. 1. weight of the body.
426 **Körpergrösze**, f. stature, size of the body.
427 **Körperhaltung**, f. attitude, deportment, carriage of the body.
428 **Körperkonstitution**, f. constitution of the body.
429 **Körperkraft**, f. bodily strength.
430 **Körperlage**, f. (fr. v. ir. liegen, to lie), position of the body.
431 **Körpermasz**, n. 1. a measure of the body.
432 **Körperschwäche**, f. debility, weakness of the body.
433 **Körperstärke**, f. physical strength.
434 **Körperübung**, f. athletics, physical exercise.
435 **Körperumfang**, m. 1. circumference of the body.
436 **Körperwärme**, f. temperature of the body.
437 **Körperzerrüttung**, f. deranged condition of the body.
438 **Körperzittern**, n. 2. tremor.
439 **Oberkörper**, m. 2. } upper part
440 **Oberleib**, m. 1. } of the body.

441 **LEBEN**, n. 2. life (from leben, to live), in compounds.
442 **Lebensart**, f. manner or mode of living.
443 **Lebensbaum**, m. 1. arbor vitæ, thuja, arbor vitæ (in cerebellum).
444 **Lebensbedürfnisse**, pl. n. 1. necessities of life, provisions.
445 **Lebensblüte**, f. prime of life.
446 **Lebensdauer**, f. } duration of life,
Lebenszeit, f. } time of life.
447 **lebensfähig**, adj. viable.
448 **Lebensfähigkeit**, f. vitality.
449 **Lebensfeuer**, n. 2. vital energy.
450 **Lebensflamme**, f. } flame or spark of
Lebensfackel, f. } life.
451 **Lebensfrische**, f. prime of life.
452 **Lebensfülle**, f. fulness of life.
453 **Lebensfunke**, m. 2. spark of life.
454 **Lebensgang**, m. 1. (fr. v. ir. gehen, to go), course of life, process of life.
455 **Lebensgefahr**, f. danger of life.
456 **Lebensgeist**, m. 1. vital spirit, pl. vital spirits.
457 **Lebensgenusz**, m. 1. enjoyment of life.
458 **Lebenshauch**, m. 1. breath (from hauchen to breathe, exhale).
459 **lebenskräftig**, adj. vital, vigorous.
460 **Lebenskraft**, f. vital power.
461 **Lebenslehre**, f. biology.
462 **lebensmüde**, adj. weary of life.
463 **Lebensmüdigkeit**, f. weariness of life.
464 **Lebensmut**, m. 1. vital energy.
465 **Lebensordnung**, f. diet, regimen.
466 **Lebensprincip**, n. 1. the soul, vital principle.
467 **Lebensregel**, f. rule or maxim of life.
468 **lebenssatt**, adj. tired of life.
469 **Lebenstrieb**, m. 1. impulse of life, vitality.
470 **Lebensüberdrusz**, m. 1. satiety of life.
471 **Lebensverlängerung**, f. prolongation of life.
472 **Lebensvorgang**, m. 1. process of life.
473 **Lebenswärme**, f. vital warmth or animal heat.
474 **Lebensweise**, f. manner or mode of life.

475 **Lebenszeichen**, n. 2. sign of life.
Lebenszeit, f. see Lebensdauer.
476 **LEIB**, m. 1. body, in compounds:
477 **Leibesbeschaffenheit**, f. condition of the body, constitution.
478 **Leibesbeschwerde**, f. bodily affection, or ailment.
479 **Leibesbewegung**, f. } physical
Leibesübung, f. } exercise.
480 **Leibesdicke**, f. corpulence.
481 **Leibesfehler**, m. 2. defect of the body.
482 **Leibesfrucht**, f. foetus.
483 **Leibesgebrechen**, n. 2. bodily defect.
484 **Leibesgestalt**, f. figure, form or shape of the body.
485 **Leibesgrösze**, f. } stature or size
486 **Leibeshöhe**, f. } of the body.
487 **Leibeshöhle**, f. abdominal cavity or cavity of the body.
488 **Leibeshülle**, f. integument.
489 **Leibeslänge**, f. stature.
490 **Leibeskraft**, f. physical strength.
491 **Leibesnahrung**, f. food, nutriment.
492 **Leibesöffnung**, f. openness of the bowels.
493 **Leibespflege**, f. care of the body.
494 **Leibesschwäche**, f. bodily weakness.
495 **Leibesstärke**, f. physical strength.
496 **Leibesstellung**, f. position, posture of the body.
497 **Leibesumfang**, m. 1. circumference of the body.
498 **leiblich**, adj. bodily, corporeal.
499 **Leibweh**, n. 1. pain in the stomach, etc.
500 **SEELE**, f. soul, mind, in compounds:
501 **Seelenadel**, m. 2. nobleness of mind or soul.
502 **Seelenangst**, f. soul trouble, anguish of soul, agony.
503 **Seelenblindheit**, f. psychic or soul blindness.
504 **Seelenforschung**, f. psychology.
505 **Seelenfrieden**, m. 2. peace of soul.
506 **Seelengrösze**, f. greatness or magnanimity of the soul.
507 **Seelengüte**, f. goodness of heart or soul.
508 **Seelenheil**, n. 1. safety or welfare of the soul,
509 **Seelenkampf**, m. 1. struggle of the soul,
510 **Seelenkraft**, f. power or faculty of the soul, mental power.
511 **seelenkrank**, adj. mentally diseased.
512 **Seelenkrankheit**, f. mental disease or disorder of the mind.
513 **Seelenkummer**, m. 2. vexation, trouble, grief of the soul.
514 **Seelenleere**, f. want of soul.
515 **Seelenleiden**, n. 2. soul trouble.
516 **seelenlos**, adj. inanimate, lifeless.
517 **Seelenlust**, f. delight of the soul.
518 **Seelenmut**, m. 1. moral courage.
519 **Seelenruhe**, peace, tranquility of the soul.
520 **Seelenschlaf**, m. 1. } sleep of the soul, refers to the interval between its separation in
521 **Seelenschlummer**, m. 2. } death from the body to their reunion at the resurrection.
522 **Seelenschmerz**, m. 1. mental grief, agony.
523 **Seelenstörung**, f. mental disturbance.
524 **seelenvergnügt**, adj. heartily content, thoroughly satisfied.
525 **Seelenvermögen**, n. 2. faculty or power of the soul or mind.
526 **seelenverwandt**, adj. congenial in soul or mind.
527 **Seelenverwandtschaft**, f. congenialty of the soul.
528 **Seelenwanderung**, f. transmigration of souls.
529 **Seelenzustand**, m. 1. state of one's soul.
530 **Seelenzwang**, m. 1. (fr. v. ir.
531 zwingen, to force), constraint of soul, etc., etc.

B. THE BODY OF MAN.

§ 6. Division of the Framework or Skeleton in Compounds.

The framework of the human body (consisting of 211 bones) called:

532 **Knochen-gebäude**, n. 1 (from bauen, to build), skeleton.
533 **Knochen-gerippe**, n. 1
534 **Knochen-gerüste**, n. 1
535 **Skelett**, n. 1. is divided into head, trunk, superior and inferior extremities, and consists of Knochen, bones; Knorpel, cartilage, knorpels; Gelenke, joints.
536 **Knochen**, m. 2. bone, in compounds:
537 **Knochenabblätterung**, f. (fr. abblättern, to scale), exfoliation, scaling of the bones.
538 **Knochenabmagerung**, f. (fr. abmagern, to emaciate, shrink), senile atrophy of bones.
539 **knochenähnlich**, adj. bony, osseous.
540 **knochenartig** adj. bone-like, bony, osseous.
541 **Knochen-anbildung**, f. (fr. anbilden, to form anew), new formation of bone.
542 **Knochenansatz**, m. 1. (fr. v. ir. ansetzen, to put on, adjoin), epiphysis.
543 **knochenbildend**, adj. ossific.
544 **Knochenbildung**, f. (fr. bilden, to build, form), formation of bone, ossification.
545 **Knochenblätterung**, f. exfoliation.
546 **Knochenbrand**, m. 1. (fr. v. ir. brennen, to burn), necrosis.
547 **knochenbrandig**, adj. necrotic.
548 **Knochenbruch**, m. 1. (fr. v. ir. brechen, to break), fracture of bone.
549 **Knochenentstehung**, f. (fr. v. ir. entstehen, to exist), ossification.
550 **Knochenerzeugung**, f. (fr. erzeugen, to produce). ossification, bone formation.
551 **Knochenfortsatz**, m. 1. (fr. fortsetzen, to continue, procede), bony process.
552 **Knochenfuge**, f. (fr. fügen, to connect, join), suture, junction of bones, symphysis, articulation.
553. **Knochengefüge**, n. 1. structure of bone.
554 **Knochengewächs**, n. 1. (fr. v. ir. wachsen, to grow), bony growth.
555 **Knochengewebe**, n. 1. (f. v. ir. weben, to weave), bony tissue.
556 **knochenhaft**, adj. bony, osseous.
557 **Knochenhaut**, f. periosteum.
558 **Knochenhautentzündung**, f. periostitis.
559 **Knochenhöhle**, f. (fr. höhlen, to hollow), bony cavity, cell.
560 **Knochenjauche**, f. pus from a bone.
561 **Knochenkapsel**, f. bony covering.
562 **Knochenkern**, m. 1. bony nucleus.
563 **Knochenknorpel**, m. 2. cartilage, where bone is developed.
564 **Knochenkopf**, m. 1. head of a bone.
565 **Knochenleim**, m. 1. gelatine.
566 **Knochenleiste**, f. ledge or ridge of bone.
567 **Knochenmark**, n. 1. bone marrow, medulla of bone.
568 **Knochenmasse**, f. osseous substance.
569 **Knochenmürbigkeit**, f. brittleness of bone.
570 **Knochennadel**, f. spicule of bone.
571 **Knochennaht**, f. suture.
572 **Knochennarbe**, f. callus.

573 **Knochenneubildung**, f. } new growth of bone.
574 **Knochenbildung**, f. }
575 **Knochenpfanne**, f. cotyloid or glenoid cavity.
576 **Knochenplatte**, f. lamella of bone.
577 **Knochenrand mit Zacken**, m. 1. (fr. zacken, to tooth), bone edge with serration.
578 **Knochenrinde**, f. cortex of bone.
579 **Knochenrisz**, m. 1. (fr. v. ir. reiszen, to tear), fissure of bone.
580 **Knochensäge**, f. bone saw.
581 **Knochensalze**, pl. n. 1. inorganic matter of bone.
582 **Knochenschaber**, m. 2. from schaben, to scrape, bone scraper, raspatory.
583 **Knochenschale**, f. osseous envelop or shell.
584 **Knochenschere**, f. bone-cutting forceps.
585 **Knochenschicht**, f. layer or plate of bone.
586 **Knochenschmerz**, m. 1. bone pain.
587 **Knochenschwiele**, f. callus.
588 **Knochenschwund**, m. 1. (from v. ir. schwinden, to diminish, shrink), atrophy, absorption of bone.
589 **Knochenspaltung**, f. (fr. spalten, to split), fissure of or in bone.
590 **Knochensplitter**, m. 2. splinter or scale of bone.
591 **Knochenstück**, n. 1. fragment or piece of bone.
592 **Knochensubstanz**, f. bony tissue.
593 **Knochensystem**, n. 1. osseous system.
594 **Knochentrennung**, f. (fr. trennen. to separate), separation of bone.
595 **Knochenverbindung**, f. (fr. v. ir.
596 verbinden, to connect, bind, join), articulation of bones;
597 **Knochenverbindung**, bewegliche or unterbrochene, movable, articulation of bone; diarthrosis;
598 **Knochenverbindung**, unbewegliche or ununterbrochene, immovable, articulation of bone, synarthrosis.
599 **Knochenverdickung**, f. thickening of a bone.
600 **Knochenverhärtung**, f. osteosclerosis.
601 **Knochenverletzung**, f. injury to a bone.
602 **Knochenverpflanzung**, f. bone grafting.
603 **Knochenverrenkung**, f. (fr. verrenken, to dislocate), dislocation of bone.
604 **Knochenverschiebung**, f. (fr. v. ir. verschieben, to dislocate, etc)., displacement of a bone.
605 **Knochenverwachsung**, f. (fr. v. ir. verwachsen, to grow together), growing together, or union of bones, or bone deformity.
606 **Knochenvorsprung**, m. 1. (fr. v. ir. vorspringen, to spring forward, project), projection of bone, or bony prominence.
607 **Knochenwand**, f. } osseous wall.
Knochenwandung, f. }
608 **Knochenwachstum**, n. 1. } growth of bone.
609 **Knochenwuchs**, m. 1. }
610 **Knochenwurm**, m. 1. spina ventosa.
611 **Knochenzange**, f. bone forceps.
612 **Knochenzerstörung**, f. (fr. zerstören, to destroy), destruction of bone.
613 **knöchericht**, adj. } bony, made of bone, osseous.
614 **knöchern**, adj. }
615 **knöchig**, adj. }
616 **Röhrenknochen**, m. 2. } hollow, long, tubular or cylindrical bone.
617 **Rohrknochen**, m 2 }
618 2. **BEIN**, n. 1. } bone, in the sense of *Knochen*, bone. in compounds:
GEBEIN, n. 1. }
619 **Bein**, felsenartiges, petrous part of temporal bone.
620 **Bein**, heiliges, os sacrum.
621 **Bein**, rundes, pisiform bone.
622 **Bein**, siebförmiges, ethmoid bone.
623 **Bein**, ungenanntes, os innominatum.
624 **Beinader**, f. a vein in the leg.
625 **beinähnlich**, adj. } bony, osseous, bone-like.
beinartig, adj. }
626 **Beinblätterung**, f. exfoliation of bone.

627 **Beinbrand**, m. 1. necrosis.
628 **Beinbruch**, m. 1. fracture.
629 **beinbrüchig**, adj. fractured.
630 **Beinchen**, n. 2. } ossicle or
Knöchlein, n. 2. } small bone.
631 **beinern**, adj. bony, osseous.
632 **Beinerzeugung**, f. ossification.
633 **Beinfügung**, f. articulation, symphysis.
634 **Beingerippe**, n. 1. }
635 **Beingerüst**, n. 1. } skeleton.
636 **Beingestell**, n. 1. }
637 **Beingewächs**, n. 1. bony growth, osteosis.
638 **beinhart**, adj. as hard as bone.
639 **Beinhaut**, f. } perios-
640 **Beinhäutchen**, n. 2. } teum.
641 **Beinhautwucherung**, f. proliferation of periosteum.
642 **Beinhöhle**, f. articular cavity or socket for a bone.
643 **beinigt**, adj. } bony, osseous.
644 **beinig**, adj. }
645 **Beinknopf**, m. 1. tuberosity at the end of bone or condyle.
646 **Beinknoten**, m. 2. tubercule or nodule of bone.
647 **Beinkopf**, m. 1. head of bone.
648 **Beinkrebs**, m. 1. cancer of bone.
649 **beinlos**, adj. boneless.
650 **Beinmark**, n. 1. marrow, medulla of bone.
651 **Beinnaht**, f. suture of bone (s).
652 **Beinnarbe**, f. callus.
653 **Beinritze**, f. fissure of bone.
654 **Beinsäge**, f. bonesaw.
655 **Beinspalte**, f. cleft or fissure of bone.
656 **Beinweh**, n. 1. bone pain, ostealgia.
657 **Beinwuchs**, m. 1. growth of bone.
658 3. **HORN**, n. 1. horn, cornu, in compounds.
659 **hornartig**, adj. }
hornicht, adj. } horn-like, horny. corneous. of horn, e. g. finger or toe-nails.
hornig, adj. }
660 **Horngewebe**, n. 1. horny or corneous tissue.
661 **hornhäutig**, adj. callous.
662 4. **KORN**, n. 1. corn, grain, granule, granulation ;
Hühnerauge, n. 1. corn (on the foot).
663 **Körnchen**, n. 2. granule (granule of medicine).
körnig, adj. granular, miliary.

664 5. **NAGEL**, m. 2. nail; onyx of the cornea.
665 **Nagel**, m. 2. Eingewachsener, ingrowing nail.
666 **Nagel**, m. 2. hysterischer, clavus hystericus.
In compounds:
667 **Nagelanlage**, f. rudiment of nail.
668 **Nagelbein**, n. 1. lachrymal bone, or unguis.
669 **Nagelbett**, n. 1. nail-bed, matrix of nail.
670 **Nagelbettentzündung**, f. onychia.
671 **Nagelbildung**, f. formation of nail.
672 **Nagelblatt**, n. 1. the nail.
673 **Nagelblüte**, f. white spot or spots on a nail.
674 **Nageleiterung**, f. suppuration under the nail.
675 **Nagelgeschwür**, n. 1. onychia, whitlow.
676 **Nagelglied**, n. 1. ungual or terminal phalanx.
677 **Nagelpilz**, m. 1. fungus attacking the nail.
678 **Nagelschwund**, m. 1. atrophy or shrinking of nail.
679 **Nagelzwang**, m. 1. ingrowing nail.
680 6. **KNORPEL**, m. 2. cartilage, in compounds :
681 **Knorpelablagerung**, f. (fr. ablagern, to deposit), deposit of cartilage.
682 **knorpelähnlich**, adj. }
683 **knorpelartig**, adj. } carti-
knorpelicht, adj. } laginous.
knorpelig, adj. }
684 **Knorpelanlage**, f. cartilaginous rudiment.
685 **Knorpelansatz**, m. 1. epiphysis.
686 **Knorpelauswuchs**, m. 1. enchondrosis.
687 **Knorpelband**, n. 1. (fr. v. ir. binden, to bind), synchondrosis.
688 **Knorpelbelag**, m. 1. } (fr. legen, to put, lay),
689 **Knorpelbeleg**, m. 1. } covering of cartilage.
690 **Knorpelbildung**, f. formation of cartilage, chondrosis.
691 **Knorpelbruch**, m. 1. (fr. v. ir. brechen, to break), rupture of cartilage.

692 **Knorpeleinfügung**, f. (fr. einfügen, to insert), synchondrosis.
693 **Knorpelentartung**, f. degeneration of cartilage.
694 **Knorpelgewächs**, n. 1. cartilaginous growth, enchondroma.
695 **knorpelhaft**, adj. cartilaginous.
696 **Knorpelhaut**, f. cartilaginous membrane, perichondrium.
697 **Knorpelhöhle**, f. cartilage cavity.
698 **Knorpelkern**, m. 1. nucleus of cartilage.
699 **Knorpelleim**, m. 1. chondrin.
700 **Knorpelüberzug**, m. 1. (fr. v. ir. überziehen, to cover), cap or covering of cartilage.
701 **Knorpelverbindung**, f. synchondrosis.
702 **Gieszbeckenknorpel**, m. 2. } arytenoid cartilage.
703 **Gieszkannenknorpel**, m. 2. } arytenoid cartilage.
704 **Zwischenknorpel**, m. 2. interarticular cartilage, etc.
705 7. **GELENK**.n. 1.(fr. lenken, to bend, turn, manage), articulation, joint, arthrosis, in compounds.
706 *Gelenk, bewegliches*, adj. movable arthrodia.
707 *Gelenk, falsches*, adj. } abnormal or false joint, pseudarthrosis.
708 *Gelenk, widernatürliches*, adj. } abnormal or false joint, pseudarthrosis.
709 *Gelenk, freies*, adj. arthrodia.
710 *Gelenk, künstliches*, adj. artificial joint.
711 *Gelenk, neues*, adj. new joint, nearthrosis.
712 *Gelenk, straffes*, adj. amphiarthrosis.
713 **Gelenkabscesz**, m. 1. joint abscess.
714 **Gelenkband**, n. 1. (fr. v. ir. binden, to bind), articular ligament, capsular ligament.
715 **Gelenkbau**, m. 1. (fr. bauen, to build), structure of a joint.
716 **Gelenkbein**, n. 1. } sesamoid bone.
717 **Gelenkbeinchen**, n. 2. } sesamoid bone.
718 **Gelenkende**, n. 1. articular end or surface of a bone.
719 **Gelenkergusz**, m. 1. (fr. v. ir. ergieszen, to overflow), effusion into a joint.
720 **Gelenkfalte**, f. crease or fold of a joint.
721 **Gelenkfläche**, f. articular surface.
722 **Gelenkflüssigkeit**, f. synovial fluid.
723 **Gelenkfortsatz**, m. 1. articular process, condyloid process.
724 **Gelenkfuge**, f. joint commissure.
725 **Gelenkfügung**, f. articulation.
726 **Gelenkgegend**, f. region of joint.
727 **Gelenkgrube**, f. (fr. v. ir. graben, to dig), articular fossa, glenoid cavity.
728 **Gelenkhaut**, f. synovial membrane.
729 **Gelenkhöcker**, m. 2. condyle.
730 **Gelenkhöckergrube**, f. condyloid fossa.
731 **Gelenkhöhle**, f. articular cavity, acetabulum.
732 **Gelenkhügelchen**, n. 2. } articular prominence, tuberosity or tubercle.
733 **Gelenkhügel**, m. 2. } articular prominence, tuberosity or tubercle.
734 **gelenkig**, adj. articulated, flexible, jointed.
735 **Gelenkkapsel**, f. articular capsule, capsular ligament.
736 **Gelenkknochen**, m. 2. bone forming part of a joint, sesamoid bone.
737 **Gelenkknopf**, m. 1. condyle.
738 **Gelenkknorpel**, m. 2. articular cartilage.
739 **gelenkknorpelartig**, adj. cartilaginous.
740 **Gelenkknorpelüberzug**, m. 1. articular cartilage.
741 **Gelenkknorren**, m. 2. condyle.
742 **Gelenkknoten**, m. 2. } loose or movable body in a joint.
743 **Gelenkkonkrement**, n. 1. } loose or movable body in a joint.
744 **Gelenkkopf**, m. 1. condyle head of bone, capitellum.
745 **Gelenkkörper**, m. 2. loose or movable body in a joint.
746 **Gelenkleim**, m. 1. synovia.
747 **Gelenklippe**, f. joint margin or rim.
748 **Gelenkmaus**, f. loose or movable body in a joint.
749 **Gelenkpfanne**, f. articular cavity or depression, glenoid cavity, acetabulum.
750 **Gelenkraum**, m. 1. articular cavity.

751 **Gelenkring**, m. 1. the rim of a joint cavity.

752 **Gelenkrolle**, f. joint condyle.

753 **Gelenksaft**, m. 1. synovia.

754 **gelenksam**, adj. flexible, pliable.

755 **Gelenkscheide**, f. joint capsula.

756 **Gelenkschienchen**, n. 2. a small articular splint.

757 **Gelenkschleim**, m. 1. synovia.

758 **Gelenkschleimhaut**, f. synovial membrane.

759 **Gelenkschmiere**, f. synovia.

760 **Gelenkschwellung**, f. (fr. v. ir. schwellen, to rise, swell), swelling of a joint.

761 **Gelenkschwund**, m. 1. (fr. v. ir. schwinden, to diminish, disappear, shrink), atrophy, wasting of a joint.

762 **Gelenkspalte**, f. joint cleft.

763 **gelenksteif**, adj. ankylosed or stiff-jointed.

764 **Gelenkstück**, n. 1. part of a joint.

765 **Gelenktasche**, f. pouch or pocket of a joint cavity.

766 **Gelenkteil**, m. 1. (fr. teilen, to divide), articular portion, condyle.

767 **Gelenkverbindung**, f. articulation.

768 **Gelenkverdickung**, f. swelling or thickening of or about a joint.

769 **Gelenkwand**, f. } joint boundary or capsule.
770 **Gelenkwandung**, f. }

771 **Gelenkwasser**, n. 2. synovia.

772 **Gelenkwirbel**, m. 2. rotatory joint.

773 **Gelenkzotte**, f. rag, villus of a joint.

774 **gelenkzottig**, adj. shaggy articulation, shaggy jointed, etc.

775 **Drehgelenk**, n. 1. (fr. drehen, to turn), pivot-joint.

776 **Fugengelenk**, n. 1. articulation, synarthrosis.

777 **Kugelgelenk**, n. 1. ball and socket-joint, enarthrosis.

778 **Rollgelenk**, n. 1. (fr. rollen, to roll), pivot-joint.

779 **Scharniergelenk**, n. 1. } hinge joint, ginglymus, ginglymoid joint.
780 **Winkelgelenk**, n. 1. }

781 **Schlottergelenk**, n. 1. loose joint or flail-like joint, etc.

782 8. **WIRBEL**, m. 2. vertebra (vertex, whorl, vertigo, giddiness), in compounds: *vertebral*.

783 **Wirbelader**, f. vertebral vein.

784 **Wirbelarterie**, f. vertebral artery.

785 **Wirbelband**, n. 1. vertebral ligament.

786 **Wirbelbein**, n. 1. vertebra.

787 **Wirbelbeinband**, n. 1. vertebral ligament.

788 **Wirbelblutader**, f. vertebral vein.

789 **Wirbelbogen**, m. 2. vertebral arch.

790 **Wirbelbruch**, m. 1. fracture of a vèrtebra.

791 **Wirbeldorn**, m. 1. spinous process of a vertebra.

792 **Wirbelfortsatz**, m. 1. process of a vertebra.

793 **Wirbelgang**, m. 1. vertebral canal.

794 **Wirbelgegend**, f. vertebral region.

795 **Wirbelgelenk**, n. 1. joint of the spine.

796 **Wirbelgeschwulst**, f. tumor of the vertebra.

797 **Wirbelhöhle**, f. } vertebral canal.
798 **Wirbelkanal**, m. 1. }

799 **Wirbelkern**, m. 1. spinal nucleus.

800 **Wirbelkernmasse**, f. primitive vertebral mass.

801 **Wirbelknochen**, m. 2. } vertebral cartilage.
802 **Wirbelknorpel**, m. 2. }

803 **Wirbelkörper**, m. 2. body of a vertebra.

804 **Wirbelkörperbruch**, m. 1. fracture of the body of a vertebra.

805 **Wirbelloch**, n. 1. vertebral foramen.

806 **wirbellos**, adj. invertebrate.

807 **Wirbelmuskel**, m. 2. spinal or vertebral muscle.

808 **wirbeln**, to whirl, rotate, to feel giddy.

809 **Wirbelpulsader**, f. vertebral artery.

810 **Wirbelquerfortsatz**, m. 1. transverse process of vertebra.

811 **Wirbelsäule**, f. vertebral column.

812 **Wirbelsäulenkrümmung**, f. } spinal curvature, scoliosis.
813 **Wirbelsäulenverbiegung**, f.
814 **Wirbelsäulenverkrümmung**, f.
815 **Wirbelschiebung**, f. (fr. v. ir. schieben, to shove, displace), spondylolithsesis.
816 **Wirbelschlagader**, f. vertebral artery.
817 **Wirbelspalte**, f. } spina bifida.
818 **Wirbelspaltung**, f.
819 **Wirbeltier**, n. 1. vertebrate.
820 **Wirbeltuberkulose**, f. tubercular disease of the vertebræ.
821 **Wirbelvereiterung**, f. suppuration of the vertebræ, etc.

§ 7. *Parts of the Head.*

822 1. **HAUPT**, n. 1. } head. In compounds.
823 **KOPF**, m. 1.
824 **Hinterhaupt**, n. 1. } occiput or hind part of the head.
825 **Hinterkopf**, m. 1.
826 **Hinterhauptbein**, n. 1. occipital bone.
827 **Hinterhauptsfontanelle**, f. posterior fontanelle.
828 **Hinterhauptsgegend**, f. occipital region.
829 **Hinterhauptsgelenk**, n. 1. alto-occipital joint.
830 **Hinterhauptshöcker**, m. 2. occipital protuberance.
831 **Hinterhauptslage**, f. occipital presentation.
832 **Hinterhauptslappen**, m. 2. occipital lobe.
833 **Hinterhauptsloch**, n. 1. occipital foramen.
834 **Hinterhauptsnaht**, f. (fr. nähen, to sew), occipital suture, lambdoid suture.
835 **Hinterhauptsstachel**, m. 2. occipital protuberance.
836 **Hinterhauptswindung**, f. occipital convolution.
837 **Hinterhauptsteil**, m. 1. occipital region.
838 **Hauptwirbel**, m. 2. } crown of the head, top, vertex
839 **Scheitel**, m. 2.
840 **Vorderhaupt**, n. 1. } forehead, sinciput.
841 **Vorderkopf**, m. 1.
842 **Vorderkopfsbein**, n. 1. frontal bone.
843 **Vorderkopfsfontanelle**, f. anterior fontanelle, etc.
844 2. **STIRN** or **STIRNE**, f. forehead, brow; in compounds, *frontal*.
845 **Stirnbein**, n 1. frontal bone.
846 **Stirnecke**, f angle of frontal bone.
847 **Stirnfontanelle**, f. anterior fontanelle.
848 **Stirnfortsatz**, m. 1. frontal process.
849 **Stirngegend**, f. frontal region.
850 **Stirnglatze**, f. bald forehead.
851 **Stirnhaut**, f. skin over the forehead.
852 **Stirnhügel**, m. 2. } frontal protuberance.
853 **Stirnwulst**, m. 1.
854 **Stirnkamm**, m. 1. } spine of frontal bone.
855 **Stirnleiste**, f.
856 **Stirnknochen**, m. 2. frontal bone.
857 **Stirnlappen**, m. 2. frontal lobe.
858 **Stirnnaht**, f. frontal suture, etc.
859 3. **SCHLÄFE**, f. temple; in compounds.
860 **Schläfenbein**, n. 1. temporal bone.
861 **Schläfenbeinfortsatz**, m. 1. process of temporal bone.
862 **Schläfenbeinfuge**, f. squamous suture.
863 **Schläfenbeingriffelfortsatz**, m. 1. styloid process of temporal bone.
864 **Schläfenbeinjochfortsatz**, m. 1. zygomatic process of temporal bone.
865 **Schläfenbeinnaht**, f. squamous suture.
866 **Schläfenbeinpyramide**, f. piramidal or petrous part of temporal bone.
867 **Schläfenbeinschuppe**, f. squamous part of temporal bone.
868 **Schläfenbeinwarzenfortsatz**, m. 1. or Zitzenecke, f. } mastoid process of temporal bone.
869 **Schläfenbeinzitzenfortsatz**, m. 1.
870 **Schläfenbinde**, f. } temporal fascia.
871 **Schläfenfascie**, f.
872 **Schläfenfläche**, f. temporal surface.
873 **Schläfenflügel**, m. 2. temporal part of great wing of sphenoid bone.
874 **Schläfenfortsatz**, m. 1. process of temporal bone.
875 **Schläfengefäsz**, n. 1. temporal vessel.
876 **Schläfengegend**, f. temporal region.

877 **Schläfengrube**, f. temporal fossa.
878 **Schläfenknochen**, m. 2. temporal bone.
879 **Schläfenlappen**, m. 2. temporal lobe.
880 **Schläfenrand**, m. 1. temporal margin.
881 **Schläfenschuppe**, f. squamous part of temporal bone.
882 **schläfenwärts**, adj. towards the temples.
883 **Schläfenwindung**, f. temporo-sphenoidal convolution.
884 **Schläfenzweig**, m. 1. temporal branch, etc.
885 4. **KEIL**, m. 1. (fr. keilen, to wedge in), wedge, embolus, in compounds:
886 **keilähnlich**, adj. ⎫ wedge-formed,
887 **keilartig**, adj. ⎬ cuneiform,
888 **keilförmig**, adj. ⎭ sphenoidal.
889 **Keilbein**, n. 1. ⎫ cuneiform bone.
890 **Keilknochen**, m. 2. ⎭ sphenoidal bone.
891 **Keilbeinflügel**, m. 2. wing of sphenoid bone.
892 **Keilbeinfontanelle**, f. sphenoidal fontanelle.
893 **Keilbeinfortsatz**, m. 1. ⎫ process of sphenoid
894 **Keilfortsatz**, m. 1. ⎭ bone.
895 **Keilbeinhöhle**, f. sphenoidal sinus.
896 **Keilbeinhorn**, n. 1. ⎫ process of sphenoid
897 **Keilbeinhörnchen**, n. 2. ⎭ bone.
898 **Keilbeinkörper**, m. 2. body of sphenoid bone.
899 **Keilbeinnaht**, f. sphenoidal suture.
900 **Keilbeinschläfenflügel**, m. 2. great wing of the sphenoid bone.
901 **Keilbeinschnabel**, m. 2. rostrum of sphenoid bone.
902 **Keilbeinspalte**, f. sphenoidal fissure.
903 **Keilschiftbeinband**, n. 1. cuneo-scaphoid ligament, etc.
904 5. **JOCH**, n. 1. yoke, in compounds:
905 **Jochbein**, n. 1. malar bone.
906 **Jochbeinnaht**, f. zygomatic suture.
907 **Jochband**, n. 1. transverse connecting ligament.
908 **Jochbogen**, m. 2. zygoma.
909 **Jochbrücke**, f. zygomatic arch.
910 **Jochfortsatz**, m. 1. zygomatic process.
911 **Jochknochen**, m. 2. malar bone.
912 **Jochmuskel**, m. 2. zygomatic muscle, etc.
913 6. **BACKEN**, m. 2. ⎫ cheek in
Backe, f. ⎭ compounds:
914 **Backenbein**, n. 1. cheek bone, malar bone, zygomatic bone.
915 **Backendrüse**, f. buccal gland.
916 **Backenfistel**, f. buccal fistula.
917 **Backenfläche**, f. buccal surface.
918 **Backengegend**, f. buccal region.
919 **Backengrübchen**, n. 2. dimple in the cheek.
920 **Backenhöhle**, f. buccal cavity.
921 **Backenknochen**, m. 2. malar bone, any bone of the cheek.
922 **Backenzahn**, m. 1. molar tooth, etc.
923 7. **WANGE**, f. cheek in compounds:
924 **Wangenbein**, n. 1. malar bone, zygoma.
925 **Wangenbildung**, f. artificial formation of the cheek.
926 **Wangendrüse** f. buccal gland.
927 **Wangenfalte**, f. buccal fold.
928 **Wangenfortsatz**, m. 1. zygoma.
929 **Wangengegend**, f. buccal or malar region.
930 **Wangengrübchen**, n. 2. dimple in the cheek.
931 **Wangenhöhle**, f. buccal cavity.
932 **Wangenknochen**, m. 2. malar bone, zygoma, etc.
933 8. **AUGE**, n. 1. eye; sight; in compounds:
934 [1] **Augapfel**, m. 2. eyeball, globe of the eye, bulbus oculi.
935 **Augapfelausrottung**, f. (fr. ausrotten, to extirpate), enucleation of the eyeball.
936 **Augapfelbinde**, f. fascia of the globe.
937 **Augapfelbindehaut**, f. ocular conjunctiva.
938 **Augapfelbrand**, m. 1. (fr. v. ir. brennen, to burn), sloughing of the globe.
939 **Augapfelhalter**, m. 2. (fr. v. ir. halten, to hold), fixation-forceps.
940 **Augapfelhäutchen**, n. 2. ocular membrane.

941 **Augapfelmuskellähmung**, f. ophthalmoplegia.
942 **Augapfelschwund**, m. 1. (fr. v. ir. schwinden, to disappear, shrink), shrunken eyeball; phthisis bulbi; atrophy of the eyeball.
943 **Augapfelvorfall**, m. 1. exophthalmos.
944 **Augapfelwand**, f. surface of the eyeball.
945 **Augapfelzucken**, n. 2. nystagmus, etc.
[1] Note 1. The **EYEBALLS** may be:
946 **contrahiert**, contracted.
947 **dilatiert**, dilated.
948 **eng zusammengezogen** (fr.
949 v. ir. **zusammenziehen**, to draw together), closely contracted.
950 **oscillierend**, in *stetiger* Bewegung, f. sein. } oscillating, to be in constant motion.
951 **rollend**, rolling.
952 **starr**, fixed.
953 in **Starrheit**, f. in fixedness, etc.
954 [2] **AUGEN**, pl. n. 1. eyes; (in compounds), ocular or ophthalmic.
955 **Augenachse**, f. axis of the eye.
956 **Augenader**, f. ophthalmic vein.
957 **Augenaderlasz**, m. 1. (fr. v. ir. lassen, to let), letting of blood from the eye.
958 **Augenarterie**, f. ophthalmic artery.
959 **Augenarzt**, m. 1. oculist, ophthalmologist.
960 **Augenast**, m. 1. ocular branch.
961 **Augenbeben**, n. 2. nystagmus.
962 **Augenbecken**, n. 2. socket of the eyeball; orbit.
963 **Augenbewegung**, f. ocular movement.
964 **Augenblase**, f. optic vesicle.
965 **Augenblutader**, f. ophthalmic vein.
966 **Augenblutflusz**, m. 1. intraocular hemorrhage.
967 **Augenblutschwamm**, m. 1. fungous growth of the eye.
968 **Augenblutunterlaufung**, f. ecchymosis of the eye.
969 **Augenbrauenausfall**, m. 1. falling out of the eyebrows' hair.
970 **Augenbrauenbogen**, m. 2. superciliary arch.
971 **Augenbrauengegend**, f. superciliary region.
972 **Augenbrauenmuskel**, m. 2. } corrugator, supercilii.
973 **Augenbrauenrunzler**, m. 2. } corrugator, supercilii.
974 **Augenbruch**, m. 1. rupture of the eyeball.
975 **Augenbutter**, f. sebum palpebrarum.
976 **Augendach**, n. 1. roof of the orbit.
977 **Augendrüse**, f. lachrymal gland.
978 **Augenfaserhaut**, f. fibrous tunic of the eye, the cornea and sclerotic.
979 **Augenfeld**, n. 1. vision field.
980 **Augenfell**, n. 1. film on eye, nebula, pannus.
981 **Augenfeuchtigkeit**, f. aqueous humor.
982 **Augenfistel**, f. lachrymal fistula.
983 **Augenflecken**, m. 2. macula corneae.
984 **Augenflimmern**, n. 2. objects (as in vertigo), flickering before the eye, (from flimmern, to flicker).
985 **Augenflusz**, m. 1. watering of the eye, epiphora, stillicidium lachrymale.
986 **Augenflüssigkeiten**, pl. f. fluids of the eye.
987 **Augenfunken**, m. 2. flashes before the eye, phosphene.
988 **Augenganglie**, f. ophthalmic ganglion.
989 **Augengefäsz**, n. 1. ophthalmic vessel.
990 **Augengegend**, f. ophthalmic region.
991 **Augengeschwulst**, f. tumor of the eye.
992 **Augengeschwür**, n. 1. ulcer of the cornea.
993 **Augengewölke**, n. 1. nebula, macula cornea.
994 **Augenglas**, n. 1. eyeglass, spectacles.
995 **Augengrund**, m. 1. fundus oculi.
996 **Augenhaut**, f. coat or tunic of the eyeball; harte or weisze, sclerotic.
997 **Augenhäutchen**, n. 2. eye-membrane, nebula, leucoma.

998 **Augenheraustreten**, n. 2. exophthalmos.
999 **Augenhintergrund**, m. 1. fundus oculi.
1000 **Augenhöhle**, f. orbital cavity.
1001 **Augenhöhlenast**, m. 1. orbital branch.
1002 **Augenhöhlenflügel**, m. 2. lesser wing of sphenoid bone.
1003 **Augenhöhlenloch**, n. 1. orbital foramen.
1004 **Augenhöhlennerv**, m. 3. orbital nerve.
1005 **Augenhöhlenrand**, m. 1. margin of the orbital cavity.
1006 **Augenhöhlenspalte**, f. orbital fissure.
1007 **Augenhöhlenteil**, m. 1. orbital portion (as frontal bone, etc.)
1008 **Augenhöhlenvene**, f. ophthalmic vein.
1009 **Augenhöhlenwand**, f. wall of orbital cavity.
1010 **Augenhornhaut**, f. } Cornea.
Cornea, f. }
1011 **Augeninnere**, n. interior of the eyeball.
1012 **Augenjucken**, n. 2. itching of the eye.
1013 **Augenkammer**, f. chamber of the eye.
1014 **Augenkammerwasser**, n. 2. aqueous humor.
1015 **Augenklappe**, f. eyelid.
1016 **Augenklappenrand**, m. 1. the eyelid's margin.
1017 **Augenklinik**, f. ophthalmic clinic.
1018 **Augenknorpel**, m. 2. tarsal cartilage.
1019 **Augenknoten**, m. 2. ophthalmic ganglion.
1020 **Augenkrankheit**, f. disease of the eyes.
1021 **Augenkrebs**, m. 1. cancer of the eye.
1022 **Augenkreis**, m. 1. the orbit.
1023 **Augenlid**, n. 1. eyelid.
1024 **Augenlidband**, n. 1. tarsal ligament.
1025 **Augenlidbindehaut**, f. palpebral conjunctiva.
1026 **Augenlidbrand**, m. 1. gangrene of the eyelid.
1027 **Augenliderdrüse**, f. meibomian gland.
1028 **Augenliderschlieszmuskel**, m. 2. orbicularis palpebrarum muscle.
1029 **Augenlidflechte**, f. herpes of the eyelid.
1030 **Augenlidgeschwulst**, f. œdemus of the eyelid.
1031 **Augenlidgriffel**, m. 2. lid-elevator.
1032 **Augenlidhacken**, m. 2. eyelid retractor.
1033 **Augenlidhalter**, m. 2. lid-elevator.
1034 **Augenlidheber**, m. 2. (fr. v. ir. heben, to lift), levator palpebræ muscle.
1035 **Augenlidknorpel**, m. 2. tarsal cartilage.
1036 **Augenlidnerv**, m. 3. palpebral nerve.
1037 **Augenlidrand**, m. 1. palpebral end or margin.
1038 **Augenlidringmuskel**, m. 2. orbicularis palpebrarum muscle.
1039 **Augenlidschlagader**, f. palpebral artery.
1040 **Augenlidspalte**, f. palpebral fissure.
1041 **Augenmuskel**, m. 2. eye muscle.
1042 **Augenmuskelkrampf**, m. 1. spasm of the eye muscle.
1043 **Augenmuskelnerv**, m. 3. oculo-motor nerve.
1044 **Augen-Nasenfurche**, f. oculonasal groove or pit.
1045 **Augennebel**, m. 2. nebula, macula cornea.
1046 **Augennetzhaut**, f. retina.
1047 **Augennerv**, m. 3. optic n. orbital n. or ophthalmic nerve.
1048 **Augennervenhaut**, f. retina.
1049 **Augenpigment**, n. 1. pigment of the eye.
1050 **Augenpol**, m. 1. pole of the globe.
1051 **Augenpunkt**, m. 1. visual point (see Gesichtspunkt).
1052 **Augenreiz**, m. 1. irritation of the eye.
1053 **Augenring**, m. 1. iris.
1054 **Augenrollmuskel**, m. 2. trochlear muscle.
1055 **Augenschere**, f. eye-scissors.
1056 **Augenschlagader**, f. ophthalmic artery.
1057 **Augenschleim**, m. 1. conjunctival mucus.
1058 **Augenschleimflusz**, m. 1. catarrhal ophthalmia.

1059 **Augenschmalz**, n. 1. sebum palpebrarum.
1060 **Augenschnupfen**, m. 2. catarrhal ophthalmia.
1061 **Augenschwamm**, m. 1. fungus growth of the eye.
1062 **Augenschwinden**, n. 2. **Augenschwund**, m. 1. } atrophy of the eyeball.
1063 **Augensperre**, f. (fr. sperren, to hinder, to close), closure of the eye.
1064 **Augenspiegel**, m. 2. ophthalmoscope.
1065 **Augenstein**, m. 1. lapis divinus.
1066 **Augenstern**, m. 1. pupil of the eye.
1067 **Augensternband**, n. 1. ciliary ligament.
1068 **Augensternerweiterung**, f. dilatation of the pupil, mydriasis.
1069 **Augensternverengerung**, f. contraction of the pupil, myosis.
1070 **Augenstreupulver**, n. 2. (fr. streuen, to disperse), powder, e. g. calomel, dusted on the eye.
1071 **Augentalg**, m. 1. sebum palpebrarum.
1072 **augentriefig**, adj. blear-eyed.
1073 **Augentripper**, m. 2. gonorrhœal ophthalmia.
1074 **Augentrockenheit**, f. xerophthalmia.
1075 **Augentropfwasser**, n. 2. guttae or drops for the eye.
1076 **Augenvene**, f. ophthalmic vein.
1077 **Augenverdunkelung**, f. obscurity of sight, amaurosis.
1078 **Augenwimper**, f. eyelash.
1079 **Augenwinkel**, m. 2. canthus.
1080 **Augenwinkelblutader**, f. angular vein.
1081 **Augenwinkelfalte**, f. epicanthus.
1082 **Augenwinkelschlagader**, f. angular artery.
1083 **Augenzahn**, m. 1. eye-tooth, canine tooth.
1084 **Augenzittern**, n. 2. (fr. zittern, to tremble), nystagmus, etc.
1085 **Augenzucken**, n. 2. (fr. zucken, to twitch), mystagmus, etc.

[2] The **EYES** may be:

1086 **eingefallen** (fr. v. ir. einfallen, to fall, sink in), injected, sunk in.
1087 **injiciert**, (fr. injicieren, to fall, sink in), injected, sunk in.
1088 **glänzend**, brilliant.
1089 **gläsern**, ein gläsernes Aussehen haben, to have a glassy look or appearance.
1090 **geschlossen** (fr. v. ir. schlieszen, to close), closed.
1091 **halb offen**, half open.
1092 **schielend**, squinting.
1093 **stierend**, staring.
1094 **thränend**, watery.
1095 **thränenvoll**, full of tears.
1096 **trüb**, dull, dim.
1097 **umgeben**, von einem dunklen Ring, surrounded by a dark ring, etc.
1098 Note 3. **STAR**, m. 1. Cataract of the eye.

a. VARIETY OF CATARACTS:

1099 ——, **baumförmiger**, arborescent cataract.
1100 ——, **diabetischer**, diabetic cataract.
1101 ——, **falscher**, false cataract, cataracta spuria.
1102 ——, **gefleckter**, spotted cataract.
1103 ——**geschrumpfter**, shrunken cataract.
1104 ——, **grauer**, gray cataract.
1105 ——, **grüner**, glau-coma.
1106 ——, **harter**, hard cataract.
1107 ——, **häutiger**, membranous cataract.
1108 ——, **Morgagnischer**, Morgagnic's cataract.
1109 ——, **punktierter**, spotted cataract, cataracta punctata.
1110 ——, **schwarzer**, black cataract, amaurosis.
1111 ——, **seniler**, senile cataract.
1112 ——, **traumatischer**, traumatic cataract.
1113 ——, **wahrer**, true, or lenticular cataract.
1114 ——, **weicher**, soft cataract.
1115 ——, **weiszer**, albugo, leucoma, etc.

b. **STAR**, in compounds:

1116 **starblind**, adj. blind from cataract.
1117 **Starblindheit**, f. blindness from cataract.
1118 **Starbrille**, f. spectacles after cataract operation.
1119 **Starentbindung**, f. (fr. v. ir. entbinden, to unbind, release), removal of cataract.
1120 **Starhaken**, m. 2. cataract hook, etc.
1121 **Thräne**, f. tear of the eye, pl.

Note 4. **THRÄNEN.**

1122 **Thränenableitung**, f. removal of the tears by the lachrymal duct.
1123 **Thränenapparat**, m. 1. lachrymal apparatus.
1124 **Thränenarterie**, f. lachrymal artery.
1125 **Thränenauge**, n. 1. watery eye.
1126 **Thränenbein**, n. 1. lachrymal bone.
1127 **Thränendrüse**, f. lachrymal gland.
1128 **Thränendrüsenentzündung**, f. inflammation of the lachrymal gland.
1129 **Thränendrüsenfistel**, f. lachrymal fistula.
1130 **Thränendrüsennerv**, m 3. lachrymal nerve.
1131 **Thränendrüsenvene**, f. lachrymal vein.
1132 **Thränendurchgang**, m. 1. lachrymal passage.
1133 **Thränenfistel**, f. lachrymal fistula.
1134 **Thränenflüssigkeit**, f. lachrymal fluid.
1135 **Thränengefäsz**, n. 1. lachrymal vessel.
1136 **Thränenkamm**, m. 1. crest of lachrymal bone.
1137 **Thränenkanal**, m. 1. }
Thränenkanälchen, n. 2 } lachrymal canal.
1138 **Thränenorgan**, n. 1. lachrymal organ.
1139 **Thränensack**, m. 1. lachrymal sack.
1140 **Thränensackwassersucht**, f. dropsy of lachrymal sack.
1141 **Thränensee**, m. 1. }
1142 **Thränenbucht**, f. } lacus lachrymalis (at the inner end or canthus).
1143 **Thränenstein**, m. 1. lachrymal calculus.
1144 **Thränenträufeln**, n. 2. epiphora.
1145 **Thränenwärzchen**, n. 2. }
1146 **Thränenwarze**, f. } caruncula lachrymalis, lachrymal papilla.
1147 **Thränenwinkelgeschwulst**, f. tumor of lachrymal sac, etc.
1148 **Thränen**, n. 2. lachrymation.
1149 9. **NASE**, f. nose, in compounds nasal.
1150 **Nasenader**, f. nasal vein.
1151 **Nasenarterie**, f. nasal artery.
1152 **Nasenatmen**, n. 2. }
Nasenatmung, f. } nasal breathing or respiration.
1153 **Nasenbein**, n. 1. nasal bone.
1154 **Nasenblutader**, f. nasal vein.
1155 **Nasendach**, n. 1. roof of nares.
1156 **Nasenfläche**, f. nasal surface.
1157 **Nasenflügel**, m. 2. wing of the nose, ala nasi.
1158 **Nasenfortsatz**, m. 1. nasal process.
1159 **Nasenfurche**, f. nasal furrow.
1160 **Nasengang**, m. 1. nasal duct.
1161 **Nasenganghaar**, n. 1. nasal vibrissa.
1162 **Nasengaumengang**, m. 1. naso-palatine canal.
1163 **Nasengaumenknoten**, m. 2. Meckel's ganglion.
1164 **Nasengewächs**, n. 1. nasal growth, polypus.
1165 **Nasengrube**, f. nasal fossa.
1166 **Nasenhaar**, n. 1. nasal vibrissa.
1167 **Nasenhaut**, f. pituitary membrane.
1168 **Nasenhöhle**, f. nasal cavity or fossa.
1169 **Nasenhöhlenscheidewand**, f. nasal septum.
1170 **Nasenkamm**, m. 1. nasal crest.
1171 **Nasenkanal**, m. 1. nasal canal.
1172 **Nasenknochen**, m. 2. nasal bone.
1173 **Nasenknorpel**, m. 2. nasal cartilage.
1174 **Nasenkuppe**, f. tip of nose.
1175 **Nasenloch**, n. 1. nostril.
1176 **Nasenlöcher**, pl. nares.
1177 **Nasenmuschel**, f. }
1178 **Nasenmuschelbein**, n. 1. } turbinated bone.
1179 **Nasennaht**, f. rhinorrhaphy.
1180 **Nasennerv**, m. 3. nasal nerve.

1181 **Nasenrachen**, m. 2. nasopharynx.
1182 **Nasenrücken**, m. 2. } bridge of the nose,
1183 **Nasenpflugschar**, f. }
1184 **Nasenpflugscharbein**, n. 1. } vomer.
1185 **Nasenschleim**, m. 1. nasal mucus.
1186 **Nasenschleimhaut**, f. nasal mucous membrane.
1187 **Nasenschlund**, m. 1. nasopharyngeal cavity.
1188 **Nasenspitze**, f. tip of nose.
1189 **Nasenstachel**, m. 2. nasal spine.
1190 **Nasenuntersuchung**, f. (fr. untersuchen, to examine), examination of the nose.
1191 **Nasenvene**, f. nasal vein.
1192 **Nasenverschlusz**, m. 1. (fr. v. ir. verschlieszen, to shut, close), occlusion of the nares.
1193 **Nasenwurzel**, f. root of the nose, etc.
1194 Note [1] **RIECHBEIN**, n. 1. ethmoid bone, in compounds :
1195 **Riechbeinloch**. n. 1. ethmoid cribriform foramen.
1196 **Riechbeinnerv**, m. 3. olfactory nerve.
1197 **Riechbeinpulsader**, f. } ethmoidal artery.
Riechbeinschlagader, f. }
1198 **Riechen**, n. 2. (from v. ir. riechen, to smell), smelling, smell, scent.
1199 **Riechhaut**, f. olfactory membrane.
1200 **Riechmittel**, n. 2. olfactory stimulant.
1201 **Riechsalz**, n. 1. carbonate of ammonia.
1202 **Riechwerkzeug**, n. 1. olfactory apparatus.
1203 **Riechzelle**, f. olfactory cell.
1204 Note [2] **SIEBBEIN**, n. 1. (fr. Sieb, n. 1. sieve), ethmoid bone, in compounds :
1205 **Siebbeinhöhle**, f. ethmoidal cavity.
1206 **Siebbeinknochen**, m. 2. ethmoid bone.
1207 **Siebbeinlabyrinth**, n. 1. turbinate process of ethmoid bone.
1208 **Siebbeinloch**, n. 1. ethmoid foramen.
1209 **Siebbeinmuschel**, f. ethmoidal turbinated bone.
1210 **Siebbeinnaht**, f. ethmoidal suture.
1211 **Siebbeinnerv**, m. 3. ethmoidal nerve.
1212 **Siebbeinplatte**, f. cribriform plate of ethmoid bone.
1213 **Siebbeinpulsader**, f. } ethmoidal artery.
Siebbeinschlagader, f. }
1214 **Siebbeinzelle**, f. ethmoidal cell, etc.
1215 10. **KIEFER**, m. 2. jaw, maxilla, in compounds :
1216 **Kieferast**, m. 1. maxillary branch, ramus of jaw.
1217 **Kieferbein**, n. 1. maxilla.
1218 **Kieferdrüse**, f. submaxillary gland.
1219 **Kieferfortsatz**, m. 1. maxillary process.
1220 **Kiefergelenk**, n. 1. temporo-maxillary joint.
1221 **Kieferknochen**, m. 2. maxillary bone.
1222 **Kieferknoten**, m. 2. maxillary ganglion.
1223 **Kieferwinkel**, m. 2. angle of jaw, etc.
1224 b. **KINN**, n. 1. chin, in compounds :
1225 **Kinnarterie**, f. mental artery.
1226 **Kinnbacken**, m. 2. jaw, maxilla.
1227 **Kinnbackenbein**, n. 1. maxillary bone.
1228 **Kinnbackengicht**, f. gout in the maxilla.
1229 **Kinnbackengrube**, f. maxilliary fossa.
1230 **Kinnbackenkanal**, m. 1. alveolar canal.
1231 **Kinnbackenkrampf**, m. 1. lockjaw, trismus.
1232 **Kinnbackenschmerz**, m. 1. neuralgia of the jaw.
1233 **Kinnbackenzahn**, m. 1. molar tooth.
1234 **Kinnlade**, f. jaw, maxilla.
1235 **Kinnnaht**, f. symphysis of the lower jaw.
1236 **Kinntuch**, n. 1. jaw bandage, etc.
1237 c. **OBERKIEFER**, m. 2. (fr. ober, superior, upper), superior maxilla, upper jaw.

1238 **Oberkieferast**, m. 1. supramaxillary branch.
1239 **Oberkieferbein**, n. 1. superior maxilla.
1240 **Oberkieferfortsatz**, m. 1. process of superior maxilla.
1241 **Oberkieferknochen**, m. 2. superior maxilla.
1242 **Oberkieferknoten**, m. 2. Meckel's ganglion.
1243 **Oberkieferkörper**, m. 2. body of superior maxilla.
1244 **Oberkieferlappen**, m. 2. pl. maxillary plates (forming the palate).
1245 **Oberkiefernerv**, m. 3. supramaxillary nerve, etc.
1246 d. **UNTERKIEFER**, m. 2. lower jaw, inferior maxilla.
1247 **Unterkieferast**, m. 1. ramus of the lower jaw.
1248 **Unterkieferbein**, n. 1. inferior maxillary bone.
1249 **Unterkieferbogen**, m. 2. arch of the lower jaw.
1250 **Unterkieferdrüse**, f. submaxillary gland.
1251 **Unterkieferfortsatz**, m. 1. process of inferior maxilla.
1252 **Unterkiefergebisz**, n. 1. the teeth of the lower jaw.
1253 **Unterkiefergegend**, f. submaxillary region.
1254 **Unterkiefergelenk**, n. 1. temporo-maxillary articulation.
1255 **Unterkieferhals**, m. 1. neck of inferior maxilla.
1256 **Unterkieferknochen**, m. 2. inferior maxillary bone.
1257 **Unterkieferknoten**, m. 2. submaxillary ganglion.
1258 **Unterkieferlähmung**, f. paralysis of the lower jaw.
1259 **Unterkieferzweig**, m. 1. ramus of the lower jaw, etc.
1260 [11] **MUND**, m. 1. mouth, in compounds:
1261 **Mundbucht**, f. oral diverticulum.
1262 **Munddrüse**, f. oral gland.
1263 **Mundgegend**, f. oral region.
1264 **Mundgrube**, f. oral diverticulum.
1265 **Mundhöhle**, f. oral cavity.
1266 **Mundöffnung**, f. oral aperture, etc.
1267 [12] **LIPPE**, f. lip, in compounds:
1268 **Lippenband**, n. 1. / **Lippenbändchen**, n. 2. } fraenum of the lips.
1269 **Lippendrüse**, f. labial gland.
1270 **Lippenfläche**, f. labial surface.
1271 **Lippenlaut**, m. 1. labial sound.
1272 **Lippenrot**, n. 1. the red portion of the lips.
1273 **Lippensaum**, m. 1. margin of the lips, etc.
1274 **Oberlippe**, f. upper lip.
1275 **Unterlippe**, f. underlip.
1276 [13] a. **OHR**, n. 1. ear, in compounds, auricular:
1277 **Ohr, äuszeres**, n. 1. auricle, pinna.
1278 **Ohr, innerstes**, n. 1. inner ear, labyrinth.
1279 **Ohr, mittleres**, n. 1. middle ear, tympanum.
1280 **Ohrast**, m. 1. auricular branch.
1281 **Ohrband**, n. 1. ear ligament.
1282 **Ohrblatt**, n. 1. pinna.
1283 **Ohrbock**, m. 1. tragus.
1284 **Ohrdrüse**, f. parotid gland.
1285 **Ohrecke, hindere**, f. antitragus.
1286 **Ohrecke, vordere**, f. tragus.
1287 **Ohrenband**, n. 1. (from Ohren, pl. see my Grammar, page 48, d.) ligament of the pinna.
1288 **Ohrengang**, m. 1. duct of parotid gland, Steno's duct.
1289 **Ohrengeflecht**, n. 1. parotid plexus.
1290 **Ohrengegend**, f. parotid region.
1291 **Ohrenhöhle**, f. aural cavity.
1292 **Ohrenknorpel**, m. 2. aural cartilage.
1293 **Ohrenschmalz**, n. 1. earwax, cerumen.
1294 **Ohrenspalte**, f. fissure of the pinna.
1295 **Ohrenstein**, m. 1. otolith.
1296 **Ohrentrommel**, f. tympanum, tympanic membrane.
1297 **Ohrflügel**, m. 2. auricle.
1298 **ohrförmig**, adj. auriform, ear-shaped.
1299 **Ohrfortsatz**, m. 1. auditory process.
1300 **Ohrgang**, m. 1. auditory canal.
1301 **Ohrgegend**, f. auricular region.
1302 **Ohrhalskanal**, m. 1. Eustachian tube.
1303 **Ohrhöhle**, f. aural cavity.

1304 **Ohrkanal**, m. 1. auricular or auditory canal.
1305 **Ohrklappe**, f. hintere, antitragus.
1306 **Ohrklappe**, f. vordere, tragus.
1307 **Ohrknöchelchen**, n. 2. auditory ossicle.
1308 **Ohrknorpel**, m. 2. auricular cartilage.
1309 **Ohrknoten**, m. 2. otic ganglion.
1310 **Ohrkrystall**, m. 1. otolith.
1311 **Ohrlabyrinth**, n. 1. ear labyrinth.
1312 **Ohrläppchen**, n. 2. ear lobe.
1313 **Ohrleiste**, f. } helix, äussere, helix; innere, antihelix.
1314 **Ohrkrempe**, f. }
1315 **Ohrloch**, n. 1. external auditory meatus.
1316 **Ohrmuschel**, f. auricle, pinna.
1317 **Ohrmuschelgrube**, f. concha.
1318 **Ohrmuschelheber**, m. 2. attollens aurem muscle.
1319 **Ohrmuschelleiste**, f. } helix.
1320 **Ohrmuschelrand**, m. 1. }
1321 **Ohrmuschelzurückzieher**, m. 2. (from v. ir. zurückziehen, to draw back), retrahens aurem muscle.
1322 **Ohrmuskel**, m. 2. ear muscle.
1323 **Ohroberfläche**, f. auricular surface.
1324 **Ohröffnung**, f. external auditory meatus.
1325 **Ohrpulsader**, f. auricular or auditory artery.
1326 **Ohrsand**, m. 1. otolith.
1327 **Ohrschläfennerv**, m. 3. auriculo-temporal nerve.
1328 **Ohrschlagader**, f. auditory artery.
1329 **Ohrschnecke**, f. cochlea.
1330 **Ohrschmalz**, n. 1. earwax, cerumen.
1331 **Ohrstein**, m. 1. } otolith.
Ohrsteinchen, n. 2. }
1332 **Ohrtrommel**, f. } tympanum, tympanic membrane.
Trommelfell, n. 1. }
1333 **Ohrtrompete**, f. Eustachian tube.
1334 **Ohrvene**, f. auricular vein.
1335 **Ohrwachs**, n. 1. cerumen.
1336 **Ohrzehe**, f. little toe, etc.
1337 b. **AMBOSZ**, m. 1. anvil, incus.
amboszförmig, adj. incudiform.
1338 **Hammer**, m. 2. hammer, malleus.
1339 **Hammeramboszgelenk**, n. 1. joint between hammer and anvil.
1340 **Hammerfalte**, f. mucous membrane fold reflected from the hammer.
1341 **Kalkimprägnierung**, f. calcification used in sklerose (sclerosis), of tympanum cavity.
1342 **Steigbügel**, m. 2. stirrup, stapes.
1343 **Steigbügelmuskel**, m. 2. stapedian muscle, stapedius.
1344 **Steigbügelplatte**, f. } base or foot of stirrup.
1345 **Steigbügeltritt**, m. 1. }
1346 **Steigbügeltour**, f. stirrup turn in bandaging the foot in a figure of an eight-bandage around the ankle, etc.
1347 4. **GESICHT**, n. 1. countenance, face, visage (from v. ir. sehen, to see).
—(for Gesicht, eyesight, sight, sense or faculty of seeing, vision, see § 18, 5, a & b).
1348 **Gesichtsarterie**, f. facial artery.
1349 **Gesichtsausdruck**, m. 1. (from ausdrücken, to express), expression of the countenance. See *Note* [2].
1350 **Gesichtsblatter**, f. } pimple, acne.
1351 **Gesichtsblätterchen**, n. 2. }
1352 **Gesichtsfarbe**, f. color of the face, complexion.
1353 **Gesichtsfläche**, f. facial surface.
1354 **Gesichtsgegend**, f. facial region.
1355 **Gesichtsgrind**, m. 1. porrigo, sycosis.
1356 **Gesichtshaut**, f. skin of the face.
1357 **Gesichtshöhlen**, f. pl. facial cavities (mouth, nose, etc.)
1358 **Gesichtsknochen**, m. 2. facial bone.
1359 **Gesichtskrampf**, m. 1. facial spasm.
1360 **Gesichtskrebs**, m. 1. cancer of the face.
1361 **Gesichtslähmung**, f. facial paralysis.
1362 **Gesichtsmuskel**, m. 2. facial muscle.
1363 **Gesichtsnerv**, m. 3. facial nerve.

1364 **Gesichtspustel**, f. facial pustule.

1365 **Gesichtsröte**, f. facial redness, blush.

1366 **Gesichtsschädel**, m. 2. facial part of the skull.

1367 **Gesichtsvene**, f. facial vein.

1368 **Gesichtszug**, m. 1. (from v. tr. ziehen, to draw) feature, lineament, mien, etc. **Gebärde** or **Geberde**, f.

Note[1] **Das Gesicht mag sein:** The countenance may be:

1369 **abgemagert**, emaciated.

1370 **blau**, blue.

1371 **blaurot**, dusty red.

1372 **bleich**, pale, pallid.

1373 **bleifarbig**, livid, leaden-hued.

1374 **dünn**, thin.

1375 **fahl**, of a sallow-hue.

1376 **gelb**, yellow.

1377 **gelblich**, yellowish.

1378 **leichenähnlich**, cadaverous, corpse-like.

1379 **leichenartig**,

1380 **leichenblasz**,

1381 **leichenhaft**,

1382 **livid**, blue, leaden-hued.

1383 **ödematös**, œdematous.

1384 **totenblasz**, **totenbleich**, deathly pale.

1385 **totenhaft**, death-like.

1386 **unverändert**, unchanged.

1387 **verändert**, changed.

1388 **vollblütig**, full-blooded, plethoric.

1389 **weichlich**, delicate, effeminate, etc.

1390 Note[2] **Der GESICHTSAUSDRUCK, mag sein:** the expression of the countenance may be:

1391 **achtlos**, inattentive, indifferent, listless.

1392 **achtsam**, attentive, watchful.

1393 **analogisch**, like, similar.

1394 **ähnlich**, resembling.

1395 **ängstlich**, **angstvoll**, anxious, disturbed.

1396 **ärgerlich**, mad.

1397 **aufgebracht**, vexatious.

1398 **aufgeregt**, excited.

1399 **ausdruckslos**, inexpressive, meaningless.

1400 **ausdrucksvoll**, expressive, impressive, e. g. not only as to character, but also as to

1401 **Schmerz**, pain, suffering, etc.

1402 **bekümmert**, troubled, filled with grief, sorrowful.

1403 **deprimiert**, depressed.

1404 **difform**, misshaped.

1405 **difformiert**, deformed.

1406 **düster**, gloomy.

1407 **einfältig**, simple, silly.

1408 **erregt**, excited, irritated.

1409 **erschreckt**, frightened, terrified.

1410 **gefaszt** (from fassen, to seize, to lay hold on), calm, composed.

1411 **gereizt**, irritated.

1412 **gleichgültig**, careless, indifferent.

1413 **intelligent**, intellectual.

1414 **irrsinnig**, insane.

1415 **kummervoll**, troubled.

1416 **leer**, vacant.

1417 **leidend**, suffering.

1418 **melancholisch**, melancholy, dejected.

1419 **mürrisch**, peevish.

1420 **niedergeschlagen**, depressed, sad.

1421 **nichtssagend**, dull, indifferent.

1422 **rasend**, raging, maniacal.

1423 **rastlos**, restless, uneasy.

1424 **rauh**, harsh.

1425 **ruhig**, quiet, tranquil.

1426 **sorglos**, careless, listless.

1427 **starr**, rigid, motionless.

1428 **stumpf**, dull, obtuse.

1429 **stupid**, dull.

1430 **teilnahmslos**, impassive.

1431 **teilnehmend**, interested.

1432 **unruhig**, restless.

1433 **unstät**, wandering.

1434 **verdreht**, **verzerrt**, distorted.

1435 **verwirrt**, confused.

1436 **verzweifelt**, desperate, in despair.

1437 **wahnsinnig**, insane.

1438 **wild**, wild, furious.

1439 **zerstreut**, absent-minded, etc.

1440 15. **GAUMEN**, m. 2. palate, in compounds:

1441 **Gaumenbein**, n. 1. palate bone.

1442 **Gaumenbogen**, m. 2. palatine arch.

1443 **Gaumendrüse**, f. palatine gland.

1444 **Gaumenfalten**, f. pl. ridges of the palate.

1445 **Gaumenflor**, m. 1. velum palati.

1446 **Gaumenflügel**, m. 2. pterygoid process.
1447 **Gaumenfortsatz**, m. 1. palatine process.
1448 **Gaumengang**, m. 1. palatine canal (from. Gang, canal).
1449 **Gaumengewölbe**, n. 1. arch of the palate.
1450 **Gaumenkeilbeingeflecht**, n. 1. spheno-palatine plexus.
1451 **Gaumenkeilbeinknoten**, m. 2. spheno- palatine ganglion.
1452 **Gaumenknochen**, m. 2. palatine bone.
1453 **Gaumenlähmung**, f. paralysis of the palate.
1454 **Gaumenleisten**, f. pl. palate ridges.
1455 **Gaumenloch**, n. 1. palatine foramen.
1456 **Gaumennaht**, f. palatine suture.
1457 **Gaumensegel**, n. 2. palate sail, velum palati.
1458 **Gaumenwurzel**, f. palatine root, etc.
1459 16. **KEHLE**, f. throat, glottis, larynx, in compounds :
1460 **Kehlbruch**, m. 1. (fr. v. ir. brechen, to break), thyrocele.
1461 **Kehldeckel**, m. 2. epiglottis.
1462 **Kehldeckelaufhängeband**, n. 1. epiglottis ligament.
1463 **Kehldeckeldrüse**, f. epiglottic gland.
1464 **Kehldeckelknorpel**, m. 2. epiglottis cartilage.
1465 **Kehldeckelkrücke**, f. epiglottic crutch.
1466 **Kehldeckelwulst**, m. 1. epiglottis cushion.
1467 **Kehldrüse**, f. thyroid gland.
1468 **Kehlgrube**, f. supra-sternal fossa.
1469 **Kehlknochen**, m. 2. hyoid bone.
1470 **Kehlknorpel**, m. 2. laryngeal cartilage.
1471 **Kehlkopf**, m. 1. larynx.
1472 **Kehlkopfband**, n. 1. laryngeal ligament.
1473 **Kehlkopfbinnenraum**, m. 1. intra-laryngeal space.
1474 **Kehlkopfbruch**, m. 1. fracture of the larynx.
1475 **Kehlkopfdrüse**, f. laryngeal gland.
1476 **Kehlkopfeingang**, m. 1. (fr. v. ir. eingehen, to go into), opening of the larynx or pharynx.
1477 **Kehlkopferöffnung**, f. (fr. er. öffnen, to open), laryngotomy.
1478 **Kehlkopferweiterung**, f. (fr. erweitern, to enlarge), dilatation of the larynx.
1479 **Kehlkopfgegend**, f. laryngeal region.
1480 **Kehlkopfgeräusch**, n. 1. (fr. rauschen, to rush, rustle), laryngeal sound or murmur (e. g. at consultation.)
1481 **Kehlkopfhaut**, f. laryngeal membrane.
1482 **Kehlkopfhöhle**, f. laryngeal cavity.
1483 **Kehlkopfknorpel**, m. 2, laryngeal cartilage.
1484 **Kehlkopfknorpelhaut**, f. larynx perichondrium.
1485 **Kehlkopfraum**, m. 1. laryngeal space.
1486 **Kehlkopftasche**, f. larynx ventricle.
1487 **Kehllaut**, m. 1. guttural sound.
1488 **Kehlloch**, n. 1. jugular foramen.
1489 **Kehlstimme**, f. guttular voice.
1490 **Kehlsucht**, f. parotitis.
1491 **Kehlzäpflein**, n. 2. uvula, etc.
1492 1493 17. **MANDEL**, f. tonsil, almond. amygdala (of brain); Mandeln, pl. f. glands of the throat, tonsils, in compounds :
1494 **Mandelabscesz**, m. 1. tonsil abscess.
1495 **Mandelabtragung**, f. tonsil removal (from v. ir. abtragen, to take or carry away or off.)
1496 **Mandelbräune**, f. angina, cynanche, tonsilitis.
1497 **Mandeldrüse**, f. tonsil.
1498 **Mandeleitergeschwulst**, f. tonsil abscess.
1499 **Mandelentzündung**, f. tonsilitis.
1500 **Mandelgeschwulst**, f. } enlarged tonsil.
1501 **Mandelhypertrophie**, f. }
1502 **Mandelschwellung**, f. }
1503 **Mandelstein**, m. 1. tonsillar calculus.

1504 18. **RACHEN**, m. 2. pharynx, fauces, throat, (for further compounds see also § 13, 6).
In compounds:
1505 **Rachenbein**, n. 1. jaw bone.
1506 **Rachenblutung**, f. pharyngeal hemorrhage.
1507 **Rachenbräune**, f. angina; pharyngitis;
1508 **Rachenbräune**, bösartige; brandige; epidemische; angina maligna or gangrenosa, diphtheria.
1509 **Rachenentzündung**, f. } pharyngitis.
1510 **Rachenschleimhautentzündung**, f. } pharyngitis.
1511 **Rachenkatarrh**, m. 1. } pharyngitis.
1512 **Rachentonsille**, f. pharyngeal tonsil.
1513 **Rachenwandung**, f. pharyngeal wall, etc.
1514 19. **ZAHN**, m. 1. tooth, in compounds:
1515 **Augenzahn**, m. 1. eye tooth, canine tooth.
1516 **Backenzahn**, m. 1. jaw tooth, molar tooth.
1517 **Milchzahn**, m. 1. milk tooth.
1518 **Milchschneidezahn**, m. 1, deciduous or milk-incisor tooth.
1519 **Mittelzahn**, m. 1. incisor tooth.
1520 **Schneidezahn**, m. 1. incisor tooth, cutter.
1521 **Vorderzahn**, m. 1. front tooth.
1522 **Weisheitszahn**, m. 1. wisdom tooth.
1523 **Zahnachse**, f. axis of a tooth.
1524 **zahnähnlich**, adj. odontoid.
1525 **Zahnanlage**, f. dental germ or rudiment.
1526 **Zahnanomalie**, f. dental anomaly.
1527 **zahnartig**, adj. odontoid.
1528 **Zahnast**, m. 1. dental branch or twig.
1529 **Zahnausbruch**, m. 1. (fr. v. ir. ausbrechen, to break forth or to come forth) dentition.
1530 **Zahnausnehmen**, n. 2. (fr. v. ir. ausnehmen, to take out) extraction of tooth.
1531 **Zahndurchbruch**, m. 1. (fr. v. ir. durchbrechen, to break through) eruption or cutting of teeth.
1532 **Zahneinpflanzung**, f. (fr. einpflanzen, to plant into) implantation of teeth.
1533 **Zahnen**, n. 2. teething, dentition.
1534 **Zahnfläche**, f. surface of a tooth.
1535 **Zahnfleisch**, n. 1. gum.
1536 **Zahnfurche**, f. dental groove.
1537 **Zahngewebe**, n. 1. dental tissue.
1538 **Zahnhals**, m. 1. neck of a tooth.
1539 **Zahnhöhle**, f. socket of a tooth, tooth cavity.
1540 **Zahnimplantation**, f. implantation of teeth.
1541 **Zahnkeim**, m. 1. } tooth germ.
1542 **Zahnkern**, m. 1. } tooth pulp.
1543 **Zahnknirschen**, n. 2. grinding of the teeth.
1544 **Zahnkrone**, f. crown of tooth.
1545 **Zahnlade**, f. jaw, tooth-socket.
1546 **Zahnlücke**, f. gap between the teeth.
1547 **Zahnrand**, m. 1. dental margin.
1548 **Zahnreihe**, f. row of teeth.
1549 **Zahnschmelz**, m. 1. tooth enamel.
1550 **Zahnstein**, m. 1. tartar of teeth.
1551 **Zahnwackeln**, n. 2. shaking or loosening of a tooth.
1552 **Zahnwechsel**, m. 2. shedding of the first so-called milk teeth.
1553 **Zahnweinstein**, m. 1. tartar on the teeth.
1554 **Zahnwurzel**, f. root of a tooth.
1555 **Zahnzelle**, f. alveolus.
1556 **Zahnausziehen**, n. 2. } (f. v. ir. ziehen, to draw) hence to draw or pull, to extract, tooth-drawing, etc.
1557 **Zahnziehen**, n. 2. } (f. v. ir. ziehen, to draw) hence to draw or pull, to extract, tooth-drawing, etc.
1558 20. **ZUNGE**, f. tongue, lingual, in compounds.
1559 **Zungenabtragung**, f. (from v. ir. abtragen, to take off, removal of the tongue.
1560 **Zungenanwachsung**, f. (from v. ir. anwachsen, to grow on) tongue-tie.
1561 **Zungenast**, m. 1. lingual branch.
1562 **Zungenbalgdrüse**, f. lingual gland.
1563 **Zungenband**, n. 1. } fraenum of the tongue.
Zungenbändchen, n. 2. } fraenum of the tongue.

1564 **Zungenbein**, n. 1. hyoid bone.
1565 **Zungenbeinbogen**, m. 2. arch of hyoid bone.
1566 **Zungenbeinbruch**, m. 1. fracture of hyoid bone.
1567 **Zungenbeingegend**, f. region of hyoid bone.
1568 **Zungenbeinhorn**, n. 1. cornu of hyoid bone.
1569 **Zungenbeinkörper**, m. 2. body of hyoid bone.
1570 **Zungenbeinzweig**, m. 1. hyoid branch.
1571 **Zungenbelag**, m. 1. } (from v. ir. belegen, to cover) fur coating or covering of the tongue.
1572 **Zungenbeleg**, m. 1. }
1573 **Zungenbeschauung**, f. (from beschauen, to look at), inspection of the tongue.
1574 **Zungenbruch**, m. 1. (from v. ir. brechen, to break), protrusion of the tongue.
1575 **Zungendrüse**, f. lingual gland.
1576 **Zungenfläche**, f. lingual surface.
1577 **Zungenfleisch**, n. 1. substance of the tongue.
1578 **zungenförmig**, adj. tongue-formed.
1579 **Zungengegend**, f. region of the tongue.
1580 **Zungengewächs**, n. 1. (from v. ir. wachsen, to grow), growth upon the tongue.
1581 **Zungengrund**, m. 1. base of the tongue.
1582 **Zungenhaut**, f. epidermis of the tongue.
1583 **Zungenknochen**, m. 2. hyoid bone.
1584 **Zungenlaut**, m. 1. lingual sound.
1585 **Zungenloch**, n. 1. foramen caecum of the tongue.
1586 **zungenlos**, adj. tongueless.
1587 **Zungenmuskel**, m. 2. lingual muscle.
1588 **Zungennaht**, f. raphé of the tongue.
1589 **Zungennerv**, m. 3. lingual nerve.
1590 **Zungenrand**, m. 1. border or edge of the tongue.
1591 **Zungenrücken**, m. 2. dorsum linguae.
1592 **Zungenspalte**, f. fissure of the tongue.
1593 **Zungenspitze**, f. tip of tongue.
1594 **Zungenüberzug**, m. 1. (from v. ir. überziehen, to cover), fur coating of the tongue.
1595 **Zungenvorfall**, m. 1. tongue prolapse.
1596 **Zungenwärzchen**, n. 2. } papilla of the tongue.
1597 **Zungenwarze**, f. }
1598 **Zungenwurzel**, f. root of tongue.
1599 **Zungenzäpfchen**, n. 2. epiglottis.
1600 **Zungenzergliederung**, f. dissection of the tongue.
1601 **Zungenzweig**, m. 1. lingual branch, etc.
1602 Note. Die **ZUNGE** mag sein: the tongue may be:
1603 **bedeckt**, } covered, loaded, e. g. with a käse-ähnlich (cheese-like), curd-like, whitish fur or exudation, whose coming off is expressed by
1604 **belegt**, }
1605 **wird abgestoszen** (from v. ir. abstoszen, to cast off, to shed), is cast off.
1606 **blasz**, pale.
1607 **braun**, brown.
1608 **dunkelbraun**, dark brown.
1609 **entzündet** (from entzünden, to inflame), inflamed.
1610 **feucht**, moist.
1611 **gallicht**, } bilious.
1612 **gallig**, }
1613 **gefurcht**, grooved.
1614 **gelb**, yellow.
1615 **geschwollen** (from v. ir. schwellen, to swell), swollen.
1616 **geschworen** (from v. ir. schwären, to ulcerate), ulcerated.
1617 **gespaltet** (from spalten, to split), cleft.
1618 **grosz**, big, large.
1619 **heisz**, hot.
1620 **kalt**, cold.
1621 **pelzig**, furred.
1622 **rein**, clean.
1623 **rissig** (from v. ir. reiszen, to tear, whence Risz, m. 1. tear, cleft, rent), chapped, fissured.
1624 **rot**, red, rötlich, reddish.
1625 **schlaff**, flabby.
1626 **trocken**, dry.
1627 **überzogen** (from v. ir. überziehen, to cover), whence
1628 **Überzug**, m. 1. cover, covering, covered.

1629 **verändert,** changed (from verändern, to change).
1630 **verbessert,** bettered, ameliorated.
1631 **vergröszert,** enlarged (from vergröszern.
1632 **verhärtet,** indurated (from verhärten).
1633 **verletzt,** injured (from verletzen).
1634 **weisz,** white, weiszlich, whitish, etc.
1635 21. **HALS,** m. 1. neck, throat, in compounds:
1636 **Halsbein,** n. 1. collar bone.
1637 **Halsbindegewebe,** n. 1. cervical connective tissue.
1638 **Halsdreieck,** n. 1. cervical triangle.
1639 **Halsdrüse,** f. cervical gland, tonsil.
1640 **Halseingeweide,** n. 1. contents of the neck.
1641 **Halsfistel,** f. cervical fistula.
1642 **Halsgefäsz,** n. 1. vessel of the neck.
1643 **Halsgeflecht,** n. 1. cervical plexus.
1644 **Halsgegend,** f. cervical region.
1645 **Halshöhle,** f. throat cavity.
1646 **Halsknoten,** m. 2. cervical ganglion.
1647 **Halsmandel,** f. tonsil.
1648 **Halsmark,** n. 1. cervical spinal cord.
1649 **Halsplatte,** f. cervical plate.
1650 **Halsröhre,** f. trachea.
1651 **Halsrückenmark,** n. 1. cervical spinal cord.
1652 **Halsspalte,** f. cervical cleft.
1653 **Halsweh,** n. 1. pain in the throat.
1654 **Halswirbel,** m. 2. } cervical vertebra.
1655 **Halswirbelbein,** n. 1. } cervical vertebra.
1656 **Halswirbeldorn,** m. 1. spinous process of cervical vertebra.
1657 **Halswirbelsäule,** f. cervical part of vertebral column.
1658 **Halswirbelsäulenfortsatz,** m. 1. spinous process of cervical vertebra.
1659 **Halswirbelzahnfortsatz,** m. 1. odontoid process.
1660 **Hals-zäpflein** or **zäpfchen,** n. 2. uvula.
1661 **Halszellgewebe,** n. 1. cervical cellular tissue, etc.
1662 22. **NACKEN,** m. 2. } nape of neck, nape, neck, nucha, cervix.
1663 **GENICK,** n. 1. } in compounds:
1664 **Nackenband,** n. 1. ligamentum nuchae.
1665 **Nackendrüse,** f. cervical gland.
1666 **Nackenfistel,** f. cervical fistula.
1667 **Nackengegend,** f. cervical region.
1668 **Nackengrube,** f. fovea nuchae, neck hollow.
1669 **Nackenkrümmung,** f. cervical curve or curvature.
1670 **Nackenlymphdrüse,** f. cervical lymphgland.
1671 **Nackenweh,** n. 1. pain in the neck.
1672 **Nackenwirbel,** m. 2. cervical vertebra.
1673 **Nackenzweig,** m. 1. cervical branch, etc.
1674 1675 § 8. **Teile des Rumpfes** und der oberen und unteren Gliedmaszen, parts of the trunk and upper and lower extremities.
1676 1. **RUMPF,** m. 1. trunk, body, in compounds:
1677 **Rumpfgegend,** f. trunk region.
1678 **Rumpfhöhle,** f. trunk cavity.
1679 **Rumpfknochen,** m. 2. bones of the trunk, etc.
1680 **ATLAS,** m. 1. } atlas, bearer, (from v. ir. tragen, to bear.)
1681 **TRÄGER,** m. 2. } atlas, bearer, (from v. ir. tragen, to bear.)
1682 2. **RÜCKEN,** m. 2. back, dorsum, in compounds *dorsal:*
1683 **Rückenader,** f. dorsal vein.
1684 **Rückenarterie,** f. dorsal artery.
1685 **Rückenast,** m. 1. dorsal branch.
1686 **Rückenband,** n. 1. dorsal ligament.
1687 **Rückenbein,** n. 1. the spine, vertebra.
1688 **Rückenblutader,** f. dorsal vein.
1689 **Rückendarre,** f. } tabes dorsalis.
Rückenmarkdarre, f. } tabes dorsalis.
1690 **Rückenfläche,** f. dorsal surface.
1691 **Rückenfurche,** f. dorsal furrow.
1692 **Rückengefäsz,** n. 1. dorsal vessel.

1693 **Rückengegend,** f. dorsal region.
1694 **Rückengelenk,** n. 1. vertebral articulation.
1695 **Rückenhaut,** f. pleura, skin of the back.
1696 **Rückenkreuz,** n. 1. lumbar region.
1697 **Rückenlendengegend,** f. lumbar spinal region.
1698 **Rückenmark,** n. 1. spinal cord.
1699 **Rückenmarkarterie,** f. spinal artery.
1700 **Rückenhalbdornmuskel,** m. 2. semi-spinalis muscle.
1701 **Rückenmarksblutader,** f. spinal vein.
1702 **Rückenmarksblutschlag,** m. 1. hemorrhage into the spinal cord.
1703 **Rückenmarkserscheinung,** f. spinal cord phenomenon.
1704 **Rückenmarkserschütterung,** f. concussion of the spinal cord.
1705 **Rückenmarkserweichung,** f. softening of the spinal cord.
1706 **Rückenmarksgefäsz,** n. 1. spinal vessel.
1707 **Rückenmarksgift,** n. 1. spinal cord poison (e. g. strychnia.)
1708 **Rückenmarksgrau,** n. 1. grey matter of spinal cord.
1709 **Rückenmarkshaut,** f. spinal meninges.
1710 **Rückenmarkskanal,** m. 1. canal of the spinal marrow.
1711 **Rückenmarkslähmung,** f. spinal paralysis.
1712 **Rückenmarksloch,** n. 1. vertebral canal.
1713 **Rückenmarksnerv,** m. 3. spinal nerve.
1714 **Rückenmarksnervengeflecht,** n. 1. spinal nerve plexus.
1715 **Rückenmarksnervenlähmung,** f. spinal nerve paralysis.
1716 **Rückenmarksnervenpaar,** n. 1. pair of spinal nerves.
1717 **Rückenmarksreizung,** f. spinal irritability.
1718 **Rückenmarksrinde,** f. medullary cortex.
1719 **Rückenmarksspalte,** f. cleft in the spinal cord (congenital).
1720 **Rückenmarksstrang,** m. 1. spinal cord..
1721 **Rückenmarksvene,** f. spinal vein.
1722 **Rückenmarksverhärtung,** f. sclerosis of the spinal cord.
1723 **Rückenmarksverletzung,** f. injury to the spinal cord.
1724 **Rückenmarkszerreiszung,** f. laceration of the spinal cord.
1725 **Rückenmuskel,** m. 2. dorsal or spinal muscle.
1726 **Rückenmuskel,** breiter, m. 2. latissimus dorsi.
1727 ——longer, m. 2. longissimus dorsi.
1728 **Rückennerv,** m. 3. dorsal nerve.
1729 **Rückennetz,** n. 1. rete dorsale.
1730 **Rückenplatte,** f. dorsal plate.
1731 **Rückenpulsader,** f. dorsal artery.
1732 **Rückensäule,** f. vertebral column.
1733 **Rückenschlagader,** f. dorsal artery.
1734 **Rückenstarre,** f. rigidity of the back.
1735 **Rückenstrang,** m. 1. spinal cord.
1736 **Rückenteil,** m. 1. dorsal portion.
1737 **Rückenwirbel,** m. 2.
1738 **Rückenwirbelbein,** n. 1. } dorsal vertebra, etc.
1739 b. **Rückgrat,** m. & n. 1. spine, vertebral column, in compounds:
1740 **rückgrätig,** adj. spinal.
1741 **Rückgratsband,** n. 1. spinal or vertebral ligament.
1742 **Rückgratsbein,** n. 1. vertebra.
1743 **Rückgratsgelenk,** n. 1. spinal articulation.
1744 **Rückgratsgicht,** f. gout of the spine.
1745 **Rückgratshöhle,** f.
1746 **Rückgratskanal,** m. 1. } spinal or vertebral canal.
1747 **Rückgratskrankheit,** f. disease of the spinal column.
1748 **Rückgratskrümmung,** f.
1749 **Rückgratsverkrümmung,** f. } curvature of the spine.
1750 **Rückgratsmuskel,** m. 2. spinal muscle.

1751 **Rückgratsnerv**, m. 3. spinal nerve.

1752 **Rückgratsschmerz**, m. 1. } pain in the

1753 **Rückgratsweh**, n. 1. } spine.

1754 **Rückgratsspalte**, f. spina bifida.

1755 **Rückgratsstrecker**, m. 2, erector spinae.

1756 **Rückgratswassersucht**, f. hydrorachis.

1757 **Rückgratswirbel**, m. 2. vertebra.

1758 **rücklaufend**, adj. } recurrent.
rückläufig, adj. }

1759 **rücklings**, adv. backwards.

1760 **Rückschritt**, m. 1. (fr.v. ir. zurückschreiten, to retrograde or to stride back, relapse, retrogression.

1761 **Rückwärtsdreher**, m. 2. supinator, etc.

1762 3. **SEITE**, f. side. mostly *lateral* in compounds :

1763 **Seitenader**, f. lateral vein.

1764 **Seitenast**, m. 1. lateral branch.

1765 **Seitenband**, n. 1. lateral ligament.

1766 **Seitenbauchlage**, f. lateral abdominal region.

1767 **Seitenbeckenbein**, n. 1. lateral bone of pelvis.

1768 **Seitenbein**, n. 1. lateral bone, parietal bone.

1769 **Seitenblutader**, f. lateral vein.

1770 **Seitenflügel**, m. 2. lateral wing.

1771 **Seitenhebel**, m. 2. lateral retractor.

1772 **Seitenhöhle**, f. lateral ventricle.

1773 **Seitenhorn**, n. 1. lateral cornu.

1774 **Seitenkopfweh**, n. 1. hemicrania.

1775 **Seitenkrampf**, m. 1. pleurodynia.

1776 **Seitenkreislauf**, m. 1. collateral circulation.

1777 **Seitenlage**, f. lateral position or presentation.

1778 **Seitenlähmung**, f. hemiplegia.

1779 **Seitenlappen**, m. 2. lateral lobe.

1780 **Seitenpulsader**, f. lateral artery.

1781 **Seitenrumpfmuskel**, m. 2. lateral trunk muscle.

1782 **Seitenschmerz**, m. 1. } pleurodynia, stitch in the side.

1783 **Seitenstechen**, n. 2. }

1784 **Seitenstrang**, m. 1. lateral fasciculus, lateral column.

1785 **Seitenteil**, m. 1. lateral portion.

1786 **Seitenventrikel**, m. 2. lateral ventricle.

1787 **Seitenverrenkung**, f. lateral dislocation.

1788 **seitlich**, adj. lateral. etc.

1789 4. **BRUST**, f. breast, chest, thorax, mamma, in compounds :

1790 **Brustader**, f. thoracic or mammary vein.

1791 **Brustaorta**, thoracic aorta.

1792 **Brustarterie**, f. thoracic or mammary artery.

1793 **Brustatmen**, n. 2. thoracic breathing.

1794 **Brustbeengung**. f. constriction or oppression about the chest.

1795 **Brustbein**, n. 1. }

1796 **Brustbeinknochen**, m. 2. } sternum.

1797 **Brustblatt**, n. 1. }

1798 **Brustschild**, n. 1. }

1799 **Brustbeinknorpel**, m. 2. xiphoid cartilage.

1800 **Brustbeinmuskel**. **dreieckiger**, m. 2. triangularis sterni.

1801 **Brustbeinrippengelenk**, n. 1. sterno-costal articulation.

1802 **Brustbeinschildknorpelmuskel**. m. 2. } sterno-thyroid muscle
Brustbeinschildmuskel, m. 2. }

1803 **Brustbeinschlüsselbeingelenk**, n. 1. } sterno-clavicular articulation.
Brustbeinschlüsselgelenk, n. 1. }

1804 **Brustbeinschlüsselverbindung**, f. }

1805 **Brustbeinschmerz**, m. 1. pain in or about the sternum.

1806 **Brustbeinspalte**, f. } sternal cleft.
Brustbeinspaltung, f. }

1807 **Brustbeinwarzenmuskel**, m. 2. sterno-mastoid muscle.

1808 **Brustbeinzungenbeinmuskel**, m. 2. sterno-hyoid muscle.

1809 **Brustbruch**, m. 1. thoracic hernia.

1810 **Brustdrüse**, f. thoracic gland, mammary gland, thymus.
1811 **Brustdrüsenanschwellung**, f. (fr. v. ir. anschwellen, to increase) swelling of the mammary gland.
1812 **Brustdrüsengegend**, f. mammary region.
1813 **Brustdrüsengeschwulst**, f. mammary tumor.
1814 **Brustdrüsengeschwür**, n. 1. mammary ulcer.
1815 **Brustdrüsengewebe**, n. 1. tissue of breast gland.
1816 **Brusteingeweide**, n. 1. thoracic viscera.
1817 **Brustfell**, n. 1. pleura.
1818 **Brustfellbruch**, m. 1. pleurocele.
1819 **Brustfellfistel**, f. fistulous opening in the pleura.
1820 **Brustfellhöhle**, f. } cavity of the pleura.
1821 **Brustfellsack**, m. 1. } cavity of the pleura.
1822 **Brustfellverwachsung**, f. pleuritic adhesion.
1823 **Brustfistel**, f. thoracic fistula.
1824 **Brustgang**, m. 1. thoracic duct.
1825 **Brustgefäsz**, n. 1. thoracic vessel.
1826 **Brustgegend**, f. thoracic region.
1827 **Brustgeschwulst**, f. thoracic tumor.
1828 **Brustgeschwür**, n. 1. empyema.
1829 **Brustglied**, n. 1. thoracic limb.
1830 **Brustgürtel**, m. 2. shoulder girdle.
1831 **Brusthaut**, f. pleura.
1832 **Brusthöhle**, f. thoracic cavity.
1833 **Brusthöhlenerweiterung**, f. fr. erweitern, to enlarge) expansion of the thoracic cavity.
1834 **Brusthöhlenverengung**, f. (fr. verengen, to narrow) contraction of the thoracic cavity.
1835 **Brusthöhlenwand**, f. thoracic wall.
1836 **Brustkasten**, m. 2. thoracic chest.
1837 **Brustkastennerv**, m. 3. thoracic nerve.
1838 **Brustknochen**, m. 2. pl. bones of the thorax.
1839 **Brustknorpel**, m. 2. costal cartilage.
1840 **Brustknoten**, m. 2. thoracic ganglion.
1841 **Brustkorb**, m. 1. thorax.
1842 **Brustkrampf**, m. 1. asthma.
1843 **Brustkrebs**, m. 1. cancer of the mammary gland.
1844 **Brustmessung**, f. measurement of the chest.
1845 **Brustmilchgang**, m. 1. thoracic duct.
1846 **Brustmuskel**, m. 2. pectoral muscle.
1847 **Brustnerv**, m. 3. thoracic nerve.
1848 **Brustpulsader**, f. thoracic artery.
1849 **Brustraum**, m. 1, thoracic cavity.
1850 **Bruströhre**, f. thoracic duct.
1851 **Brustsaft**, m. 1. linctus.
1852 **Brustsarkom**, n. 1. mammary sarcoma.
1853 **Brustschild**, n. 1. sternum.
1854 **Brustschildknorpelmuskel**, m. 2. sterno-thyroid muscle.
1855 **Brustschlagader**, f. thoracic artery.
1856 **Brustschlüsselbeinzitzenfortsatzmuskel**, m. 2. sterno-cleido-mastoid muscle.
1857 **Brustschulterblutader**, f. acromio-thoracic vein.
1858 **Brustschulterschlagader**, f. acromio-thoracic artery.
1859 **Brustschwamm**, m. 1. fungus growth of mamma.
1860 **Brustscirrhus**, m. 1. scirrhus of mamma.
1861 **Brustspalte**, f. congenital fissure of sternum.
1862 **Brustsprache**, f. thoracic voice.
1863 **Bruststich**, m. 1. paracentesis.
1864 **Bruststimme**, f. chest voice.
1865 **Brustton**, m. 1. (pectoriloquy), chest voice.
1866 **Brustumfang**, m. 1. chest circumference.
1867 **Brustvene**, f. thoracic vein.
1868 **Brustwand**, f. } thoracic wall.
Brustwandung, f. } thoracic wall.
1869 **Brustwarze**, f. } nipple.
Brustzitze, f. } nipple.
1870 **Brustwarzendeckel**, m. 2. nipple shield.
1871 **Brustwarzenhof**, m. 1. } areola of the nipple.
1872 **Brustwarzenkreis**, m. 1. } areola of the nipple.

1873 **Brustwasser**, n. 2. accumulated fluid in the chest.
1874 **Brustwirbel**, m. 2. thoracic vertebra.
1875 **Brustwirbelgegend**, f. dorsal region.
1876 **Brustwirbelsäule**, f. dorsal or thoracic spine.
1877 **Brustzungenbeinmuskel**, m. 2. sterno-hyoid muscle.
1878 **auskultieren**, v. to auscultate.
1879 **Auskultationsschall**, m. 1. auscultation sound.
1880 **Resonantz**, f. resonance, heard in percussion.
rumpelnd, adj. rumpling (from rumpeln, to rumple).
Wiederhall, m. 1. / **Widerhall**, m. 1. } resonance (as in percussion).
1881 5. **BAUCH**, m. 1. / **Unterleib**, m. 1. } belly, abdomen, epigastrium. *abdominal* in compounds:
1882 **Bauchaorta**, f. abdominal aorta.
1883 **Bauchaortengeflecht**, n. 1. abdominal aortic plexus.
1884 **Baucharterie**, f. abdominal artery.
1885 **Bauchatmen**, n. 2. abdominal respiration.
1886 **Bauchauftreibung**, f. abdominal distention.
1887 **Bauchbedeckung**, f. / **Bauchdeckung**, f. } abdominal covering or parietes
1888 **Bauchbeschauung**, f. abdominal inspection.
1889 **Bauchblatt**, n. 1. lamina ventralis.
1890 **Bauchbruch**, m. 1. abdominal or ventral hernia.
1891 **Bauchdecken**, lit. belly covering, in compounds: epigastric, e. g.
1892 **Bauchdeckenarterie**, f. epigastric artery.
1893 **Bauchdeckenblutader**, f. epigastric vein.
1894 **Bauchdeckennaht**, f. suture of abdominal wall.
1895 **Baucheingeweide**, n. 1. abdominal viscera.
1896 **Bauchfell**, n. 1. peritoneum.
1897 **Bauchfellband**, n. 1. peritoneal ligament.
1898 **Bauchfellblatt**, n. 1. layer of peritoneum.
1899 **Bauchfellbucht**, f. recess of the peritoneum.
1900 **Bauchfellfalte**, f. fold of peritoneum.
1901 **Bauchfellfortsetzung**, f. process of peritoneum.
1902 **Bauchfellhöhle**, f. peritoneal cavity.
1903 **Bauchfellplatte**, f. layer of peritoneum.
1904 **Bauchfellsack**, m. 1. peritoneal sac.
1905 **Bauchfelltasche**, f. peritoneal pouch.
1906 **Bauchfellverwachsung**, f. adhesion of peritoneum.
1907 **Bauchfistel**, f. abdominal fistula.
1908 **Bauchfläche**, f. surface of the abdomen.
1909 **Bauchgeflecht**, n. 1. abdom. plexus.
1910 **Bauchgegend**, f. abdom. region.
1911 **Bauchhaut**, f. peritoneum.
1912 **Bauchhöhle**, f. peritoneal cavity.
1913 **Bauchhöhleneileiterschwangerschaft**, f. tubo-abdominal pregnancy.
1914 **Bauchhöhlenschwangerschaft**, f. / **Bauchschwangerschaft**, f. } abdominal pregnancy.
1915 **Bauchklopfen**, n. 2. abdominal pulsation.
1916 **Bauchkrampf**, m. 1. abdominal spasm, colic.
1917 **Bauchlinie**, f. linea alba.
1918 **Bauchmitte**, f. mesogastrium, umbilical region.
1919 **Bauchmündung**, f. abdominal aperture.
1920 **Bauchmuskel**, m. 2. abdominal muscle.
1921 **Bauchnabel**, m. 2. umbilicus.
1922 **Bauchnaht**, f. abdom. suture.
1923 **Bauchnerv**, m. 3. abdom. nerve.
1924 **Bauchpulsader**, f. / **Bauchschlagader**, f. } abdominal aorta.
1925 **Bauchraum**, m. 1. abdom. cavity.
1926 **Bauchring**, m. 1. abdom. inguinal ring.
1927 **Bauchspeichel**, m. 2. pancreatic juice.
1928 **Bauchspeichelausführungsgang**, m. 1. pancreatic duct.

1929 **Bauchspeicheldrüse**, f. pancreas.
1930 **Bauchspeicheldrüsengang**, m. 1. pancreatic duct.
1931 **Bauchspeicheldrüsenkopf**, m. 1. head of the pancreas.
1932 **Bauchspeicheldrüsensaft**, m. 1. pancreatic juice.
1933 **Bauchspeicheldrüsenschwanz**, m. 1. tail of the pancreas.
1934 **Bauchspeicheldrüsenverstopfung**, f. obstruction of the pancreatic duct.
1935 **Bauchspeicheldrüsenzwölffingerdarmpulsader**, f. pancreatico-duodenal artery.
1936 **Bauchteil**, m. 1. abdominal portion.
1937 **Bauchvene**, f. abdominal vein.
1938 **Bauchwand**, f. } abdominal wall.
Bauchwandung, f. }
1939 **Bauchweichen**, pl. f. lateral wall of the abdomen, groin.
1940 **Bauchwindsucht**, f. tympanitis.
1841 **Bauchwirbel**, m. 2. lumbar vertebra.
1942 **Bauchwirbelsäule**, f. lumbar vertebral column.
1943 **Bauchzwang**, m. 1. tenesmus, etc.
1944 6. **NABEL**, m. 2. navel, umbilicus, *umbilical* in compounds:
1945 **Nabelader**, f. umbilical vein.
1946 **Nabelarterie**, f. umbilical artery.
1947 **Nabelband**, n. 1. round ligament of the liver.
1948 **Nabelbinde**, f. umbilical binder.
1949 **Nabelbläschen**, n. 2. } umbilical vesicle.
Nabelblase, f. }
1950 **Nabelblutflusz**, m. 1. } hemorrhage from the umbilicus.
Nabelblutung, f. }
1951 **Nabelbruch**, m. 1. umbilical hernia.
1952 **Nabelbruchband**, n. 1. umbilical truss.
1953 **Nabeldarmfistel**, f. omphalo-intestinal fistula.
1954 **nabelförmig**, adj. umbilicated.
1955 **Nabelgrube**, f. umbilical fossa.
1956 **Nabelkrankheit**, f. disease of the umbilicus.
1957 **Nabelöffnung**, f. umbilical aperture.
1958 **Nabelringbruch**, m. 1. acquired umbilical hernia.
1959 **Nabelschnitt**, m. 1. section of umbilical cord.
1960 **Nabelschnur**, f. umbilical cord.
1961 **Nabelschnurbändchen**, n. 1. thread for tying umbilical cord.
1962 **Nabelschnurknoten**, m. 2. knot of umbilical cord.
1963 **Nabelschnurvorfall**, m. 1. prolapse of umbililical cord.
1964 **Nabelstrang**, m. 1. umbilical cord.
1965 **Nabeltuch**, n. 1. umbilical cloth.
1966 **Nabelvene**, f. umbilical vein.
1967 **Nabelvenenentzündung**, f. omphalo-phlebitis, inflammation of umbilical vein.
1968 **Nabelverband**, m. 1. dressing for navel.
1969 **Nabelwassergeschwulst**, f. umbilical oedema, etc.
1970 7. **GLIED**, n. 1, limb, member (penis), in compounds:
1971 **Gliedabnehmung**, f. } amputation of a limb.
1972 **Gliedabsetzung**, f. }
1973 **Gliederfuge**, f. articulation, joint.
1974 **gliederig**, adj. limbed.
1975 **Gliederknöchel**, m. 2. joint, knuckle.
1976 **Gliederschwund**, m. 1. (fr. v. ir. schwinden, to disappear), withering of limbs.
1977 **gliederstärkend**, adj. strengthening the limbs, tonic.
1978 **Gliedmaszen**, pl. limbs, extremities, members of the body.
1979 **Gliedmaszen**, oberen, pl. upper extremities.
1980 **Gliedmaszen**, unteren, pl. lower extremities.
1981 **Gliedmaszenband**, n. 1. ligament of the limbs, etc.
1982 8. **ACHSEL**, f. axis, axilla, in compounds:
1983 **Achselader**, f. } axillary vein.
Achselblutader, f. }
1984 **Achselarterie**, f. axillary artery.
1985 **Achselband**, n. 1. shoulder strap.

1986 **Achselbein**, n. 1. scapula.
1987 **Achseldrüse**, f. axillary gland.
1988 **Achselfalte**, f. axillary fold.
1989 **Achselgefäsz**, n. 1. axillary vessel.
1990 **Achselgrube**, f. armpit, axilla.
1991 **Achselhaar**, n. 1. axillary hair.
1992 **Achselhöhle**, f. armpit, axilla.
1993 **Achselnervengeflecht**, n. 1. axillary plexus.
1994 **achsical**, adj. axial, etc.
1995 9. **RIPPE**, f. rib, in compounds:
1996 **Rippenabdruck**, m. 1. cast of ribs, impression of ribs.
1997 **Rippenarterie**, f. intercostal artery.
1998 **Rippenblutader**, f. intercostal vein.
1999 **Rippenbruch**, m. 1. fracture of a rib.
2000 **Rippenbrustbeingelenk**, n. 1. costo-sternal articulation.
2001 **Rippenfell**, n. 1. costal pleura.
2002 **Rippenfurche**, f. costal furrow.
2003 **Rippengegend**, f. costal region.
2004 **Rippenhals**, m. 1. neck of a rib.
2005 **Rippenhalsband**, n. 1. costo-transverse ligament.
2006 **Rippenhaut**, f. pleura.
2007 **Rippenhöckergelenk**, n. 1. costo-transverse articulation.
2008 **Rippenknochen**, m. 2. bony part of a rib.
2009 **Rippenknorpel**, m. 2. costal cartilage.
2010 **Rippenknorpelverknöcherung**, f. ossification of costal cartilage.
2011 **Rippenköpfchen**, n. 2. head of a rib.
2012 **Rippenpfanne**, f. costal fossa e. g. (on vertebra).
2013 **Rippenweiche**, f. hypochondriac region.
2014 **Rippenwinkel**, m. 2. angle of a rib.
2015 **Rippenwirbel**, m. 2. } dorsal or costal vertebra.
2016 **Rippenwirbelbein**, n. 1. } dorsal or costal vertebra.
2017 **Rippenzwischenraum**, m. 1. intercostal space, etc.
2018 10. **SCHULTER**, f. shoulder, humerus, in compounds.
2019 **Schulterband**, n. 1. ligament of the shoulder-joint.
2020 **Schulterbein**, n. 1. } scapula.
2021 **Schulterblatt**, n. 1. } scapula.
2022 **Schulterknochen**, m. 2. } scapula.
2023 **Schulterblattband**, n. 1. scapular ligament.
2024 **Schulterblattgegend**, f. scapular region.
2025 **Schulterblattgelenkfortsatz**, m. 1. glenoid process of scapula.
2026 **Schulterblattgelenkgrube**, f. } glenoid cavity of scapula.
2027 **Schulterblattgrube**, f. } glenoid cavity of scapula.
2028 **Schulterblattgräte**, f. } spine of scapula.
2029 **Schultergräte**, f. } spine of scapula.
2030 **Schulterblatthals**, m. 1. neck of scapula.
2031 **Schulterblattkopf**, m. 1. head of scapula.
2032 **Schulterblattpfanne**, f. glenoid cavity.
2033 **Schulterecke**, f. } acromion process.
2034 **Schulterend**, n. 1. } acromion process.
2035 **Schultergelenk**, n. 1. shoulder joint.
2036 **Schultergelenkkapsel**, f. capsular ligament of the shoulder joint.
2037 **Schultergelenklippe**, f. margin of glenoid cavity.
2038 **Schultergelenkpfanne**, f. glenoid cavity of scapula.
2039 **Schultergürtel**, m. 2. shoulder girdle.
2040 **Schulterhacken**, m. 2. coracoid process.
2041 **Schulterhackenschlüsselbeinband**, n. 1. coraco-clavicular ligament.
2042 **Schulterhöhle**, f. acromion.
2043 **Schulterkamm**, m. 1. spine of the scapula.
2044 **Schulterknochen**, m. 2. scapula.
2045 **Schulterpfanne**, f. glenoid cavity of scapula.
2046 **Schulterschnabel**, m. 2. coracoid process.
2047 **Schulterwinkel**, m. 2. angle of the scapula, etc.
2048 11. a. **ARM**, m. 1. arm, in compounds.
2049 **Armader**, f. vein of the arm.
2050 **Armarterie**, f. artery of the arm.

2051 **Armbein**, n. 1. humerus, bone of the arm.

2052 **Armbeinbruch**, m. 1. } fracture of the arm or of the humerus.
2053 **Armbruch**, m. 1. }

2054 **Armbeuge**, f. (fr. v. ir. biegen, to bend) elbow or bend of the arm.

2055 **Armblutader**, f. vein of the arm.

2056 **Armgeflecht**, n. 1. brachial plexus.

2057 **Armgelenk**, n. 1. brachial articulation.

2058 **Armheber**, m. 2. deltoid muscle.

2059 **Armhöhle**, f. armpit.

2060 **Armknochen**, m. 2. humerus, a bone of the arm.

2061 **Armmuskel**, m. 2. brachial muscle.

2062 **Armnerv**, m. 3. brachial nerve.

2063 **Armpulsader**, f. brachial artery.

2064 **Armschlinge**, f. armsling.

2065 **Armspeiche**, f. } radius.
2066 **Armspindel**, f. }

2067 **Armvene**, f. brachial vein, etc.

2068 b. **Oberarm**, m. 1. upper arm.

2069 **Oberarmbein**, n. 1. humerus.

2070 **Oberarmbeingelenkkopf**, m. 1. head of the humerus.

2071 **Oberarmbeinhals**, m. 1. neck of the humerus.

2072 **Oberarmbeinkopf**, m. 1. **Oberarmbeinköpfchen**, m. 2. } head of the humerus.

2073 **Oberarmdreieck**, n. 1. brachial triangle.

2074 **Oberarmgegend**, f. humeral region.

2075 **Oberarmgelenk**, n. 1. shoulder joint.

2076 **Oberarmgelenkgrube**, f. glenoid fossa of scapula.

2077 **Oberarmgrube**, f. hintere, olecranon fossa of humerus.

2078 **Oberarmgrube**, f. vordere, coronoid fossa of humerus.

2079 **Oberarmknochen**, m. 2. humerus.

2080 **Oberarmknorren**, m. 2. condyle of humerus.

2081 **Oberarmkopf**, m. 1. head of humerus.

2082 **Oberarmmuskel**, m. 2. muscle of the upper arm.

2083 **Oberarmpulsader**, f. **Oberarmschlagader**, f. } brachial artery.

2084 **Oberarmverrenkung**, f. dislocation of the humerus, etc.

2085 c. **UNTERARM**, m. 1. } forearm.
2086 **VORDERARM**, m. 1. }

2087 **Vorderarmgegend**, f. region of the forearm.

2088 **Vorderarmgelenk**, n. 1. articulation of the forearm.

2089 **Vorderarmknochen**, m. 2. bone of the forearm.

2090 **Vorderarmknockenband**, n. 1. interosseous ligament of the forearm, etc.

2091 12. **ELLBOGEN** or **ELLENBOGEN**, m. 2. elbow (fr. Elle, f. yard, and Bogen, m. 2. arch, bow, fr. v. ir. biegen, to bend), in compounds:

2092 **Ellbogenbein**, n. 1. } ulna.
2093 **Ellbogenbeinknochen**, m. 2. }

2094 **Ellbogenknochenkopf**, m. 1. olecranon.

2095 **Ellbogenbeuge**, f. } bend of the elbow
2096 **Ellbogenbug**, m. 1. }

2097 **Ellbogenfortsatz**, m. 1. olecranon process.

2098 **Ellbogengegend**, f. ulnar region.

2099 **Ellbogengelenk**, n. 1. elbow joint.

2100 **Ellbogengrube**, f. hollow of the elbow (anterior aspect), antecubital fossa, etc.

2101 13. **SPEICHE**, f. radius, in compounds:

2102 **Speichenarterie**, f. radial artery.

2103 **Speichenbeuger**, m. 2. biceps; der Hand, flexor carpi radialis.

2104 **Speichenblutader**, f. radial vein.

2105 **Speichenende**, n. 1. extremity of radius.

2106 **Speichengriffelfortsatz**, m. 1. styloid process of radius.

2107 **Speichenknochen**, m. 2. radius.

2108 **Speichenköpfchen**, n. 2. head of the radius.

2109 **Speichenmuskel**, m. 2. radius muscle.

2110 **Speichennerv**, m. 3. radial nerve.
2111 **Speichenpulsader**, f. radial artery.
2112 **Speichenrand**, m. 1. border or side of radius.
2113 **Speichenschlagader**, f. radial artery.
2114 **Speichenstrecker**, m. 2. radial extension.
2115 **Speichenvorsprung**, m. 1. radial eminence, thenar eminence of the hand, etc.
2116 14. **HAND**, f. hand.
2117 ——, flache, the palm of the hand.
2118 ——, hohle, the hollow of the hand, in compounds:
2119 **Handbad**, n. 1. handbath.
2120 **Handballen**, m. 2. ball of the hand.
2121 **Handband**, n. 1. ligament of the hand.
2122 **Handbein**, n. 1. bone of the hand.
2123 **Handbeugung**, f. flexion of the wrist.
2124 **Handfläche**, f. palm of the hand.
2125 **Handflechte**, f. tendon of the hand.
2126 **Handgelenk**, n. 1. wrist joint.
2127 **Handknöchel**, m. 2. knuckle.
2128 **Handknochen**, m. 2. bone of the hand.
2129 **Handrücken**, m. 2. back or dorsum of the hand.
2130 **Handrückenband**, n. 1. dorsal ligament of the hand.
2131 **Handrückengegend**, f. dorsal region of the hand.
2132 **Handsehne**, f. tendon of the hand.
2133 **Handwurzel**, f. wrist, carpus.
2134 **Handwurzelband**, n. 1. carpal ligament, annular ligament.
2135 **Handwurzelbein**, n. 1. carpal bone.
2136 **Handwurzelgegend**, f. carpal region.
2137 **Handwurzelkanal**, m. 1. passage for flexortendons beneath the annular ligament.
2138 **Handwurzelknochen**, m. 2. carpal bone.
2139 **Handwurzelknochenband**, n. 1. transverse carpal ligament, etc.
2140 **MITTELHAND**, f. metacarpus, palm.
2141 **Mittelhandbein**, n. 1. } metacarpal bone.
2142 **Mittelhandknochen**, m. 2. } metacarpal bone.
2143 **Mittelhandgegend**, f. metacarpal region.
2144 **Mittelhandgelenk**, n. 1. metacarpal joint, etc.
2145 15. **FINGER**, m. 2. finger, *digital*, in compounds:
2146 **Fingerband**, n. 1. digital ligament.
2147 **Fingerbein**, n. 1. } phalanx.
2148 **Fingerknochen**, m. 2. } phalanx.
2149 **Fingerbeuger**, m. 2. flexor of the finger.
2150 **Fingercarpalgelenk**, n. 1. metacarpo-carpal joint.
2151 **fingerförmig**, adj. digitate.
2152 **Fingergelenk**, n. 1. phalangeal joint.
2153 **Fingerglied**, n. 1. phalanx.
2154 **Fingergrube**, f. digital cavity or fossa.
2155 **Fingerkuppe**, f. fingertip.
2156 **Fingernagel**, m. 2. fingernail.
2157 **Fingernerv**, m. 3. digital nerve.
2158 **Fingersehne**, f. digital tendon.
2159 **Fingerspitze**, f. tip of finger.
2160 **Fingerverwachsung**, f. webbed fingers.
2161 **Mittelfinger**, m. 2. middle finger.
2162 **Ohrfinger**, m. 2. little or ear finger.
2163 **Ringfinger**, m. 2. ring finger.
2164 **Zeigefinger**, m. 2. (fr. zeigen, to show, to point), forefinger, index.
2165 16 **DAUMEN**, m. 2. thumb, in compounds:
2166 **Daumenballen**, m. 2. thenar eminence.
2167 **Daumenfläche**, f. surface of the thumb.
2168 **Daumengegend**, f. thenar region.
2169 **Daumenglied**, n. 1. phalanx of thumb.
2170 **Daumennagelglied**, n. 1. terminal phalanx of thumb.
2171 **Daumenrand**, m. 1. radial border, etc.

2172 17. **HÜFTE**, f. hip, in compounds:
(Lende, f. loins, hip.)
2173 **Hüftbein**, n. 1. } os innominatum, ilium.
2174 **Hüftknochen**, m. 2. } os innominatum, ilium.
2175 **Hüftbeinblatt**, n. 1. ilium.
2176 **Hüftbeinfuge**, f. symphysis pubis.
2177 **Hüftbeingrube**, f. venter of the ilium.
2178 **Hüftbeinkamm**, m. 1 } crest of the ilium.
2179 **Hüftkamm**, m. 1. } crest of the ilium.
2180 **Hüftbeinlendenband**, n. 1. ilio-lumbar ligament.
2181 **Hüftbeinloch**, n. 1. obturator foramen.
2182 **Hüftbeinlochfurche**, f. } obturator canal.
2183 **Hüftbeinlochkerbe**, f. } obturator canal.
2184 **Hüftbeinstachel**, m. 2. spine of the ilium.
2185 **Hüftbeuge**, f. } from v. ir. biegen, to bend) flexor of the thigh, on trunk.
2186 Hüftbug, m. 1. } from v. ir. biegen, to bend) flexor of the thigh, on trunk.
2187 **Hüftblatt**, n. 1. ilium.
2188 **Hüftgeflecht**, n. 1. sacral plexus.
2189 **Hüftgegend**, f. the thigh region.
2190 **Hüftgelenk**, n. 1. hip joint.
2191 **Hüftgelenkband**, n. 1. hip joint ligament.
2192 **Hüftgelenkkapsel**, f. capsule of the hip.
2193 **Hüftgelenkpfanne**, f. acetabulum.
2194 **Hüftkreuzbeinband**, n. 1. ilio-sacral ligament.
2195 **Hüftkreuzbeinfuge**, f. } sacro iliac sychondrosis.
2196 **Hüftkreuzfuge**, f. } sacro iliac sychondrosis.
2197 **Hüftlendenband**, n. 1. ilio-lumbar ligament.
2198 **Hüftloch**, n. 1. obturator foramen.
2199 **Hüftlochband**, n. 1. obturator membrane.
2200 **Hüftlochgefäsze**, n. 1. pl. obturator vessels.
2201 **Hüftlochkerbe**, f. obturator canal.
2202 **Hüftnervengeflecht**, n. 1. sacral plexus.
2203 **Hüftpfanne**, f. acetabulum, cotyloid cavity.
2204 **Hüftschenkelband**, n. 1. ilio-femoral ligament, etc.
2205 18. **BECKEN**, n. 2. pelvis, in compounds:
2206 **Beckenabschnitt**, m. 1. (fr. v. ir. abschneiden, to cut off, separate), section of pelvis.
2207 **Beckenabweichung**, f. (fr. v. ir. abweichen, to deviate) pelvic deformity.
2208 **Beckenachse**, f. pelvic-axis.
2209 **Beckenapertur**, f. aperture of pelvis.
2210 **Beckenausgang**, m. 1. (fr. v. ir. ausgehen, to go out), pelvic outlet, inferior aperture of pelvis.
2211 **Beckenband**, n. 1. pelvic ligament.
2212 **Beckenbauchfell**, n. 1. pelvic peritoneum.
2213 **Beckenbein**, n. 1. os innominatum.
2214 **Beckenbinde**, f. pelvic fascia.
2215 **Beckenbindegewebe**, n. 1. pelvic connective tissue.
2216 **Beckenboden**, m. 2. pelvic floor.
2217 **Beckenbucht**, f. superior aperture of pelvis, pelvic inlet.
2218 **Beckendach**, n. 1. roof of pelvis.
2219 **Beckendarmhöhle**, f. pelvic intestinal cavity.
2220 **Beckendrüse**, f. pelvic gland.
2221 **Beckendurchmesser**, m. 2. } pelvic diameter.
2222 **Beckendiameter**, m. 2. } pelvic diameter.
2223 **Beckeneingang**, m. 1. (fr. v. ir. eingehen, to enter) superior aperture of pelvis, inlet.
2224 **Beckeneingangsebene**, f. plane of pelvic inlet.
2225 **Beckeneingeweide**, n. 1. pelvic viscera.
2226 **Beckenenge**, f. smallest part of pelvic cavity.
2227 **Beckenfascie**, f. pelvic fascia.
2228 **Beckenfehler**, m. 2. pelvic deformity.
2229 **Beckengefäsz**, n. 1. pelvic vessel, pl. vessels.
2230 **Beckengeflecht**, n. 1. pelvic plexus.
2231 **Beckengegend**, f. pelvic region.
2232 **Beckengelenk**, n. 1. pelvic articulation.
2233 **Beckengrube**, f. iliac fossa.
2234 **Beckengurt**, m. 1. } pelvic girdle.
2235 **Beckengürtel**, m. 2. } pelvic girdle.

2236 **Beckenhalbring**, m. 1. half of pelvic girdle.
2237 **Beckenhöhle**, f. pelvic cavity.
2238 **Beckenhöhlenfläche**, f. surface of pelvic cavity.
2239 **Beckenkanal**, m. 1. pelvic canal.
2240 **Beckenknochen**, m. 2. os innominatum.
2241 **Beckenkrümmung**, f. pelvic curvature.
2242 **Beckenmasz**, n. 1. measure of pelvis.
2243 **Beckenneigung**, f. (fr. neigen, to incline) pelvic inclination.
2244 **Beckenöffnung**, f. (fr. öffnen, to open) pelvic aperture.
2245 **Beckenplatte**, f. pelvic layer.
2246 **Beckenrand**, m. 1. pelvic rim.
2247 **Beckenraum**, m. 1. pelvic space.
2248 **Beckenring**, m. 1. pelvic girdle or circumference.
2249 **Beckenschaufel**, f. pelvic hollow of os sacrum.
2250 **Beckenumfang**, m. 1. pelvic circumference.
2251 **Beckenwand**, f. / **Beckenwandung**, } wall of pelvis.
2252 **Beckenweichteile**, m. 1. pl. soft parts of pelvis.
2253 **Beckenweite**, f. the widest part of the pelvic cavity.
2254 **Beckenzellgewebe**, n. 1. pelvic connective tissue.
2255 **Beckenzwerchfell**, n. 1. pelvic diaphragm, etc.
2256 19. **SITZBEIN**, n. 1.
2257 *Gesäsz* or *Gesäszbein*, n. 1. } (fr. v. ir. sitzen, to sit) nates, buttocks, ischium, fundament, in compounds.
2258 **Sitzbeinhöcker**, m. 2.
2259 **Sitzbeinknorren**, m. 2. } tuber ischii.
2260 **Sitzbeinstachel**, m. 2. spine of ischium.
2261 **Sitzhöckerkreuzbeinband**, n. 1. sacro-sciatic ligament, etc.
2262 **KREUZ**, n. 1. cross, back, loins.
2263 **Kreuzband**, n. 1. crucial ligament.
2264 **Kreuzbein**, n. 1. sacrum.
2265 **Kreuzbeinaushöhlung**, f. (fr. aushöhlen, to excavate) hollow of the sacrum.
2266 **Kreuzbeinfläche**, f. surface of the sacrum.
2267 **Kreuzbeinflügel**, m. 2. ala of the sacrum.
2268 **Kreuzbeinhorn**, n. 1. process of the sacrum.
2269 **Kreuzbeinkanal**, m. 1. sacral canal.
2270 **Kreuzbeinloch**, n. 1. sacral foramen.
2271 **Kreuzbeinneigung**, f. inclination of the sacrum.
2272 **Kreuzbeinwirbel**, m. 2. sacral vertebra.
2273 **kreuzförmig**, adj. cruciform.
2274 **Kreuzgeflecht**, n. 1. sacral plexus.
2275 **Kreuzgegend**, f. sacral region.
2276 **Kreuzknochen**, m. 2. sacrum.
2277 **Kreuzknorrenband**, n. 1. sacro-sciatic ligament.
2278 **Kreuzknoten**, m. 2. sacral ganglion.
2279 **Kreuzstachelband**, n. 1. lesser sacro-sciatic ligament.
2280 **Kreuzsteiszband**, n. 1.
2281 **Kreuzsteiszbeinband**, n. 1. } sacrococcygeal ligament.
2282 **Kreuzsteiszbeingegend**, f. sacro-coccygeal region.
2283 **Kreuzsteiszbeinverbindung**, f. sacro-coccygeal articulation.
2284 **kreuzweise**, adj. crucial.
2285 **Kreuzwirbel**, m. 2. sacral vertebra, etc.
2286 21. **SCHAM**, f. (fr. v. refl. sich schämen, to be ashamed), shame, in compounds:
2287 **Scham** or **Schamteile, männliche**, f. male pudenda.
2288 **Scham or Schamteile, weibliche**, f. female pudenda.
2289 **Schamband**, n. 1. / **Schambändchen**, n. 2. } frænum clitoridis.
2290 **Schambein**, n. 1. os pubis.
2291 **Schambeinband**, n. 1. ligamentum pubis.
2292 **Schambeinblasenband**, n. 1. vesico-pubic ligament.
2293 **Schambeinbogen**, m. 2. pubic arch.
2294 **Schambeinfuge**, f. pubic symphysis.
2295 **Schambeinhöcker**. m. 2. crest or spine of os pubis.

2296 **Schambeinkamm**, m. 1. crest of os pubis.
2297 **Schambeinknorpel**, m. 2. interpubic disk.
2298 **Schambeinrand**, m. 1. margin of os pubis.
2299 **Schambeinstachel**, m. 2. spine of os pubis.
2300 **Schamberg**, m. 1. } mons veneris.
2301 **Venusberg**, m. 1. }
2302 **Schamhügel**, m. 2. }
2303 **Schamblutader**, f. pubic vein.
2304 **Schambogen**, m. 2. pubic arch.
2305 **Schambogenscheitel**, m. 2. vertex of pubic arch.
2306 **Schambogenschenkel**, m. 2. ramus of pubic arch.
2307 **Schambug**, m. 1. the groin.
2308 **Schamdrüse**, f. inguinal gland.
2309 **Schamfuge**, f. symphysis pubis.
2310 **Schamfugenkante**, f. edge of symphysis pubis.
2311 **Schamfugenknorpel**, m. 2. cartilage of symphysis pubis.
2312 **Schamgang**, m. 1. (fr. v. ir. gehen, to go), vagina.
2313 **Schamgegend**, f. pubic region.
2314 **Schamglied, männliches**, n. 1. penis.
2315 **Schamglied, weibliches**, n. 1. vulva.
2316 **Schamhaar**, n. 1. pubic hair.
2317 **Schamhügel**, m. 2. mons veneris.
2318 **Schamknochen**, m. 2. os pubis.
2319 **Schamlefze**, f. nympha,
2320 labium pudendi (or Schamlippe).
2321 **Schamlefzenbändchen**, n. 2. ligament or frenum of labium pudendi.
2322 **Schamlefzennaht**, f. (fr. nähen, to sew), labial suture.
2323 **Schamlefzenscheidenbruch**, m. 1. labio-vaginal hernia.
2324 **Schamleiste**, f. the groin.
2325 **Schamlippe**, f. labium pudendi.
2326 **Schamlippenbändchen**, n. 2. ligament, or frænum of labium pudendi.
2327 **Schamöffnung**, f. entrance of vulva.
2328 **Schamrinne**, f. } rima vulvæ.
2329 **Schamritze**, f. }
2330 **Schamseite**, f. inguinal region or the groin.
2331 **Schamspalte**, f. (fr. spalten, to split) rima vulvæ.
2332 **Schamteile**, m. 1. pl. pudenda.
2333 **Schamwinkel**, m. 2. angle of os pubis.
2334 **Schamzüngelchen**, n. 2. } clitoris, glans clitoridis (Kitzlerdrüse) etc. (from kitzeln, to tickle) hence Kitzel or Kitzeln, tickling.)
Clitoris, **tickler**, }
Clitoriseichel, f. }
Kitzler, m. 2. }
2335 **STEISZ**, m. 1. } rump, buttocks, nates, breech.
2336 **Hintere**, m. 3. } In compounds:
2337 **Steiszbein**, n. 1. coccyx.
2338 **Steiszbeinband**, n. 1. coccygeal ligament.
2339 **Steiszbeinhöcker**, m. 2 cornu of coccyx.
2340 **Steiszbeinknoten**, m. 2. coccygeal ganglion.
2341 **Steiszbeinspitze**, f. tip of the coccyx.
2342 **Steiszbeinwirbel**, m. 2. coccygeal vertebra.
2343 **Steiszdrüse**, f. coccygeal gland.
2344 **Steiszfistel**, f. fistula in ano.
2345 **Steiszgegend**, f. region of the nates.
2346 **Steiszknochen**, m. 2. coccyx.
2347 **Steiszlage**, f. breech presentation.
2348 **Steiszwirbel**, m. 2. coccygeal vertebra.
2349 **Steiszzange**, f. breech forceps, etc.
2350 23. **SCHENKEL**, m. 2. leg, thigh, crus, peduncle; in compounds:
2351 **Schenkelband**, n. 1. crural or femoral ligament.
2352 **Schenkelbein**, n. 1. femur.
2353 **Schenkelbeinhals**, m. 1. neck of the femur.
2354 **Schenkelbeuge**, f. the fold of the groin.
2355 **Schenkelbinde**, f. crural fascia or fascia of the thigh.
2356 **Schenkelbindefortsatz**, m. 1. process of crural fascia.
2357 **Schenkelbogen**, m. 2. crural arch, so-called Poupart's ligament.
2358 **Schenkelfuge**, f. the fold of the groin.
2359 **Schenkelgegend**, f. crural or femoral region.

2360 **Schenkelgelenk**, n. 1. hip-joint.
2361 **Schenkelgrube**, f. crural fossa.
2362 **Schenkelhals**, m. 1. neck of the femur.
2363 **Schenkelhernia**, f. femoral hernia.
2364 **Schenkelkanal**, m. 1. crural or femoral canal.
2365 **Schenkelknochen**, m. 2. the femur.
2366 **Schenkelknorren**, m. 2. condyle of the femur.
2367 **Schenkelkopf**, m. 1. head of the femur, etc.
2368 **OBERSCHENKEL**, m. 2. upper part of the lower limb, the thigh, in compounds:
2369 **Oberschenkelanzieher**, m. 2. abductor muscle of the femur.
2370 **Oberschenkelarterie**, f. femoral artery.
2371 **Oberschenkelbein**, n. 1. } femur.
2372 **Oberschenkelknochen**, m. 2. } femur.
2373 **Oberschenkelbeuger**, m. 2. flexor of the thigh.
2374 **Oberschenhelblutader**, f. femoral vein.
2375 **Oberschenkelbruch**, m. 1. femoral hernia; fracture of femur.
2376 **Oberschenkelfläche**, f. surface of the thigh.
2377 **Oberschenhelhalsbruch**, m. 1. fracture of the femur's neck.
2378 **Oberschenkelmuskel**, m. 2. muscle of the thigh, etc.
2379 24. **KNIE**, n. 1. knee, in compounds:
2380 **Knieband**, n. 1. knee ligament.
2381 **Kniebeuge**, f. knee-bend, popliteal space.
2382 **Kniebügel**, m. 2. knee-cap.
2383 **Kniefiechse**, f. hamstring.
2384 **knieförmig**, adj. geniculate.
2385 **Kniegelenk**, n. 1. knee-joint.
2386 **Kniegelenkgegend**, f. region of the knee-joint.
2387 **Kniegelenkkapsel**, f. capsule of the knee-joint.
2288 **Kniegelenkmaus**, f. loose body of the knee-joint.
2389 **Kniegrube**, f. popliteal space.
2390 **Kniehöcker**, m. 2. corpus geniculatum.
2391 **Kniekappe**, f. knee-cap.
2392 **Kniekapsel**, f. knee-capsule.
2393 **Kniekehle**, f. popliteal space.
2394 **Kniehkehlenpulsader**, f. popliteal artery.
2395 **Knieknochen**, m. 2. bone of the knee.
2396 **Kniescheibe**, f. patella, etc.
2397 25. **SCHIENBEIN**, n. 1. } tibia.
2398 **Schienbeinknochen**, m. 2. } tibia.
2399 **Schienbeinfläche**, f. tibial surface.
2400 **Schienbeingräte**, f. spine of the tibia.
2401 **Schienbeinkante**, f. } crest of the tibia.
2402 **Schienbeinleiste**, f. } crest of the tibia.
2403 **Schienbeinrand**, m. 1. } crest of the tibia.
2404 **Schienbeinkopf**, m. 1. head of the tibia.
2405 **Schienbeinröhre**, f. tibia.
2406 **Schienbeinstachel**, m. 2. spine of the tibia.
2407 **Schienbeinvene**, f. tibial vein.
2408 26. **WADE**, f. calf of the leg, in compounds:
2409 **Wadenbein**, n. 1. fibula.
2410 **Wadenbeinkopf**, m. 1. } head of the fibula.
Wadenbeinköpfchen, n. 2. } head of the fibula.
2411 **Wadenbeinköpfchenband**, n. 1. ligament of the head of the fibula.
2412 **Wadenbeinschienbeinband**, n. 1. tibio-fibular ligament.
2413 **Wadenbeinschienbeingelenk**, n. 1. tibio-fibular articulation.
2414 **Wadenknochen**, m. 2. fibula, etc.
2415 27. **FUSZ**, m. 1. foot, basis, pes, in compounds:
2416 **Fuszballen**, m. 2. ball of the foot.
2417 **Fuszbänder**, n. 1. pl. foot ligaments.
2418 **Fuszbeuge**, f. } instep.
2419 **Fuszbiege**, f. } instep.
2420 **Fuszblatt**, n. 1. sole of the foot.
2421 **Fuszgelenk**, n. 1. articulation or joint of the foot.
2422 **Fuszgelenkband**, n. 1. foot ligament or ankle-joint.

2423 **Fuszgewölbe**, n. 1. arch of the foot.
2424 **Fuszknöchel**, m. 2. malleolus, ankle bone.
2425 **Fuszknochen**, m. 2. bone of the foot.
2426 **Fuszknorren**, m. 2. malleolus.
2427 **Fuszrücken**, m. 2. dorsum of the foot.
2428 **Fuszrückenbogen**, m. 2. dorsal arch of the foot.
2429 **Fuszsohle**, f. sole of the foot.
2430 **Fuszwurzelband**, n. 1. (from **Fuszwurzel**, f. tarsus), tarsal ligament.
2431 **Fuszwurzelbein**, n. 1. tarsal bone.
2432 **Fuszwurzelmittelfuszband**, n. 1. (from **Mittelfusz**, m. 1. metatarsus), tarso-metatarsal ligament.
2433 **Fuszzehe**, f. toe of the foot.
2434 **Vorderfusz**, m. 1. metatarsus and phalanges, etc.
2435 28. **KNÖCHEL**, m. 2. malleolus, knuckle, knuckle-joint, in compounds:
2436 **Knöchelanschwellung**, f. swelling about the ankle.
2437 **Knöchelband**, n. 1. ligament of the ankle.
2438 **Knöchelbein**, n. 1. bone of the ankle.
2439 **Knöchelchen**, n. 2. ossicle.
2440 **Knöchelgelenk**, n. 1. ankle joint.
2441 **Knöchelgelenkband**, n. 1. ankle ligament.
2442 **Knöchlein**, n. 2. little or small bone, ossicle, etc.
2443 29. **FERSE**, f. heel, in compounds:
2444 **Fersenbein**, n. 1. os calcis.
2445 **Fersenflechse**, f. tendo Achillis.
2446 **Fersenhöcker**, m. 2. tuberosity of os calcis.
2447 **Fersenknochen**, m. 2. os calcis.
2448 30. **ZEHE**, f. toe, in compounds:
2449 **Zehengelenk**, n. 1. joint of the toe.
2450 **Zehenglied**, n. 1. phalanx of the toe.
2451 **Zehenknochen**, m. 2. bone of the toe.
2452 **Zehennagel**, m. 2. toe-nail.
2453 **Zehenspitze**, f. point of the toe, etc.
2454 §9. **Die Fasern, Flechsen, Sehnen, Muskeln**, the fibres, tendons, sinews, muscles, in compounds:
2455 **FASER**, f. fibre, filament, thread, string.
2456 **Faserband**, n. 1. accessory ligament.
2457 **Faserbildung**, f. fibrous formation.
2458 **Faserbündel**, m. 2. bundle of fibres.
2459 **Fäserchen**, n. 2. fibrilla.
2460 **faserförmig**, adj. filiform.
2461 **Fasergewebe**, n. 1. fibrous tissue.
2462 **Fasergewirr**, n. 1. a maze of fibres.
2463 **Faserhaut**, f. fibrous membrane.
2464 **Faserhülle**, f. fibrous capsule.
2465 **faserig**, adj. fibrous, fibrinous, filamentous, fasciculate.
2466 **faserig-elastisch**, adj. fibro-elastic.
2467 **faserig-knorpelig**, adj. fibro-cartilaginous.
2468 **Faserkapsel**, f. fibrous capsular ligament.
2469 **Faserknorpel**, m. 2. fibro-cartilage.
2470 **faser-knorpelig**, adj. fibro-cartilaginous.
2471 **Faser-knorpel-schicht**, f. (from schichten, to heap up in layers or strata) fibro-cartilaginous layer.
2472 **Faserkreuzung**, f. crossing of fibres.
2473 **Faserlücke**, f. interfibrillar interstice.
2474 **Fasernetz**, n. 1. network of fibres.
2475 **Fasernetzknorpel**, m. 2. fibrous cartilage.
2476 **Faserring**, m. 1. fibrous ring.
2477 **Faserringband**, n. 1. fibrous annular ligament.
2478 **Fasersarkom**, n. 1. fibro-sarcoma.
2479 **Faserschicht**, f. fibrous layer.
2480 **Faserstoff**, m. 1. fibrin.
2481 **Faserstoffablagerung**, f. deposit of fibrin.
2482 **Faserstoffanhäufung**, f. accumulation of fibrin.
2483 **faserstoffarm**, adj. poor in fibrin.
2484 **faserstoffartig**, adj. fibrinous.

2485 **Faserstoffauflagerung**, f. deposit of fibrin.
2486 **Faserstoffgerinsel**, n. 2. fibrinous coagulum.
2487 **faserstoffig**, adj. fibrinous.
2488 **Faserstoffniederschlag**, m. 1. (from niederschlagen, to beat down), fibrinous precipitation.
2489 **Faserstoffpfropf**, m. 1. thrombus of fibrin.
2490 **Faserstoffscholle**, f. layer or stratum of fibrin.
2491 **Faserstoffzotte**, f. fibrinous tuft.
2492 **Faserstrang**, m. 1. fasciculus.
2493 **Fasersubstanz**, f. fibrinous substance.
2494 **Faserung**, f. fibrillation.
2495 **Faserursprung**, m. 1. fibrous origin.
2496 **Faserverlauf**, m. 1. course or direction of fibres.
2497 **Faserzelle**, f. fibre cell.
2498 **Faserzug**, m. 1. fasciculus of fibres.
2499 **fasciieren**, v. to bandage.
2500 **Fasciation**, f. envelopment with bandages.
2501 **Fascie**, f. fascia.
2502 **Fascienblatt**, n. 1. layer of fascia.
2503 **Fascikel**, m. 2. fasciculus, etc.
2504 2. **FLECHSE** f. } tendon, sinew, in compounds.
2505 **SEHNE**, f. }
2506 **flechsenähnlich**, adj. } tendinous.
flechsenartig, adj. }
2507 **Flechsenhaut**, f. aponeurosis.
2508 **flechsig**, adj. tendenous, aponeurotic.
2509 3. **SEHNE**, f. tendon, sinew, in compounds.
2510 **Sehnenabscesz**, m. 1. thecal abscess.
2511 **Sehnenausbreitung**, f. aponeurosis.
2512 **Sehnenband**, n. 1. tendinous ligament.
2513 **Sehnenbein**, n. 1. sesamoid bone.
2514 **Sehnenblatt**, n. 1. tendinous layer or fascia.
2515 **Sehnenbogen**, m. 2. tendinous arch.
2516 **Sehnenfaden**, m. 2. } tendinous fibre or cord.
2517 **Sehnenfaser**, f. }
2518 **Sehnenflecken**, m. 2. macua lactea, milk spot (of serous surfaces).
2519 **Sehnengewebe**, n. 1. tendon tissue.
2520 **Sehnenhaube**, f. cranial aponeurosis.
2521 **Sehnenhaut**, f. tendinous membrane or covering.
2522 **Sehnenknöchelchen**, n. 2. sesamoid bone.
2523 **Sehnennaht**, f. the suturing of a tendon.
2524 **Sehnennarbe**, f. cicatrix of a tendon.
2525 **Sehnenring**, m. 1. annulus tendineus of membrana tympani.
2526 **Sehnenrisz**, m. 1. rupture of a tendon.
2527 **Sehnensack**, m. 1. synovial sack about tendons.
2528 **Sehnenscheide**, f. sheath of a tendon.
2529 **Sechnenverwachsung**, f. adhesion of a tendon.
2530 **sehnig**, adj. tendinous, sinewy.–
2531 **Achillessehne**, f. } tendon of Achilles, etc.
2532 **Achillesflechse**, f. }
2533 4. **MUSKEL**, m. 2. muscle, in compounds:
2534 **Muskeln, gegenwirkende**, pl. counteracting muscles.
2535 **Muskeln, unwillkürliche**, pl. involuntary muscles.
2536 **Muskeln, willkürliche**, pl. voluntary muscles.
2537 **Muskeln, zusammenwirkende**, pl. together working as coöperative muscles.
2538 **Muskeln, zusammenziehende**, pl. constrictors.
2539 **Muskelabspannung**, f. relaxation of a muscle.
2540 **Muskelansatz**, m. 1. muscular insertion.
2541 **Muskelanspannung**, f. stretching of a muscle, muscular tension.
2542 **Muskelband**, n. 1. muscle bundle or fasciculus.
2543 **Muskelbau**, m. 1. muscular structure.
2544 **Muskelbauch**, m. 1. belly of a muscle.
2545 **Muskelbewegung**, f. action or movement of a muscle.
2546 **Muskelbinde**, f. fascia or aponeurosis of a muscle.
2547 **Muskelblatt**, n. 1. muscular layer.

2548 **Muskeldruck**, m. 1. pressure of a muscle.

2549 **Muskelfaser**, f. } muscular fibre.
Muskelfäserchen, n. 2. }

2550 **Muskelfiber**, f. muscular fibril.

2551 **Muskelfleisch**, n. 1. muscular tissue or substance.

2552 **Muskelfortsatz**, m. 1. muscular process.

2553 **Muskelgeräusch**, n. 1. muscular murmur.

2554 **Muskelgitter**, n. 2. muscular meshwork of interlacing fibres (e. g. in tongue.)

2555 **Muskelgruppe**, f. group of muscles.

2556 **muskelhaft**, adj. } muscular, i. e. strong in muscle.
2557 **muskelig**, adj. }
2558 **muskelkräftig**, adj. }

2559 **Muskelhaut**, f. muscular coat.

2560 **Muskelhülle**, f. muscular coat or sheath.

2561 **Muskelkern**, m. 1. nucleus of muscle fibre.

2562 **Muskelkopf**, m. 1. head of a muscle.

2563 **Muskelkörper**, m. 2. body of a muscle.

2564 **Muskelkurve**, f. muscle-curve.

2565 **Muskellage**, f. } muscular layer.
Muskellager, n. 2. }

2566 **Muskel-platte**, f. muscle plate.

2567 **Muskelton**, m. 1. muscle sound.

2568 **Muskeltrieb**, m. 1. muscular movement.

2569 **Muskelverdichtung**, f. induration of a muscle.

2570 **Muskelwulst**, f. muscular elevation or swelling.

2571 **musculär**, adj : } muscular, i. e. strong in muscle, etc.
2572 **musculös**, adj : }

5. In compounds with **muskel** at the close :

2573 **Abzieher-Muskel**, m. 2. abductor-muscle (fr. v. ir. abziehen, to draw off or away.)

2574 **Anzieher-muskel**, m. 2. adductor muscle (fr. v. ir. anziehen, to adduce.)

2575 **Auswärtsdreher-muskel**, m. 2. } supinator muscle.
2576 **Auswärtsroller-muskel**, m. 2. }
2577 **Auswärtswender-muskel**, m. 2. }
2578 **Augenlidschliesz-muskel**, m. 2. } orbicularis palpebrarum muscle.

2579 **Augenmuskel**, m. 2. muscle of the eye.

2580 **Backenmuskel**, m. 2. baccinator muscle.

2581 **Beckenmuskel**, m. 2. pelvis muscle.

2582 **Bauchmuskel**, m. 2. abdominal muscle.

2583 **Beugermuskel**, m. 2. (fr. biegen, beugen, to bend), flexor muscle.

2584 **Brustmuskel**, m. 2. thoracic muscle.

2585 **Deltamuskel**, m. 2. deltoid muscle.

2586 **Einwärtsdreher-muskel**, m. 2. } pronator muscle.
2587 **Einwärtsroller-muskel**, m. 2. }
2588 **Einwärtswender-muskel**, m. 2. }

2589 **Fuszmuskel**, m. 2. muscle of the foot.

2590 **Gefäszmuskel**, m. 2. vascular muscle.

2591 **Gesichtsmuskel**, m. 2. facial muscle.

2592 **Halsmuskel**, m. 2. cervical muscle.

2593 **Handmuskel**, m. 2. muscle of the hand.

2594 **Hohlmuskel**, m. 2. hollow muscle.

2595 **Kaumuskeln**, m. 2. pl. masseters muscles (from kauen, to chew, masticate.)

2596 **Kopfmuskeln**, m. 2. pl. muscles of the head.

2597 **Mundmuskeln**, m. 2. pl. muscles of the mouth.

2598 **Nackenmuskel**, m. 2. cervicular muscle.

2599 **Nasenmuskel**, m. 2. nasal muscle.

2600 **Niederzieher**, m. 2. depressor muscle.

2601 **Oberarmmuskel**. m. 2. brachial muscle.
2602 **Oberschenkelmuskel**, m. 2. femoral muscle.
2603 { **Ringmuskel**, m. 2. circular muscle. **Rollermuskel**, m. 2. rotator muscle.
2604 **Rückenmuskel**, m. 2. dorsal muscle.
2605 **Rumpfmuskel**, m. 2. trunk muscle.
2606 **Rutenmuskel**, m. 2. erector penis.
2607 **Schädelmuskel**, m. 2. cranial muscle.
2608 **Schlieszmuskel**, m. 2. sphincter or constrictor muscle.
2609 **Schultermuskel**, m. 2. } scapular muscle.
2610 **Schulterblattmuskel**, m. 2. } scapular muscle.
2611 **Streckermuskel**, m. 2. extensor muscle.
2612 **Unterschenkelmuskel**, m. 2. muscle of the leg.
2613 **Vorderarmmuskel**, m. 2. forearm muscle.
2614 **Wadenmuskel**, m. 2. peroneal muscle, etc.
2615 §10. **Das Nervensystem**, the nervous system.
2616 1. **GEHIRN**. n. 1. brain, encephalon, in compounds:
2617 **gehirnartig**, adj. brain-like, encephaloid.
2618 **Gehirnbalken**, m. 2. corpus callosum.
2619 **Gehirnband**, n. 1. commissure of the brain.
2620 **Gehirnbehälter**, m. 2. cranium, skull.
2621 **Gehirnbewegung**, f. cerebral movement (pulsation.)
2622 **Gehirnbläschen**, n. 2. } cerebral vesicle.
2623 **Gehirnblase**, f. } cerebral vesicle.
2624 **Gehirnblutflusz**, m. 1. } sanguineous apoplexy.
2625 **Gehirnblutschlag**, m. 1. } sanguineous apoplexy.
2626 **Gehirnblutung**, f. cerebral hemorrhage, apoplexy.
2627 **Gehirnbruch**, m. 1. hernia cerebri, encephalocele.
2628 **Gehirnbrücke**, f. pons Varolii.
2629 **Gehirndruck**, m. 1. brain-compression.
2630 **Gehirneinschnitt**, m. 1. cerebral fissure.
2631 **Gehirnerscheinung**, f. cerebral phenomenon.
2632 **Gehirnerschütterung**, f. } concussion of the brain.
2633 **Gehirnerstarrung**, f. } concussion of the brain.
2634 **Gehirnerweichung**, f. softening of the brain.
2635 **Gehirnfalte**, f. fold of the brain.
2636 **Gehirnfett**, n. 1. cerebrin.
2637 **Gehirngefäsz**, n. 1. cerebral vessel.
2638 **Gehirngewicht**, n. 1. weight of the brain.
2639 **Gehirngewölbe**, n. 1. fornix cerebri.
2640 **Gehirngrund**, m. 1. base of the brain.
2641 **Gehirngrundfläche**, f. surface of the base of the brain.
2642 **Gehirnhäutchen**, n. 2. } cerebral meninges.
2643 **Gehirnhaut**, f. } cerebral meninges.
2644 **Gehirnhaut**, f. harte (hard), dura mater.
2645 **Gehirnhaut**, f. mittlere (middle), arachnoid.
2646 **Gehirnhaut**, f. weiche (soft), pia mater.
2647 **Gehirnhöhle**, f. cerebral ventricle.
2648 **Gehirnhülle**, cerebral meninges.
2649 **Gehirninsel**, f. island of Reil.
2650 **Gehirnkammer**, f. cerebral ventricle.
2651 **Gehirnkern**, m. 1. cerebral nucleus.
2652 **Gehirnklappe**, f. valve of Vieussens.
2653 **Gehirnknoten**, m. 2. cerebral ganglion.
2654 **Gehirnkrümmung**, f. cerebral convolution, gyrus.
2655 **Gehirnlappen**, m. 2. cerebral lobe.
2656 **gehirnlos**, adj. brainless.
2657 **Gehirnmangel**, m. 2. absence or want of brain.
2658 **Gehirnmark**, n. 1 medulla cerebri.
2659 **Gehirnmarkhügel**, m. 2. corpus mammillare.
2660 **Gehirnmiszbildung**, f. malformation of brain.
2661 **Gehirnödem**, n. 1. œdema of the brain.
2662 **Gehirnreiz**, m. 1. cerebral irritation.

2663 **Gehirnrinde**, f. cerebral cortex.
2664 **Gehirnsand**, n. 1. brainsand, acervulus cerebri.
2665 **Gehirnsaum**, m. 1. fimbria hippocampi, taenia semicircularis.
2666 **Gehirnschädel**, m. 2. } cranium,
2667 **Gehirnschale**, f. } skull.
2668 **Gehirnscheidewand**, f. septum lucidum.
2669 **Gehirnschenkel**, m. 2. cerebral peduncle.
2670 **Gehirnschlag**, m. 1. } cerebral
Gehirnschlagflusz, m. 1. } apoplexy.
2671 **Gehirnschwiele**, f. corpus callosum.
2672 **Gehirnspalte**, f. cerebral fissure.
2673 **Gehirnstamm**, m. 1. primary cerebral peduncle.
2674 **Gehirnstiel**, m. 1. crus cerebri.
2675 **Gehirnvorfall**, m. 1. hernia cerebri.
2676 **Gehirnwasser**, n. 2. cerebrospinal fluid.
2677 **Gehirnwassererergusz**, m. 1. serous apoplexy.
2678 **Gehirnwulst**, f. hippocampus major.
2679 **Gehirnzelt**, n. 1. tentorium cerebelli.
2680 **Mittelgehirn**, n. 1. mid-brain mesocephalon, etc.
2681 2. **HIRN**, n. 1. brain. encephalon, in compounds:
2682 (**Gehirn** gives often the same or other compounds).
2683 **Hirnabmagerung**, f. cerebral atrophy.
2684 **Hirnanhang**, m. 1. hypophysis cerebri, pituitary gland.
2685 **Hirnarterienring**, m. 1. circle of Willis.
2686 **Hirnbalken**, m. 2. corpus callosum.
2687 **Hirnbläschen**, n. 2. } cerebral
Hirnblase, f. } vesicle.
2688 **Hirnblasen**, n. 2. pl. } cephalic
2689 **Hirnblasengeräusch**, n. 1. } bellows
2690 **Hirnblasenschall**, m. 1. } sound.
2691 **Hirnblatt**, n. 1. fontanelle.
2692 **Hirnblutader**, f. cerebral vein.
2693 **Hirnblutergusz**, m. 1. } sanguineous apoplexy.
2694 **Hirnblutflusz**, } cerebral hemorrhage, apo-
2695 **Hirnblutung**, f. } plexy.
2696 **Hirnblutleiter**, m. 2. cerebral sinus.
2697 **Hirnbruch**, m. 1. hernia cerebri.
2698 **Hirnbrücke**, f. pons Varolii.
2699 **Hirndeckel**, m. 2. cranium.
2700 **Hirndruck**, m. 1. compression of the brain.
2701 **Hirnerscheinung**, f. cerebral phenomenon.
2702 **Hirnerschütterung**, f. concussion of the brain.
2703 **Hirnerweichung**, f. softening of the brain.
2704 **Hirnfaser**, f. brain fibre.
2705 **Hirnfell**, n. 1. pia mater.
2706 **Hirnfett**, n. 1. cerebrin.
2707 **Hirnfinne**, f. cysticercus in the brain.
2708 **Hirnfläche**, f. surface of the brain.
2709 **Hirnform**, f. shape of the brain.
2710 **Hirnfurche**, f. cerebral sulcus.
2711 **Hirnfusz**, m. 1. base of the brain.
2712 **Hirnganglie**, f. cerebral ganglion.
2713 **Hirngefäsz**, n. 1. cerebral vessel.
2714 **Hirngeschwulst**, f. cerebral tumor.
2715 **Hirngeschwür**, n. 1. fungus cerebri.
2716 **Hirngewölbe**, n. 1. fornix cerebri.
2717 **Hirngezelt**, see Hirnzelt.
2718 **Hirnhalbkugel**, f. cerebral hemisphere.
2719 **Hirnhaut**, f. cerebral meninges.
2720 **Hirnhautblutleiter**, m. 2. meningeal sinus, sinus of the dura mater.
2721 **Hirnhautblutung**, f. meningeal hemorrhage.
2722 **Hirnhautpulsader**, f. } meningeal
2723 **Hirnhautschlagader**, f. } artery.
2724 **Hirnhautschwamm**, m. 1. fungus of the dura mater.
2725 **Hirnhöhle**, f. cerebral ventricle.

2726 **Hirnhülle,** f. cerebral membrane.
2727 **Hirnkammer,** f. cerebral ventricle.
2728 **Hirnkapsel,** f. cranium.
2729 **Hirnkern,** m. 1. cerebral nucleus.
2730 **Hirnklappe,** f. valve of Vieussens.
2731 **Hirnknöpfchen,** n. 2. corpus mammillare.
2732 **Hirnknoten,** m. 2. cerebral ganglion, pons Varolii.
2733 **Hirnkörper,** m. 2. corpus striatum.
2734 **Hirnlähmung,** f. paralysis of the brain (Paresis f. incomplete paralysis of the mind, etc.)
2735 **Hirnlappen,** m. 2. cerebral lobe.
2736 **hirnlos,** adj. brainless.
2737 **Hirnmantel.** m. 2. the cortex of the cerebrum.
2738 **Hirnmark,** n. 1. medullary substance of brain.
2739 **Hirnmarkhügel,** m. 2. corpus mammillare.
2740 **Hirnmarksegel,** n. 2. medullary velum.
2741 **Hirnmasse,** f. brain substance.
2742 **Hirnnerv,** m. 3. cerebral nerve.
2743 **Hirnnervenpaar,** n. 1. pair of cerebral nerves.
2744 **Hirnnervenschwäche,**f. neurasthenia cerebralis.
2745 **Hirnpfanne,** f. cranium, skull.
2746 **Hirnquetschung,** f. contusion of the brain.
2747 **Hirnrantengrube,** f. fossa rhomboidalis, fourth ventricle.
2748 **Hirnrinde,** f. cerebral cortex.
2749 **Hirnrückenmark,** n. 1. cerebro-spinal medulla.
2750 **Hirnrückenmarknerv,** m. 3. cerebro-spinal nerve.
2751 **Hirnsand,** m. 1. brainsand, acervulus cerebri.
2752 **Hirnschädel,** m. 2. cranium, skull.
2753 **Hirnschädelbeinmark,** n. 1. diploë.
2754 **Hirnschädelbruch,** m. 1. fracture of the skull.
2755 **Hirnschädeldach,** n. 1. vertex of the skull.
2756 **Hirnschädelfuge,** f. cranial suture.
2757 **Hirnschädelgewölbe.** n. 1. vault of the cranium.
2758 **Hirnschädelhaut,** f. pericranium.
2759 **Hirnschädelknochen,** m. 2. cranial bone.
2760 **Hirnschädelnaht,** f. cranial suture.
2761 **Hirnschädelschwamm,** m. 1. fungus of the cranial bones.
2762 **Hirnschale,** f. cranium, skull.
2763 **Hirnschalenmuskel,** m. 2. occipito-frontalis muscle.
2764 **Hirnscheidewand,** f. septum lucidum.
2765 **Hirnschenkel,** m. 2. cerebral peduncle.
2766 **Hirnschlag,** m. 1. cerebral apoplexy.
2767 **Hirnschlagader,** f. cerebral artery.
2768 **Hirnschlagflusz,** m. 1. cerebral apoplexy.
2769 **Hirnschlitz,** m. 1. cerebral fissure.
2770 **Hirnschwamm,** m. 1. fungus cerebri, hernia cerebri.
2771 **Hirnschwiele,** f. corpus callosum.
2772 **Hirnschwund,** m. 1. atrophy of the brain.
2773 **Hirnsichel,** f. falx cerebri or cerebelli.
2774 **Hirnspalte,** f. cerebral fissure.
2775 **Hirnspinnengewebe,** n. 1. arachnoid membrane.
2776 **Hirnstamm,** m. 1. caudex cerebri.
2777 **Hirnstein,** m. 1. concretion in the brain.
2778 **Hirnstiel,** m. 1. crus cerebri.
2779 **Hirnventrikel,** m. 2. cerebral ventricle.
2780 **Hirnvorfall,** m. 1. protrusion of the brain.
2781 **Hirnwasserbruch,** m. 1. encephalocele.
2782 **Hirnwindung,** f. cerebral convolution, gyrus.
2783 **Hirnzelt,** n. 1. tentorium cerebelli, etc.
2784 3. **NERV,** m. 3. **Nerve,** f. } nerve, in compounds beginning the words:
2785 **Nervdrücken,** n. 2. nerve compression.

2786 **Nerven,** in compounds: neuro—or nerve:

2787 **nervenartig,** adj. nerve-like, plexiform.

2788 **Nerven-arznei,** f. nervine medicine or remedy.

2789 **Nervenast,** m. 1. nerve-branch.

2790 **Nervenatrophie.** f. atrophy or shrinking of a nerve.

2791 **Nervenaufregung,** f. nerve excitation.

2792 **Nervenausbreitung,** f. distribution of nerves.

2793 **Nervenaussatz,** m. 1. anaesthetic leprosy.

2794 **Nervenbahn,** f. nerve tract.

2795 **Nervenbau,** m. 1. nerve structure.

2796 **Nervenbindegewebsscheide,** f. neurilemma, nerve sheath.

2797 **Nervenbündel,** n. 2. nerve fasciculus.

2798 **Nervenbüschel,** n. 2. nerve bundle.

2799 **Nervencentralorgan,** n. 1. central nerve organ.

2800 **Nervencentrum,** n. 1. nerve centre.

2801 **Nervendehnung,** f. nerve stretching.

2802 **Nervendruck,** m. 1. pressure on a nerve.

2803 **Nerveneinrichtung,** f. arrangement of nerves.

2804 **Nervenelongation,** f. nerve elongation or stretching.

2805 **Nervenendigung,** f. nerve termination.

2806 **Nervenendknospe,** f. terminal nerve-bud.

2807 **Nervenendplatte,** f. terminal nerve plate.

2808 **Nervenerregung,** f. nerve excitation.

2809 **Nervenerschütterung,** f. concussion of a nerve.

2810 **Nervenerweichung,** f. softening of a nerve.

2811 **Nervenevolution,** f. tearing out of a nerve by torsion.

2812 **Nervenfädchen,** n. 2. }
Nervenfaden, m. 2. } nerve fila-
2813 **Nervenfaser,** f. } ment.
Nervenfäserchen, n. 2. }

2814 **Nervenfasernetz,** n. 1. reticulum of nerve fibres.

2815 **Nervenfaserschicht,** f. nerve-fibre layer.

2816 **Nervenfett,** n. 1. nerve-fat, protogon.

2817 **Nervenfortsatz,** m. 1. nerve process.

2818 **Nervenfurche,** f. furrow or space for nerves.

2819 **Nervengebiet,** n. 1. } nervous
2820 **Nervengeflecht,** n. 1. } plexus.

2821 **Nervengewebe,** n. 1. nerve tissue.

2822 **Nervengitter,** n. 2. nerve plexus.

2823 **Nervengrenzstrang,** m. 1. chief nerve cord.

2824 **Nervenhaut,** f. neurilemma, retina.

2825 **Nervenherd,** m. 1. nerve centre.

2826 **Nervenhügel,** m. 2. nerve-bulb-end organ.

2827 **Nervenhülle,** f. nerve sheath, neurilemma.

2828 **Nervenkern,** m. 1. nerve nucleus.

2829 **Nervenknospe,** f. nerve-bud or end-organ.

2830 **Nervenknoten,** m. 2. nerve ganglion.

2831 **nervenknotig,** adj. ganglionic.

2832 **Nervenkörperchen,** n. 2. nerve corpuscle.

2833 **Nervenkrebs,** m. 1. cancer of a nerve.

2834 **Nervenkugel,** f. nerve ganglion.

2835 **Nervenlähmung,** f. neuroparalysis.

2836 **Nervenlauf,** m. 1. course or tract of a nerve.

2837 **Nervenlèben,** n. 2. nerve-life, nerve-nutrition.

2838 **nervenlos,** adj. nerveless, weak.

2839 **Nervenmark,** n. 1. nerve medulla.

2840 **Nervenmasse,** f. nerve substance.

2841 **Nervenmittel,** n. 2. nervine remedy.

2842 **Nervennaht,** f. suture of nerves.

2843 **Nervennarbe,** f. nerve-scar.

2844 **Nervennetz,** n. 1. nerve plexus, network of nerves.

2845 **Nervenpaar,** n. 1. pair of nerves.

2846 **Nervenpaarung,** f. division of nerves in pairs.

2847 **Nervenpapille**, f. nerve papilla.
2848 **Nervenplastik**, f. nerve union by suture.
2849 **Nervenreflex**, m. 1. nervous reflex or reflex of nerves.
2850 **nervenreich**, adj. rich in nerves.
2851 **Nervenreiz**, m. 1. nerve irritant.
2852 **Nervenreizmittel**, n. 2. nervine excitement.
2853 **Nervenreizung**, f. nerve irritation.
2854 **Nervenröhre**, f. nerve fibre or tube.
2855 **Nervenscheide**, f. neurilemma, nerve sheath.
2856 **Nervenschicht**, f. nervous layer.
2857 **Nervenschlag**, m. 1. } apoplexy.
2858 **Nervenschlagflusz**, m. 1. } apoplexy.
2859 **nervenschwach**, adj. nervous, neurasthenic.
2860 **Nervenstamm**, m. 1. nerve trunk.
2861 **nervenstärkend**, adj. nervine, tonic.
2862 **Nervenstarre**, f. nervous rigor.
2863 **Nervenstich**, m. 1. nerve puncture.
2864 **Nervenstrang**, m. 1. nervous strang, cord, or trunk.
2865 **Nervenstrom**, m. 1. nervous current.
2866 **Nervensubstanz**, f. nerve tissue.
2867 **Nervensystem**, n. 1. nervous system.
2868 **Nerventhätigkeit**, f. nerve activity.
2869 **Nervenwärzchen**, n. 2. } nerve papilla.
2870 **Nervenwarze**, f. } nerve papilla.
2871 **Nervenwerk**, nervous system.
2872 **Nervenwurzel**, f. } nerve root.
2873 **Nervenwürzelchen**, n. 2. } nerve root.
2874 **Nervenzelle**, f. nerve-cell.
2875 **Nervenzellenfortsatz**, m. 1. nerve-cell process.
2876 **Nervenzellensäule**, f. nerve-cell column (of spinal cord.)
2877 **Nervenzellenschicht**, f. ganglionic cell-layer.
2878 **Nervenzittern**, n. 2. nervous tremor, twitching.
2879 **Nervenzuckung**, f. nervous spasm, convulsion.
2880 **Nervenzufall**, m. 1. nervous attack.
2881 **Nervenzweig**, m. 1. nerve branch
2882 **nervicht**, adj. } nervous, sinewy.
2883 **nervig**, adj. } nervous, sinewy.
2884 **nervös**, adj. nervous.
2885 **Nervosismus**, m. 1. } neurasthenia.
2886 **Nervosität**, f. } neurasthenia.
2887 Compounds with *nerv*, nerve closing the word.
2888 **Achsel-nerv**, m. 3. axillary nerve.
2889 **Augen-nerv**. m. 3. optic nerve, orbital nerve, ophthalmic nerve.
2890 **Augenhöhlennerv**, m. 3. orbital nerve.
2891 **Augenlidnerv**, m. 3. palpebral nerve.
2892 **Augenmuskelnerv**, m. 3. oculo-motor nerve.
2893 **Bauchnerv**, m. 3. pelvic nerve.
2894 **Beinnerv**, m. 3. accessory nerve.
2895 **Brustnerv**, m. 3. thoracic nerve.
2896 **Darmnerv**, m. 3. intestinal nerve.
2897 **Drüsennerv**, m. 3. gland-nerve.
2898 **Eingeweidenerv**, m. 3. splanchnic nerve.
2899 **Eingeweidenervensystem**, splanchnic nervous system.
2900 **Fingernerv**, m. 3. digital nerve.
2901 **Fusznerv**, m. 3. nerve of the foot.
2902 **Gangliennervensystem**, n. 1. ganglionic nervous system.
2903 **Gaumenkeilbeinnerv**, m. 3. spheno-palatine nerve.
2904 **Gaumennerv**, m. 3. palatine nerve.
2905 **Gebärmutternerv**, m. 3. uterine nerve.
2906 **Gefäsznerv**, m. 3. vascular nerve.
2907 **Gefühlsnerv**, m. 3. sensory nerve.
2908 **Gehirnnerv**, m. 3. cerebral nerve.
2909 **Gehirnnervenpaar**, n. 1. pair of cerebral nerves.
2910 **Gehörnerv**, m. 3. auditory nerve.

2911 **Gekrösnerv**, m. 3. mesenteric nerve.
2912 **Geruchsnerv**, m. 3. olfactory nerve.
2913 **Gesäsznerv**, m. 3. gluteal nerve (from Gesäsz, n. 1. buttocks).
2914 **Geschmacksnerv**, m. 3. gustatory nerve; glosso-pharyngeal nerve.
2915 **Gesichtsnerv**, m. 3. facial nerve.
2916 **Haarnerv**, m. 3. ciliary nerve.
2917 **Halsnerv**, m. 3. cervical nerve.
2918 **Handnerv**, m. 3. nerve of the hand.
2919 **Hautnerv**, m. 3. cutaneous nerve.
2920 **Herznerv**, m. 3. cardiac nerve.
2921 **Hirnrückenmarksnerv**, m. 3. cerebro-spinal nerve.
2922 **Hodennerv**, m. 3. spermatic nerve.
2923 **Hohlhandfinger-nerv**, m. 3. } palmar nerve.
2924 **Hohlhandnerv**, m. 3. } palmar nerve.
2925 **Hörnerv**, m. 3. auditory nerve.
2926 **Hörnervenloch**, n. 1. auditory nerve foramen.
2927 **Hörnervenstamm**, m. 1. auditory nerve trunk.
2928 **Hüftbeinloch-nerv**, m. 3. } obturator nerve.
2929 **Hüftloch-nerv**, m. 3 } obturator nerve.
2930 **Hüftnerv**, m. 3. sciatic nerve.
2931 **Jochwangennerv**, m. 3. temporo-malar nerve.
2932 **Kaumuskelnerv**, m. 3. } masseteric nerve.
2933 **Kaunerv**, m. 3. } masseteric nerve.
2934 **Kehlkopfnerv**, m. 3. laryngeal nerve.
2935 **Kiefermuskelnerv**, m. 3. masseteric nerve.
2936 **Kieferzungenbein-muskelnerv**, m. 3. } mylo-hyoid nerve.
2937 **Kieferzungennerv**, m. 3. } mylo-hyoid nerve.
2938 **Kinnnerv**, m. 3. mental nerve.
2939 **Kitzlernerv**, m. 3. } nerve of the clitoris, tickler-nerve.
Clitorisnerv, m. 3. } nerve of the clitoris, tickler-nerve.
2940 **Kniekehlennerv**, m. 3. popliteal nerve.
2941 **Kopfnerv**, m. 3. cranial nerve.
2942 **Kreuzbeinnerv**, m. 3. } sacral nerve.
2943 **Kreuznerv**, m. 3. } sacral nerve.
2944 **Lebernerv**, m. 3. hepatic nerve.
2945 **Lendenleistennerv**, m. 3. } lumbar nerve.
2946 **Lendennerv**, m. 3. } lumbar nerve.
2947 **Linsennervenknoten**, m. 2. (from
2948 **Linse**, f. lentil, lens) lenticular ganglion.
2949 **Lungenmagennerv**, m. 3. pneumo-gastric nerve.
2950 **Lungennerv**, m. 3. pulmonary nerve.
2951 **Magennerv**, m. 3. gastric nerve.
2952 **Mammarnerv**, m. 3. mammary nerve.
2953 **Mastdarmnerv**, m. 3. haemorrhoidal nerve.
2954 **Mäuschen**, n. 2. funny bone (ulnar nerve at elbow joint).
2955 **Mesenterialnerv**, m. 3. mesenteric nerve.
2956 **Milznerv**, m. 3. splenic nerve.
2957 **Mittelarmnerv**, m. 3. } median nerve.
2958 **Mittelnerv**, m. 3. } median nerve.
2959 **Muskelnerv**, m. 3. muscular nerve.
2960 **Nackennerv**, m. 3. cervical nerve.
2961 **Nasengaumennerv**, m. 3. naso-palatine nerve.
2962 **Nasennerv**, m. 3. nasal nerve.
2963 **Nebennerv**, m. 3. accessary nerve.
2964 **Nierennerv**, m. 3. renal nerve.
2965 **Oberaugenhöhlennerv**, m. 3. supra-orbital nerve.
2966 **Oberbauchnervengeflecht**, n. 1. epigastric plexus.
2967 **Oberkiefernerv**, m. 3. supra-maxillary nerve.
2968 **Oberrollnerv**, m. 3. supra-trochlear nerve.
2969 **Oberschlüsselbeinnerv**, m. 3. supra-clavicular nerve.
2970 **Oberschulterblattnerv**, m. 3. supra-capsular nerve.
2971 **Ohrennerv**, m. 3. } auditory nerve.
Ohrnerv, m. 3. } auditory nerve.
2972 **Radialnerv**, m. 3. radial nerve.
2973 **Riechnerv**, m. 3. olfactory nerve.

2974 **Rollmuskelnerv**, m. 3. } fourth cranial
2975 **Rollnerv**, m. 3. } nerve.
2976 **Rückenmarksnerv**, m. 3. spinal nerve.
2977 **Rückenmarksnervengeflecht**, n. 1. spinal nerve plexus.
2978 **Rückenmarksnervenlähmung**, f. spinal nerve paralysis.
2979 **Rückenmarksnervenpaar**, n. 1. pair of spinal nerves.
2980 **Rückennerv**, m. 3. dorsal nerve.
2981 **Rückgratsnerv**, m. 3. spinal nerve.
2982 **Rumpfnervensystem**, n. 1. sympathetic nervous system.
2983 **Rutennerv**, m. 3. nerve of the penis.
2984 **Samennerv**, m. 3. spermatic nerve.
2985 **Samenstrangnerv**, m. 3. nerve of spermatic cord.
2986 **Schamnerv**, m. 3. pubic nerve.
2987 **Schamschenkelnerv**, m. 3. genito-crural nerve.
2988 **Schenkelnerv**, m. 3. nerve of the thigh.
2989 **Schienbeinnerv**, m. 3. tibial nerve.
2990 **Schläfennerv**, m. 3. temporal nerve.
2991 **Schlundkopfnerv**, m. 3. } pharyngeal
2992 **Schlundnerv**, m. 3. } nerve.
2993 **Schneckennerv**, m. 3. cochlear nerve.
2994 **Schulterblattnerv**, m. 3. } scapular
2995 **Schulternerv**, m. 3. } nerve.
2996 **Sehnerv**, m. 3. optic nerve.
2997 **Siebbeinnerv**, m. 3. ethmoidal nerve.
2998 **Sinnesnerv**, m. 3. nerve of sense.
2999 **Sitzbeinnerv**, m. 3. sciatic nerve.
3000 **Sohlennerv**, m. 3. plantar nerve.
3001 **Speichennerv**, m. 3. radial nerve.
3002 **Spinalnerv**, m. 3. spinal nerve.
3003 **Spinalnervensystem**, n. 1. spinal nervous system.
3004 **Steiszbeinnerv**, m. 3. } coccygeal
3005 **Steisznerv**, m. 3. } nerve.
3006 **Stimmnerv**, m. 3. laryngeal nerve.
3007 **Stirnnerv**, m. 3. frontal or supra-orbital nerve.
3008 **Strahlennerv**, m. 3. ciliary nerve.
3009 **Thränendrüsennerv**, m. 3. lachrymal nerve.
3010 **Trommelnerv**, m. 3. nerve of the tympanum.
3011 **Unteraugenhöhlennerv**, m. 3. infra-orbital nerve.
3012 **Unterkiefernerv**, m. 3. inferior dental nerve.
3013 **Unterleibsnerv**, m. 3. abdominal nerve.
3014 **Unterlippennerv**, m. 3. inferior labial nerve.
3015 **Unterrollnerv**, m. 3. infratrochlear nerve.
3016 **Unterschenkelnerv**, m. 3. saphenous nerve.
3017 **Unterschulterblattnerv**, m. 3. subscapular nerve.
3018 **Unterzungennerv**, m. 3. hypoglossal nerve.
3019 **Vorhofsnerv**, m. 3. (from
3020 **Vorhof**, m. 1. vestibule) vestibular nerve.
3021 **Wadenbeinnerv**, m. 3. external popliteal nerve.
3022 **Wadennerv**, m. 3. peroneal nerve.
3023 **Wangennerv**, m. 3. nerve of the cheek.
3024 **Zahnhöhlennerv**, m. 3. } dental
3025 **Zahnnerv**, m. 3. } nerve
3026 **Zehennerv**, m. 3. digital nerve of the toe.
3027 **Zungenbeinkiefernerv**, m. 3. mylo-hyoid nerve.
3028 **Zungenfleischnerv**, m. 3. hypoglossal nerve.
3029 **Zungenmagennerv**, m. 3. pneumo-gastric nerve.
3030 **Zungennerv**, m. 3. gustatory nerve.
3031 **Zungenschlundkopfnerv**, m. 3. } glosso-pharyngeal
3032 **Zungenschlundnerv**, m. 3. } nerve.
3033 **Zwergfellnerv**, m. 3. (from
3034 **Zwergfell**, n. 1. diaphragm) phrenic nerve.
3035 **Zwischenknochennerv**, m. 3. interosseous nerve.

3036 **Zwischenrippennerv**, m. 3. intercostal nerve, etc.

3037 **Der Rumpf und seine Bestandteile.** The Thorax and its contents.

3038 § 11. **Die Atmungswerkzeuge**, the respiratory organs.

3039 1. **ATMEN**, n. 2.
3040 **ATMUNG**, f. } (from atmen, to breathe, inhale, respire) breathing, respiration, inspiration, in compounds:

3041 **atmig**, adj. respiring.

3042 **Atmungsbedürfnis**, n. 1. necessity of breathing.

3043 **Atmungsbeklemmung**, f.
3044 **Atmungsbeschwerde**, f. } difficulty or oppression of breathing, dyspnoea.

3045 **Atmungscentrum**, n. 1. respiratory centre.

3046 **atmungsfähig**, adj. capable of respiring.

3047 **Atmungsgeräusch**, n. 1. respiratory murmur or sound.

3048 **Atmungsgymnastik**, f. respiratory gymnastics or exercises.

3049 **Atmungslähmung**, f. paralysis of respiration.

3050 **Atmungsmuskel**, m. 2. respiratory muscle.

3051 **Atmungsmuskulatur**, f. muscular apparatus for respiration.

3052 **Atmungsnerv**, m. 3. respiratory nerve.

3053 **Atmungspforte**, f. opening or orifice of respiratory passage.

3054 **Atmungsprozesz**, m. 1. process of respiration.

3055 **Atmungsschleimhaut**, f. respiratory mucous membrane.

3056 **Atmungsstörung**, f. disturbance in respiration.

3057 **Atmungsstrom**, m. 1. respiratory stream (of atmosphere.)

3058 **atmungsunfähig**, adj. incapable of respiration.

3059 **Atmungsvorgang**, m. 1. process of breathing.

3060 **Atmungswerkzeug**, n. 1. respiratory organ.

3061 2. **ATEM**, m. 1. (from atmen, to breathe), breath, breathing, respiration.

3062 **Atem holen or schöpfen**, to draw breath.

3063 **aufatmen**, to recover breath.

3064 **Atem tiefheraufholen**, to draw a deep, long breath.

3065 **Atem an sich halten**, to hold one's breath.

3066 **atembar**, adj. respirable, in compounds:

3067 **Atembeklemmung**, f. (from beklemmen, to hinder), dyspnoea, oppression in breathing.

3068 **Atembeschwerde**, f. dyspnoea, difficulty in respiration.

3069 **Atembewegung**, f. (from bewegen, v. ir. to move) respiratory movement.

3070 **Atemgeräusch**, n. 1. respiratory murmur or sound.

3071 ——, **abgeschwächtes**, weakened, diminished breath-sound, feeble vesicular murmur;

3072 ——, **amphorisches**, amphoric breath-sound;

3073 ——, **bronchiales**, bronchial or tubular breath-sound;

3074 ——, **mangelndes**, suppressed or defective breath-sound;

3075 ——, **saccadiertes**, interrupted or jerky breath-sound;

3076 ——, **unbestimmtes**, harsh subtubular breath-sound;

3077 ——, **verlängertes**, prolonged breath-sound;

3078 ——, **verschärftes**, exaggerated quick puerile or compensatory breath-sound.

3079 **Atemgeruch**, m. 1. smell of the breath.

3080 **Atemkrampf**, m. 1. respiratory spasm.

3081 **atemlos**, adj. breathless, out of breath.

3082 **Atemmuskel**, m. 2. respiratory muscle.

3083 **Atemnot**, f. dyspnoea.

3084 **Atemorgan**, n. 1. organ of respiration.

3085 **Atemzug**, m. 1. breath, respiration, inspiration.

3086 **Atemzünglein**, n. 2. epiglottis.

3087 **Ausatmung**, f. (from ausatmen, to exhale), exhalation.

3088 **Einatmung**, f. (from einatmen, to inhale, inspire), respiration.

3089 **Engatmigkeit**, f. | shortness of breath, from kurz, short.
3090 **Kurzatmigkeit**, f. |

3091 **Mundatmen**, n. 2. oral respiration, to respire through the mouth.

3092 **Nasenatmen**, n. 2. nasal respiration, to respire through the nose.

3093 **Rippenatmen**, n. 2. costal respiration.

3094 **Röhrenatmen**, n. 2. tubal respiration, to respire through a tube, etc.

3095 3. **LUFT**, f. air, atmosphere, in compounds.

3096 **Luftansammlung**, f. (from
3097 **ansammeln**, to collect), Collection of air (e. g. in pneumothorax).

3098 **Luftbehälter**, m. 2. (from v. ir. behalten, to keep), to keep air-e. g. the lungs.

3099 **Luftbeschaffenheit**, f. air condition.

3100 **Luftbläschen**, n. 2. } air vesicle, pulmonary
Luftblase, f. } vesicle.

3101 **Luftbrust**, f pneumothorax.

3102 **Luftdruck**, m. 1. atmospheric pressure.

3103 **luftführend**, adj. air carrying (as the trachea, etc).

3104 **Luftgefäsz**, n. 1. air vessel, pl., the lungs.

3105 **Lufthunger**, m. 2. anxiety for air, breath.

3106 **lufthungrig**, adj. anxious for air or breath.

3107 **Luftkanal**, m. 1. air passage.

3108 **Luftkeim**, m. 1. micro-organism of the air.

3109 **Luftmangel**, m. 2. want of air, etc.

3110 4. **LUFTRÖHRE**, f. trachea, in compounds:

3111 **Luftröhrenast**, m. 1. bronchus.

3112 **Luftröhrendeckel**, m. 2. epiglottis.

3113 **Luftröhrendrüse**, f. bronchial gland.

3114 **Luftröhrengefäsz**, n. 1. a vessel of the trachea.

3115 **Luftröhrengegend**, f. tracheal region.

3116 **Luftröhrenknorpel**, m. 2. tracheal cartilage.

3117 **Luftröhrenkopf**, m. 1. larynx.

3118 **Luftröhrenring**, m. 1. tracheal or bronchial ring.

3119 **Luftröhrenschleimhaut**, f. mucous membrane of trachea or bronchus.

3120 **Luftröhrenschnitt**, m. 1. tracheotomy.

3121 **Luftröhrenspalte**, f. rima glottidis.

3122 **Luftröhrenstein**, m. 1. tracheal or bronchial concretion.

3123 **Luftröhrenverengerung**, f. stenosis of the trachea.

3124 **Luftröhrenwand**, f. wall of the trachea, etc.

3125 **Luftschöpfen**, n. 2. respiration, inhalation.

3126 **Luftstrom**, m. 1. current of air.

3127 **Luftweg**, m. 1. air passage.

3128 **Luftzelle**, f. air vesicle or alveolus.

3129 **Luftzug**, m. 1. air current.

3130 **Ventilation**, f. (from ventilieren, to ventilate), ventilation.

3131 5. **LUNGE**, f. lung (pulmonary) in compounds:

3132 **Lungenabscesz**, m. 1. pulmonary abscess, vomica.

3133 **Lungenabschnitt**, m. 1. part or section of the lung.

3134 **Lungenader**, f. pulmonary vein.

3135 **Lungenarterie**, f. pulmonary artery.

3136 **Lungenarterienast**, m. 1. branch of pulmonary artery.

3137 **Lungenarterienklappe**, f. pulmonary valve.

3138 **Lungenarterienstamm**, m. 1. trunk of pulmonary artery.

3139 **Lungenatmung**, f. } pulmonary respiration.
Lungenatmen, n. 2. }

3140 **Lungenatmungsgeräusch**, n. 1. breathing sound or sound of respiration.

3141 **Lungenatrophie**, f. atrophy or wasting of the lung.

3142 **Lungenaufblähung**, f. distention of the lung.

3143 **Lungenauswurf**, m. 1. sputum.

3144 **Lungenband**, n. 1. pulmonary ligament.

3145 **Lungenblähung**, f. inflation of the lung, emphysema of the lung.
3146 **Lungenbläschen**, n. 2. **Lungenblase**, f. } vesicle, alveolus of the lung.
3147 **Lungenblatt**, n. 1. lobe of the lung.
3148 **Lungenblutader**, f. pulmonary vein.
3149 **Lungenblutflusz**, m. 1. hemorrhage from the lungs.
3150 **Lungenblutung**, f. bleeding from the lungs.
3151 **Lungenblutsturz**, m. 1. violent hemoptysis.
3152 **Lungenbruch**, m. 1. pneumocele.
3153 **Lungendrüse**, f. bronchial gland.
3154 **Lungeneinschnitt**, m. 1. fissure of the lung.
3155 **Lungenerweiterung**, f. emphysema of the lung.
3156 **Lungenfell**, n. 1. pleura pulmonalis.
3157 **Lungenfeuchtigkeit**, f. pulmonary moisture.
3158 **Lungenfistel**, f. pulmonary fistula.
3159 **Lungenflügel**, m. 2. lobe of the lung.
3160 **Lungenfurche**, f. fissure of the lung.
3161 **Lungengefäsz**, n. 1. pulmonary vessel.
3162 **Lungengeflecht**, n. 1. pulmonary plexus.
3163 **Lungengewebe**, n. 1. tissue of the lung.
3164 **Lungenhaut**, f. pleura pulmonalis.
3165 **Lungenhernie**, f. hernia of the lung.
3166 **Lungenherz**, n. 1. right side of the heart.
3167 **Lungenherzkammer**, f. right ventricle.
3168 **Lungenhöhle**, f. pulmonary cavity.
3169 **Lungeninfarkt**, m. 1. (obsolete) pulmonary infarction, filling, obstruction.
3170 **Lungenkreislauf**, m. 1. pulmonary circulation.
3171 **Lungenläppchen**, n. 2. lobule of the lung.
3172 **Lungenlappen**, m. 2. lobe of the lung.
3173 **Lungenmagennerv**, m. 3. pneumo-gastric nerve.
3174 **Lungennerv**, m. 3. pulmonary nerve.
3175 **Lungenpigment**, n. 1.
3176 **Lungenfarbenstoff**, m. 1. } lung pigment.
3177 **Lungenpulsader**, f. pulmonary artery.
3178 **Lungenpulsaderklappe**, f. pulmonary valve.
3179 **Lungenschall**, m. 1. pulmonary sound.
3180 **Lungenschlag**, m. 1. pulmonary apoplexy, oedema of the lung.
3181 **Lungenschlagader**, f. pulmonary artery.
3182 **Lungenschleimhaut**, f. mucous membrane of the lung.
3183 **Lungenschrumpfung**, f. (from schrumpfen, to contract), contraction or induration of the lung.
3184 **Lungenschwiele**, f. pulmonary callosity (following filling or infarct).
3185 **Lungenspitze**, f. apex of the lung.
3186 **Lungensplenisation**, f. splenization of the lung.
3187 **Lungenstein**, m. 1. pulmonary concretion.
3188 **Lungensucht**, f. consumption.
3189 **lungensüchtig**, adj. consumptive.
3190 **Lungenvene**, f. pulmonary vein.
3191 **Lungenvenensack**, m. 1. left auricle.
3192 **Lungenvorfall**, m. 1. protrusion of the lung.
3193 **Lungenwassersucht**, f. oedema of the lung.
3194 **Lungenwurzel**, f. root of the lung.
3195 **Lungenzelle**, f. pulmonary vesicle, etc.
3196 § 12 **Das Gefäszsystem**, the vascular system.
3197 1. **ADER**, f. a vein.
3198 **goldne** or **güldne**, haemorrhoidal vein, haemorrhoids or piles, (see for other compounds in Vene, vein. In compounds.
3199 **Aderbein**, n. 1. varicose vein in the leg.

3200 **Aderbinde**, f. } bandage, liga-
Ligatur, f. } ture.
3201 **Aderbruch**, m. 1. rupture of a vein, varicocele.
3202 **Äderchen**, n. 2. a little vein, venule.
3203 **Aderentzündung**, f. phlebitis.
3204 **Adergebäude**, n. 1. vascular, venous system.
3205 **Adergeflecht**, n. 1. vascular plexus; plexus of veins.
3206 **Adergewebe**, n. 1. venous tissue.
3207 **Aderhaut**, f. } choroid
Aderhäutchen, n. 2. } membrane.
3208 **Aderhautentzündung**, f. choroiditis.
3209 **Aderhautgeflecht**, n. 1. choroid plexus.
3210 **Aderhautschwinden**, n. 2. } atrophy of the
3211 **Aderhautschwund**, m. 1. } choroid.
3212 **Aderhautspalt**, m. 1. } coloboma of the cho-
3213 **Aderhautspaltung**, f. } roid.
3214 **Aderhautspanner**, m. 2. ciliary muscle.
3215 **aderig**, adj. venous.
3216 **Aderknopf**, m. 1. } varicose vein,
3217 **Aderknoten**, m. 2. } varix.
3218 **Aderlaszen**, n. 2. } phlebotomy,
3219 **Aderlasz**, m. 1. } venesection.
3220 **Aderlaszanhänger**, m. 2. advocate of bleeding.
3221 **Aderlaszbäuschchen**, n. 2. compress applied after bloodletting.
3222 **Aderlaszbecken**, n. 2. basin used at bloodletting.
3223 **Aderlaszgerät**, n. 1. } instrument for
3224 **Aderlaszzeug**, n. 1. } bleeding,
3225 **Aderlaszkunst**, f. } art of blood-
3226 **Aderlaszlehre**, f. } letting.
3227 **Aderlaszlanzette**, f. bleeding lancet.
3228 **Aderlasznarbe**, f scar after the wound of bloodletting is healed.
3229 **aderlos**, adj. veinless.
3230 **Adernetz**, n. 1. venous network.
3231 **Adernetzschlagader**, f. choroid artery (lateral ventricle of brain.)
3232 **aderreich**, adj. venous, rich in veins.
3233 **Aderschlag**, m. 1. pulse, pulsation.
3234 **Aderschlagmesser**, n. 2. pulsimeter.
3235 **Aderstrang**, m. 1. venous chord or plexus.
3236 **Adersystem**, n. 1. vascular system.
3237 **Aderwasser**, n. 2. blood-serum, etc.
3238 2. **AORTA**, f. } or grosze Pulsader, or grosze Schlagader, f.
3239 **HERZRÖHRE**, } aorta, great, main artery of the body.
3240 **Aorta, absteigende**, descending aorta.
3241 **Aorta, aufsteigende**, ascending aorta, in compounds:
3242 **Aortenausdehnung**, f. dilatation of the aorta.
3243 **Aortenbogen**, m. 2. arch of the aorta.
3244 **Aortengeflecht**, n. 1. aortic plexus.
3245 **Aortenherz**, n. 1. the left side of the heart.
3246 **Aortenkammer**, f. left ventricle of the heart.
3247 **Aortenklappe**, f. aortic valve.
3248 **Aortenklappenfehler**, m. 2. defect of aortic valve.
3249 **Aortenschlitz**, m. 1. aortic opening (in diaphragm.)
3250 **Aortenspalte**, f. aortic opening (in diaphragm.)
3251 **Aortenstenosengeräusch**, n. 1. murmur of aortic stenosis.
3252 **Aortenton**, m. 1. aortic sound.
3253 **Aortenwurzel**, f. root of the aorta.
3254 **Aortenzwiebel**, f. bulbus aortæ.
3255 3. **ARTERIE**, f. artery.
3256 **Arterie, ungenannte**, innominate artery.
3257 **Arteriektasis**, f. aneurism.
3258 **arteriell**, adj. arterial.
3259 **Arterienast**, m. 1. arterial branch.
3260 **Arterienblut**, n. 1. arterial blood.
3261 **Arterieneröffnung**, f. arteriotomy.
3262 **Arterienerweiterung**, f. dilatation of an artery, aneurism.

3263 **Arteriengeräusch**, n. 1. arterial murmur.
3264 **Arterienrohr**, n. 1. arterial tube.
3265 **Arterienscheide**, f. sheath of artery.
3266 **Arterienverengerung**, f. narrowing of an artery.
3267 **Arterienverletzung**, f. injury to an artery.
3268 **Arterienverschlieszung**, f. occlusion of an artery.
3269 **Arterienverzweigung**, f. arterial ramification, etc.
3270 **Arterienwand**, f. arterial wall, etc.
3271 4. **BLUT**, n. 1. (from bluten, to bleed), blood.
3272 **Blutabgang**, m. 1. (from v. ir. abgehen, to go away, depart), hemorrhage, loss of blood, menstruation.
3273 **Blutader**, f. vein.
3274 **Blutaderblut**, n. 1. venous blood.
3275 **Blutadergeflecht** n. 1. venous plexus.
3276 **Blutadergeschwulst**, f. } varix, varicose swelling.
3277 **Blutaderknoten**, m. 2. }
3278 **Blutadernetz** n. 1. venous plexus.
3279 **Blutalbumin**, n. 1. blood albumin.
3280 **Blutandrang**, m. 1. (from v. ir. andringen, to press on), congestion, active hyperaemia.
3281 **Blutanhäufung**, f. (from anhäufen, to accumulate), accumulation of blood, congestion, plethora, engorgement.
3282 **Blutansammlung**, f. (from ansammeln, to gather), accumulation of blood.
3283 **Blutanschoppung**, f. engorgement, hemorrhagic infarct.
3284 **Blutarmut**, f. anaemia, poverty of the blood.
3285 **blutausleerend**, adj. depletive.
3286 **Blutaustretung**, f. extravasation of blood.
3287 **Blutaustritt**, m. 1. (from v. ir. austreten, to step out), extravasation of blood.
3288 **Blutauswurf**, m. 1. (from v. ir. auswerfen, to throw out), sputum with blood.
3289 **Blutbahn**, f. blood passage, blood vessel.
3290 **Blutbehälter**, m. 2. blood vessel, sinus.
3291 **Blutbereitung**, f. (from bereiten, to make, prepare), haematopoesis, blood formation.
3292 **Blutbeschaffenheit**, f. condition of blood.
3293 **Blutbestandteil**, m. 1. constituent part of blood.
3294 **Blutbeule**, f. haematoma.
3295 **Blutbewegung**, f. circulation or movement of the blood.
3296 **Blutbilder**, m. 2. blood producer, albumin, protein.
3297 **Blutblase**, f. haematoma, haematocystis.
3298 **Blutbrechen**, n. 2. haematemesis.
3299 **Blutbruch**, m. 1. (from v. ir. brechen, to break), haematocele.
3300 **Blutcyste**, f. encysted blood, sanguineous cyst.
3301 **Blutdrüse**, f. vascular gland.
3302 **Blutegel**, m. 2. leech.
3303 **bluten**, to bleed.
3304 **Blutentartung**, f. blood degeneration.
3305 **blutenthaltend**, adj. bloody, sanguineous, blood containing.
3306 **Blutentleerung**, f. artificial bleeding.
3307 **Blutentmischung**, f. disintegration of blood, infection of blood (in syphilis).
3308 **Blutentwickelung**, f. development of blood.
3309 **blutentziehend**, adj. drawing blood, haemagogic.
3310 **Blutentziehung**, f. artifical bleeding.
3311 **Blutfarbe**, f. blood color.
3312 **blutfarbig**, adj. blood colored.
3313 **Blutfarbstoff**, m. 1. haemoglobin, haematoglobulin, haematocrystallin.
3314 **Blutfaserstoff**, m. 1. fibrin.
3315 **Blutfäule**, f. septicaemia, pyaemia.
3316 **Blutflecken**, m. 2. blood stain, blood spot, purpuric spot.
3317 **Blutflusz**, m. 1. (from v. ir. fleszen, to flow), hemorrhage, haematorrhoea.
3318 **blutflüssig**, adj. hemorrhagic.

3319 **Blutfülle**, f. plethora, hyperaemia.
3320 **Blutgang**, m. 1. (from v. ir. gehen, to go), flow of blood, menses.
3321 **Blutgefäsz**, n. 1. blood vessel.
3322 **Blutgefäszausbreitung**, f. vascular distribution.
3323 **Blutgefäszbindegewebe**, n. 1. connective tissue of a blood vessel.
3324 **Blutgefäszgeräusch**, n. 1. vascular rustling, noise, sound.
3325 **Blutgefäszgeschwulst**, f. angioma.
3326 **Blutgefäszknäuel**, m. 2. convolution or tuft of blood vessels, glomerulus.
3327 **Blutgefäsznetz**, n. 1. network of blood vessels.
3328 **Blutgefäszstamm**, m. 1. vascular trunk.
3329 **Blutgefäszton**, m. 1. vascular tone.
3330 **Blutgefäszverknöcherung** f. calcification of blood vessels.
3331 **Blutgefäszverstopfung**, f. obstruction of blood vessels.
3332 **Blutgefäszwand**, f. wall of a blood vessel.
Blutgehalt, m. 1. (see 3337).
3333 **Blutgeräusch**, n. 1. haemic murmur.
3334 **Blutgerinnung**, f. (from v. ir. rinnen, to flow, to drop. [gerinnen, to coagulate], coagulation of blood.
3335 **Blutgerinsel**, n. 2. blood coagulum.
3336 **Bluthaargefäsz**, n. 1. capillary blood vessel.
3337 **Blutgehalt**, m. 1. blood contents.
bluthaltig, adj. containing blood.
3338 **Blutharnen**, n. 2. haematuria.
3339 **Blutherd**, m. 1. blood centre.
3340 **Bluthof**, m. 1. area sanguinea.
3341 **Bluthöhle**, f. haematic or blood cavity.
3342 **Bluthusten**, m. 2. haemoptysis.
3343 **blutig**, adj. bloody, sanguineous.
3344 **Blutinsel**, f. infarct.
3345 **Blutklumpen**, m. 2. blood clot, coagulum.
3346 **Blutknoten**, m. 2. hemorrhagic infarct.
3347 **Blutkörnchen**, n. 2. blood granule.
3348 **Blutkreislauf**, m. 1. (from v. ir. laufen, to run), circulation of the blood.
3349 **Blutkrystall**, m. 1. blood crystal.
3350 **Blutkuchen**, m. 2. blood coagulum.
3351 **Blutkügelchen**, n. 2. blood corpuscle.
3352 **Blutlauf**, m. 1. blood circulation.
3353 **blutleer**, adj. bloodless, exsanguine.
3354 **Blutleiter**, m. 2. sinus.
3355 **blutlos**, adj. bloodless, ex-sanguine.
3356 **Blutlosigkeit**, f. anaemia, bloodlessness.
3357 **blutmachend**, adj. blood-forming, haematopoetic.
3358 **Blutmal**, n. 1. birth mark, naevus.
3359 **Blutmangel**, m. 2. anaemia, need or want of blood.
3360 **Blutmasse**, f. mass or quantity of blood.
3361 **Blutmauser**, f. } retrogressive metamorphosis of the blood.
3362 **Blutmauserung**, f. }
3363 **Blutpfropf**, m. 1. thrombus, hemorrhagic infarct.
3364 **Blutpilz**, m. 1. boletus satanas (poisonous fungus); in bacteriology micrococcus prodigiosus.
3365 **Blutplasma**, n. 1. blood plasma.
3366 **Blutplättchen**, n. 2. blood disc.
3367 **Blutprobe**, f. blood testing.
3368 **blutreich**, adj. rich in blood, plethoric.
3369 **Blutreichtum**, n. 1, plethora, vascularity.
3370 **blutreinigend**, adj. purifying the blood.
3371 **blutrot**, adj. bloodred.
3372 **Blutrot**, n. 1. coloring matter of the blood, haematin.
3373 **Blutruhr**, f. bloody flux.
3374 **blutrünstig**, adj. bloody, black and blue (in contusion or bruise).
3375 **Blutschlag**, m. 1. (from v. ir. shlagen, to beat), apoplexy.

3376 **Blutschlagflusz,** m. 1. } apoplexy.
3377 **Blutflusz,** m. 1. }
3378 **Blutschorf,** m. 1. crust formed of blood clot.
3379 **Blutschwamm,** m. 1. fungus haematodes (as in cancer.)
3380 **Blutschwär,** m. 1. } boil, furuncle.
3381 **Blutschwären,** m. 2. }
3382 **Blutschweisz,** m. 1. } bloody sweat.
3383 **Blutschwitzen,** n. 2. }
2384 **Blutserum,** n. 1. blood serum.
3385 **Blutspeien,** n. 2. } haemoptysis.
3386 **Blutspuken,** n. 2. }
3387 **Blutspur,** f. trace of blood, blood mark.
3388 **Blutstauung,** f. vascular engorgement.
3389 **Blutstillen,** n. 2. blood stopping, styptic.
3390 **blutstillend,** adj. styptic, haemostatic.
3391 **Blutstillstand,** m. 1. blood stasis.
3392 **Blutstockung,** f. passive hyperaemia, engorgement.
3393 **Blutstuhl,** m. 1. bloody stool.
3394 **Blutsturz,** m. 1. violent hemorrhage or haemoptysis.
2395 **Blutverwandtschaft,** f. consanguinity.
3396 **Bluttausch,** f. transfusion of blood.
3397 **Blutteilchen,** n. 2. blood corpuscle.
3398 **Bluttröpfeln,** n. 2. the dropping of blood, stillicidium sanguinis.
3399 **Blutüberfüllung,** f. } hyperaemia, congestion, plethora.
3400 **Blutüberladung,** f. }
3401 **Blutumlauf,** m. 1. circulation of the blood.
3402 **——groszer,** greater.
3403 **——kleiner,** lesser circulation through the system (lungs).
3404 **Blutung,** f. bleeding, hemorrhage.
3405 **Blutungsquelle,** f. source of bleeding.
3406 **Blutungszuckung,** f. anaemic convulsion.
3407 **blutunterlaufen,** adj. bloodshot.
3408 **Blutunterlaufung,** f. suggillation, ecchymosis, vibex.
3409 **Blutveränderung,** f. blood change.
3410 **Blutverarmung,** f. impoverishment of the blood.
3411 **Blutverdickung,** f. thickening of the blood.
3412 **Blutverdünnung,** f. reduction (from verdünnen, to attenuate), dilution of the blood.
3413 **Blutvergiftung,** f. blood poisoning.
3414 **Blutverirrung,** f. deviation of the blood (from verirren, to deviate).
3415 **Blutverlust,** m. 1. loss of blood.
3416 **Blutvermehrung,** f. increase of the quantity of blood.
3417 **Blutverminderung,** f. decrease in the quantity of the blood.
3418 **Blutverteilung,** f. blood distribution.
3419 **Blutverwandlung,** f. blood metamorphosis.
3420 **Blutvorrat,** m. 1. supply of blood.
3421 **Blutwallung,** hyperaemia, engorgement, congestion.
3422 **Blutwärme,** f. blood heat.
3423 **Blutwarze,** f. birth mark.
3424 **Blutwasser,** m. 2. serum sanguinis.
3425 **Blutwassergefäsz,** n. 1. lymphatic vessel.
3426 **blutwässerig,** adj. serous, lymphatic.
3427 **Blutwassermangel,** m. 2. deficiency of serum in the blood, anaemydria.
3428 **Blutwelle,** f. bloodwave.
3429 **Blutwurzel,** f. tormentil root.
3430 **Blutzelle,** f. blood cell.
3431 **Blutzuflusz,** m. 1. supply of blood, flow of blood.
3432 **Blutzufuhr,** f. blood supply.
3433 **Blutzwang,** m. 1. blood flux, dysentery, etc.
3434 **Geblüt,** n. 1. blood, is used to denote, generally, all the blood in the body.
3435 **verbluten,** to bleed to death.
3436 **Verblutung,** f. bleeding to death.
3437 Note 1. The *arterial* blood is
3438 **hellrot,** light red.
3439 The *venous* blood is **dunkelrot,** dark red.

3440 5. **GEFÄSZ**, n. 1. vessel, tube, canal. In compounds.
3441 **Gefäszanfüllung**, f. vascular engorgement.
3442 **Gefäszast**, m. 1. branch of a vessel.
3443 **Gefäszausbreitung**, f. vascular distribution.
3444 **Gefäszausdehnung**. f. vascular dilatation.
3445 **Gefäszbahn**, f. vascular passage.
3446 **Gefäszbezirk**, n. 1. vascular region.
3447 **Gefäszbildung**, f. formation of vessels.
3448 **Gefäszblatt**, n. 1. vascular layer.
3449 **Gefäszbündel**, n. 2. vascular bundle.
3450 **Gefäszbüschel**, m. or n. 2. vascular tuft.
3451 **Gefäszchen**, n. 2. a small vessel.
3452 **Gefäszdruck**, m. 1. pressure on a vessel.
3453 **Gefäszdrüse**, f. vascular gland.
3454 **Gefäszeinmündung**, f. anastomosis.
3455 **Gefäszendothel**, n. 2. endothelium of vessels.
3456 **Gefäszentzündung**, f. inflammation of vessels.
3457 **Gefäszerweichung**, f. softening of vessels.
3458 **gefäszerweiternd**, adj. dilating vessels.
3459 **Gefäszerweiterung**, f. telcangiectasis.
3460 **Gefäszfurche**, f. space for vessels.
3461 **Gefäszgallenfistel**, f. circulatory biliary fistula.
3462 **Gefäszgeflecht**, n. 1. plexus of vessels.
3463 **Gefäszgeräusch**, n. 1. vascular murmur.
3464 **Gefäszgeschwür**, n. 1. ulcer of a blood vessel.
3465 **Gefäszgewebe**, n. 1. vascular tissue.
3466 **Gefäszhauptstamm**, m. 1. principal trunk of a vessel.
3467 **Gefäszhaut**, f. vascular membrane, tunica vasculosa.
3468 **Gefäszhof**, m. 1. vascular area.
3469 **Gefäszhöhle**, f. lumen of a vessel.
3470 **gefäszig**, adj. vascular.
3471 **Gefäszigkeit**, f. vascularity.
3472 **Gefäszkanälchen**, n. 2. vascular canaliculus.
3473 **Gefäszknäuel**, m. 2. vascular coil, glomerulus.
3474 **Gefäszknoten**, m. 2. ligature of a vessel.
3475 **Gefäszkrampf**, m. 1. vascular spasm.
3476 **Gefäszkranz**, m. 1. } corona
3477 **Gefäszkreis**, m. 1. } vascularis.
3478 **Gefäszkropf**, m. 1. struma vasculosa, vascular gôitre.
3479 **Gefäszlähmung**, f. paralysis of vessels.
3480 **Gefäszleere**, f. emptiness of vessels.
3481 **Gefäszlehre**, f. angiology.
3482 **Gefäszmal**, n. 1. vascular naevus.
3483 **Gefäszverbindung**, f. (from v. ir. verbinden, to connect), vascular connection.
3484 **Gefäszmündung**, f. orifice of a vessel.
3485 **Gefäszmuskelhaut**, f. muscular coat of vessels.
3486 **Gefäsznarbe**, f. vascular cicatrix.
3487 **Gefäsznerv**, m. 3. vascular nerve.
3488 **Gefäsznetz**, n. 1. vascular network.
3489 **Gefäszöffnung**, f. vascular aperture.
3490 **Gefäszpapille**, f. vascular papilla.
3491 **Gefäszrohr**, n. 1. lumen of a vessel.
3492 **Gefäszschall**, m. 1. vascular murmur.
3493 **Gefäszscheide**, f. sheath of a vessel.
3494 **Gefäszscheidenbahn**, f. track of sheath of a vessel.
3495 **Gefäszschicht**, f. vascular layer.
3496 **Gefäszschlinge**, f. vascular loop.
3497 **Gefäszschwamm**, m. 1. angioma, fungus haematodes.
3498 **Gefäszspalt**, m. 1. space occupied by vessels.
3499 **Gefäszstamm**, m. 1. trunk of a vessel.
3500 **Gefäszstrang**, m. 1. vascular cord.

5

3501 **Gefäszsystem,** n. 1. vascular system.
3502 **Gefäszthätigkeit,** f. activity of the vessels.
3503 **Gefäsztonus,** m. 1. vascular tone.
3504 **Gefäszüberfüllung,** f. vascular engorgement.
3505 **Gefäszveränderung,** f. vascular change.
3506 **Gefäszverbreitung,** f. vascular distribution.
3507 **Gefäszverengerung,** f. narrowing of vessels, angiosternosis.
3508 **Gefäszverknöcherung,** f. ossification of vessels.
3509 **Gefäszverschwärung,** f. ulceration of a blood vessel.
3510 **Gefäszverstopfung,** f. blocking or plugging of vessels.
3511 **Gefäszverzweigung,** f. ramification of vessels.
3512 **Gefäszwand,** f. } wall of
Gefäszwandung. f. } a vessel.
3513 **Gefäszwärzchen,** n. 2. vascular papilla.
3514 **Gefäszwucherung,** f. angioma, proliferation of vessels.
3515 **Gefäszzergliederung,** f. dissection of vessels.
3516 **Gefäszzerreiszung,** f. laceration of vessels.
3517 **Gefäszzone,** f. vascular area.
3518 **Gefäszzweig,** m. 1. branch of a vessel, etc.
3519 6. **HERZ,** n. 1. heart (soul, spirit, courage), *cardiac*, in compounds.
3520 **Herzabscesz,** m. 1. cardiac abscess.
3521 **Herzader,** f. cardiac or coronary vein.
3522 **Herzanlage,** f. rudiment of the heart.
3523 **Herzarterie,** f. cardiac artery.
3524 **Herzatrophie,** f. atrophy of the heart.
3525 **Herzaufregung,** f. cardiac excitement.
3526 **Herzbalken,** m. 2. columna carnea.
3527 **Herzbeben** (zittern), n. 2. palpitation of the heart.
3528 **Herzbeklemmung,** f. } from v. tr. beklemmen, to oppress, pinch, oppression of the heart.
3529 **Herzbeklommenheit,** f. }
3530 **herzberuhigend,** adj. quieting or soothing the heart.
3531 **Herzbeschleunigung,** f. (from beschleunigen, to hasten), heart acceleration.
3532 **Herzbeutel,** m. 2. pericardium.
3533 **Herzbeuteldämpfung,** f. pericardial dulness.
3534 **Herzbeutelhöhle,** f. cavity of the pericardium.
3535 **Herzbeutelverdickung,** f. thickening of the pericardium.
3536 **Herzbeutelverwachsung,** f. pericardial growth or adhesion.
3537 **Herzbeutelwasser,** n. 2. pericardial fluid.
3538 **Herzbewegung,** f. motion of the heart.
3539 **Herzblatt,** n. 1. sternum.
3540 **Herzblut,** n. 1. the blood in or of the heart.
3541 **Herzblutader,** f. coronary vein.
3542 **Herzbrand,** m. 1. } heart-
3543 **Herzbrennen,** n. 2. } burn.
3544 **Herzbruch,** m. 1. cardiocele.
3545 **Herzbuckel,** m. 2. praecordial prominence.
3546 **Herzdämpfung,** f. cardiac dulness.
3547 **Herzdegeneration,** f. degeneration of the heart (fatty or waxy).
3548 **Herzdilatation,** f. dilatation of the heart.
3549 **Herzdrücken,** n. 2. cardialgia, oppression of the heart.
3550 **Herzdrüse,** f. cardiac gland.
3551 **Herzensangst,** f. anguish.
3552 **Herzensruhe,** f. } perisy-
3553 **Herzensstillstand,** m. 1. } stole.
3554 **Herzzurückstosz,** m. 1. diastolic impulse of the heart.
3555 **Herzerschlaffung,** f. diastole.
3556 **Herzerweichung,** f. softening of the heart.
3557 **Herzerweiterung,** f. dilatation of the heart.
3558 **Herzfell,** n. 1. pericardium.
3559 **Herzfiber,** f. fibre of the heart.
3560 **Herzfleisch,** n. 1. cardiac muscle, myocardium.
3561 **Herzfleischschwund,** m. 1. atrophy of the walls of the heart.

3562 **herzförmig,** adj. cordi-form, heart-shaped or heart-formed.
3563 **Herzganglien,** pl. m. 1. cardiac ganglia.
3564 **Herzgefäsz,** n. 1. vessel of the heart.
3565 **Herzgeflecht,** n. 1. cardiac plexus.
3566 **Herzgegend,** f. cardiac region.
3567 **Herzgegendwölbung,** f. precordial prominence.
3568 **Herzgekröse,** n. 1. mesocardium.
3569 **Herzgeräusch,** n. 1. cardiac murmur, heart sound.
3570 **Herzgerinsel,** n. 2. heart clot.
3571 **Herzgeschwulst,** f. cardiac tumor.
3572 **Herzgeschwür,** n. 1. ulcer of the heart.
3573 **Herzgespann,** n. 1. sense of epigastric distention with disturbance of the heart.
3574 **Herzgewebe,** n. 1. tissue of the heart.
3575 **Herzgrübchen,** n. 2. } **Herzgrube,** f. } pit of the stomach.
3576 **Herzhaut,** f. äuszere, pericardium.
3577 **Herzhaut,** f. innere, endocardium.
3578 **Herzhemmungscentrum,** n. 1. cardio-inhibitory centre.
3579 **Herzhemmungsnerv,** m. 3. cardio-inhibitory nerve.
3580 **Herzhöhle,** f. heart cavity.
3581 **Herzhöhlenverengung,** f. heart-cavity contraction.
3582 **Herzhypertrophie,** f. cardiac or heart-hypertrophy.
3583 **Herzimpuls,** m. 1. impulse of the heart.
3584 **Herzinsufficienz,** f. cardiac insufficiency.
3585 **Herzkammer,** f. heart ventricle.
3586 **Herzkammerpulsadermündung,** f. arterial orifice of the ventricle.
3587 **Herzkammerscheidewand,** f. ventricular septum.
3588 **Herzkammerwand,** f. ventricular wall.
3589 **Herzklappe,** f. cardiac valve.
3590 **Herzklopfen,** n. 2. palpitation of the heart.
3591 **Herzknorpel,** m. 2. sternum.
3592 **Herzknoten,** m. 2. cardiac ganglion.
3593 **Herzkrampf,** m. 1. angina pectoris.
3594 **Herzkranzarterie,** f. coronary artery of the heart.
3595 **Herzläppchen,** n. 2. } **Herzlappen,** m. 2. } appendix auriculae.
3596 **Herzluftbeutel,** m. 2. pneumo-pericardium.
3597 **Herzlungengeräusch,** n. 1. cardio-pulmonary murmur or sound.
3598 **Herzmangel,** m. 2. absence of the heart.
3599 **Herzmattheit,** f. }
3600 **Herzmattigkeit,** f. } faintness, weakness of the heart.
3601 **Herzmiszbildung,** f. deformity of the heart, cardiac deformity.
3602 **Herzmündung,** f. heart orifice.
3603 **Herzmuskel,** m. 2. cardiac muscle, myocardium.
3604 **Herznebenkammer,** f. auricle.
3605 **Herznerv,** m. 3. cardiac nerve.
3606 **Herznervengeflecht,** n. 1. cardiac nerve plexus.
3607 **Herzohr,** n. 1. } **Herzöhrchen,** n. 2. } auricle.
3608 **Herzostien,** pl. n. 1. (fr. ostium. n. 1. orifice), orifices of the heart.
3609 **Herzpochen,** n. 2. palpitation of the heart.
3610 **Herzpolyp,** m. 1. clot or clod in the heart.
3611 **Herzpuls,** * m. 1. cardiac impulse or pulse of the heart.
3612 **Herzpulsader,** f. cardiac artery, aorta.
3613 **Herzreiz,** m. 1. cardiac stimulant.
3614 **Herzreizung,** f. cardiac irritation.
3615 **Herzröhre,** f. aorta.
3616 **Herzruptur,** f. heart rupture.
3617 **Herzsack,** m. 1. pericardium.
3618 **Herzscheidewand,** f. septum of the heart.
3619 **Herzschlag,** m. 1. impulse of beating of the heart, paralysis of the heart.
3620 **Herzschlagader,** f. aorta or cardiac artery.
3621 **Herzschwäche,** f. feebleness of the heart.

3622 **Herzschwiele**, f. hardening or induration or callosity of the heart.
3623 **Herzschwund**, m. 1. atrophy of the walls of the heart.
3624 **Herzspitze**, f. apex of the heart.
3625 **herzstärkend**, adj. strengthening the heart.
3626 **Herzstillstand**, m. 1. cessation of the heart's action.
2627 **Herzstosz**, m. 1. shock or impulse of the heart.
3628 **Herzthätigkeit**, f. action of the heart.
3629 **Herztod**, m. 1. stoppage, death of the heart.
3630 **Herzton**, m. 1. cardiac sound.
3631 **Herzvene**, f. cardiac or coronary vein.
3632 **Herzveränderung**, f. change in the heart.
3633 **Herzvergröszerung**, f. hypertrophy or enlargement of the heart.
3634 **Herzverhärtung**, f. hardening or induration of the heart.
3635 **Herzverknöcherung**, f. ossification of the heart.
3636 **Herzvorhof**, m. 1. auricle.
3637 **Herzvorhofsscheidewand**, f. auricular septum of the heart.
3638 **Herzvorkammer**, f. auricle.
3639 **Herzwand**, f. / **Herzwandung**, f. } cardiac wall.
3640 **Herzwasser**, n. 2. liquor pericardii.
3641 **Herzzittern**, n. 2. palpitation of the heart.
3642 **Herzzufall**, m. 1. cardiac attack.
3643 **Herzzusammenziehung**, f. systole, etc.
3644 *(Note) **Der Puls, Pulsschlag mag sein**: The pulse may be.
3645 **aussetzend**, adj. intermittent (from aussetzen, to set out, stop, suspend, here in the sense of omitting some pulsations).
3646 **doppelschlägig**, adj. double
3647 beating (from v. ir, schlagen, to beat and double, doppel), dicrotic.
3648 **drahtförmig**, adj. wiry.
3649 **erhaben**, adj. high, lofty.
3650 **fadenförmig**, adj. thready.
3651 **fieberhaft**, adj. feverish.
3652 **frequent**, adj. frequent.
3653 **geschwind**, adj. quick.
3654 **gespannt**, adj. tense.
3655 **grosz**, adj. large.
3656 **hart**, adj. hard.
3657 **heftig**, adj. vehement, violent.
3658 **hüpfend**, adj. jerking.
3659 **jagend**, adj. galloping.
3660 **kaum fühlbar**, adj. scarcely perceptible.
3661 **klein**, adj. small.
3662 **kurz**, adj. short.
3663 **langsam**, adj. slow.
3664 **mäszig stark**, adj. moderately strong.
3665 **nachgebend**, adj. yielding.
3666 **nicht fühlbar**, adj. not perceptible.
3667 **rasch**, adj. quick, rapid.
3668 **regelmäszig**, adj. regular(ly).
3669 **regelwidrig**, adj.* abnormal, irregular.
3670 **reichlich**, adj. richly.
3671 **schnellend**, adj. bounding under the touch.
3672 **schwach**, adj. weak.
3673 **schwächerwerdend**, adj. diminishing in strength, sinking.
3674 **schwankend**, adj. undulating.
3675 **schwirrend**, adj. vibrating.
3676 **selten**, adj. seldom ; seltener, (compar.) infrequent.
3677 **stillstehend**, adj. standing still, ceasing, arrest of pulsation.
3678 **stockend**, adj. ceasing to pulsate.
3679 **träge** or **träg**, adj. slow.
3680 **unregelmäszig**, irregular.
3681 **unterbrochen**, adj. interrupted or intermittent.
3682 **weich**, adj. soft.
3683 **zweischlägig** adj. double beating, dicrotic, etc.
3684 7. **LYMPHE**, f. lymph (clear fluid, blood-water.)
3685 **Saugader**, f. (from v. ir. saugen, to absorb, to suck), lymphatic vessel, in compounds.
3686 **lymphähnlich**, adj. / 3687 **lymphatisch**, adj. } lymphatic.
3688 **Lymphbahn**, f. lymph passage.
3689 **Lymphbahnanlage**, f. rudimentary lymph passage.

3690 **Lymphbahnstörung,** f. changes or disturbance in the lymph passages.

3691 **Lymphbehälter,** m. 2. lymph-reservoir.

3692 **Lymphcapillaren** or **Lymphkapillaren** } pl. (from singular:

3693 **Kapillar,** n. 1. Haarader or Haargefäsz), lymph-capillaries.

3694 **Lymphdrüse,** f. lymphatic gland.

3695 **lymphdrüsenähnlich,** adj. lymphatic, gland-like.

3696 **Lymphdrüsengeschwulst,** f. swelling of a lymphatic gland, lymphoma.

3697 **Lymphdrüsensystem,** n. 1. lymphatic gland system.

3698 **Lymphflusz,** m. 1. lymphorrhoea.

3699 **Lymphgefäsz,** n. 1. lymphatic vessel.

3700 **Lymphgefäszgeflecht,** n. 1. plexus of lymphatics.

3701 **Lymphgefäsznetz,** n. 1. lymphatic plexus.

3702 **Lymphgefäszstamm,** m. 1. lymphatic trunk.

3703 **Lymphgefäszsystem,** n. 1. lymphatic system.

3704 **Lymphgefäszverengerung,** f. narrowing of lymphatic vessels.

3705 **Lymphgefäszverschliezung,** f. occlusion of lymphatic vessels.

3706 **Lymphgefäszwundernetz,** n. 1. lymphatic rete mirabile.

3707 **Lymphgeschwulst,** f. lymphoma.

3708 **Lymphherz,** n. 1. lymph heart.

3709 **Lymphknötchen,** n. 2. solitary lymph follicle (e. g. in intestine.)

3710 **Lymphknoten,** m. 2. lymphatic gland.

3711 **Lymphkörnchen,** n. 2. lymph granule.

3712 **Lymphkörper,** m. 2. } lymph corpuscle.
3713 **Lymphkörperchen,** n. 2. }

3714 **Lymphkuchen,** m. 2. lymph coagulum.

3715 **Lymphkugel,** f. } lymph corpuscle.
3716 **Lymphkügelchen,** n. 2. }

3717 **Lymphom,** n. 1. lymphoma, glandular swelling.

3718 **Lymphorrhagie,** f. } lymphorrhoea.
3719 **Lymphorrhöe,** f. }

3720 **Lymphose,** f. formation of lymph in the lymphatic vessels.

3721 **Lymphröhrchen,** n. 2. } lymph tube or lymph passage.
3722 **Lymphröhre,** f. }

3723 **Lymphsack,** m. 1. lymph sac.

3724 **Lymphscheide,** f. lymph channel or sinus in lymph gland.

3725 **Lymphsee,** m. 1. large lymph space.

3726 **Lymphspalte,** f. lymph space.

3727 **Lymphstämmchen,** n. 2. lymphatic trunk.

3728 **Lymphstauung,** f. (from stauen, to dam, stem) lymph stasis.

3729 **Lymphstrom,** m. 1. lymph-stream.

3730 **Lymphweg,** m. 1. lymph passage.

3731 **Lymphzelle,** f. lymph cell, etc.

3732 8. **PFORTE,** f. door, gate, opening, orifice, porta. In compounds:

3733 **Pfortader,** f. port or portal vein, mesenteric vein, cystic vein, vena porta.

3734 **Pfortaderblut,** n. 1. portal blood.

3735 **Pfortadergebiet,** n. 1. portal region.

3736 **Pfortaderkrebs,** m. 1. cancer of the portal vein.

3737 **Pfortadersystem,** n. 1. portal venous system.

3738 **Pfortaderverschlieszung,** f. } occlusion of the portal vein.
3739 **Pfortaderverstopfung,** f. }

3740 **Pfortaderverzweigung,** f. ramification of the portal vein.

3741 **Pfortaderwurzel,** f. radicle of the portal vein.

3742 **Pfortaderzweig,** m. 1. branch of the portal vein.

3743 **PFÖRTNER,** m. 2, pylorus orifice of the stomach, mouth of the stomach.

3744 **Pförtnergegend**, f. pyloric region.
3745 **Pförtnerklappe**, f. pyloric sphinxter or valve.
3746 **Pförtnervene**, f. pyloric vein, etc.
3747 9. **VENE**, f. vein, in compounds:
3748 **Venenast**, m. 1. branch of a vein
3749 **Venenblut**, n. 1. venous blood.
3750 **Venenbruch**, m. 1. varix varicocele.
3751 **Venenerweiterung**, f. venous distention.
3752 **Venengefäsz**, n. 1, vein.
3753 **Venengefäszstamm**, m. 1. venous trunk.
3754 **Venengeflecht**, n. 1. venous plexus.
3755 **Venengeräusch**, n. 1. venous murmur, souffle.
3756 **Venenkanal**, m. 1. lumen of a vein.
3757 **Venenklappe**, f. valve of a vein.
3758 **Venenkranz**, m. 1. corona venosa, venous circle.
3759 **Venennetz**, n. 1. venous plexus or network.
3760 **Venenpfropfen**, m. 2, thrombus in a vein.
3761 **Venenrohr**, n. 1. lumen of a vein.
3762 **Venensack**, m. 1. vein-sac (e. g. arterio-venous aneurysm).
3763 **Venensausen**, n. 2. venous hum.
3764 **Venenscheide**, f. sheath of a vein.
3765 **Venenunterbindung**, f. venous ligation.
3766 **Venenverschlieszung**, f. } occlusion of a vein.
3767 **Venenverstopfung**, f. }
3768 **Venenzweig**, m. 1. branch of a vein.
3769 { **venerial**, adj. } venous.
{ **venerisch**, adj. }
3770 **venös**, adj. }
3771 §13. **Die Verdauungswerkzeuge.** The organs of digestion. In compounds:
3772 1. **BREI**, m. 1. broth, gruel, pap, pulp.
3773 **breiähnlich**, adj. } pappy, pulpy, atheromatous.
3774 **breiartig**, adj. }
3775 **breiicht**, adj. }
3776 **breiig**, adj. }
3777 **breiweich**, adj. pulpy, soft.
3778 2. **CHYMUS**, m. 1. } chyme.
3779 **Magenbrei**, m. 1. }
3780 **Speisebrei**, m. 1. }
3781 3. **Chylus**, m. 1. } chyle.
3782 **Speisesaft**, m. 1. }
3783 **chylös**, adj. chylous.
3784 **Chylusbahn**, f. chyle track.
3785 **Chylusgefäsz**, n. 1. lacteal vessel.
3786 **Chyluskörnchen**, n. 2. } chyle or lymph corpuscle.
3787 **Chyluskörperchen**, n. 2. }
3788 4. **NÄHREN**, n. 2. feeding (from nähren, to feed, nourish, nurture.)
3789 **nährend**, adj. nourishing, nutritive.
3790 **Nährgang**, m. 1. alimentary canal.
3791 **Nährgeschäft**, n. 1. nutrition work.
3792 **nahrhaft**, adj. nourishing, nutritious.
3793 **nahrhaftlos**, adj. non-nutritive.
3794 **Nährklystier**, n. 1. nutritious enema.
3795 **Nährkraft**, f. nourishing power.
3796 **nahrlos**, adj. non-nutritive.
3797 **Nährmutter**, f. fostermother.
3798 **Nährsaft**, m. 1. chyle.
3799 **Nährstoff**, m. 1. nourishing food or material.
3800 5. **NAHRUNG**, f. food, nourishment, nutrition.
3801 **Nahrungsaufnahme**, f. absorption.
3802 **Nahrungsbeschaffenheit**, f. dietetic conditions of food.
3803 **Nahrungsbrei**, m. 1. chyme.
3804 **Nahrungsdotter**, m. 2. food-yolk.
3805 **Nahrungsentziehung**, f. deprivation of food.
3806 **Nahrungsflüssigkeit**, f. chyle.
3807 **Nahrungskanal**, m. 1. alimentary canal.
3808 **Nahrungsklystier**, n. 1. nutrient enema.
3809 **Nahrungsmangel**, m. 2. poverty of food.
3810 **Nahrungsmilk**, f. chyle.
3811 **Nahrungsmittel**, n. 2. food, nutriment.
3812 **Nahrungsröhre**, f. alimentary tube.

3813 **Nahrungssaft**, m. 1. chyle.

3814 **nahrungssaftenthaltend**, adj. chyliferous.

3815 **Nahrungsscheu**, f. aversion for food.

3816 **Nahrungsschlauch**, m. 1. alimentary canal, gullet.

3817 **Nahrungsstoff**, m. 1. food, nutritive materials.

3818 **Nahrungsverweigerung**, f. refusal to take food.

3819 **Nahrungsvorschrift**, f. dietetics, rules of diet.

3820 **Nahrungsweg**, m. 1. food passage.

3821 **Nahrungszufuhr**, f. supply of food, etc.

3822 6. **RACHEN**, m. 2. pharynx, fauces, throat, (for further compounds see also §7. 18.)

3823 **Racheneingang**, m. 1. } (from v. ir. gehen, to go) isthmus of fauces, pharyngeal opening.
3824 **Rachenenge**, f. }

3825 **Rachenhaut**, f. pharyngeal membrane.

3826 **Rachenhöhle**, f. pharyngeal cavity.

3827 **Rachenmündung**, f. } pharyngeal opening, isthmus of fauces.
3828 **Rachenöffnung**, f. }

3829 **Rachenmuskel**, m. 2. pharyngeal muscle.

3830 **Rachenraum**, m. 1. pharyngeal space.

3831 **Rachenschleimhaut**, f. pharyngeal mucous membrane.

3832 **Rachenspalte**, f. isthmus of the fauces.

3833 **Rachentonsille**, f. pharyngeal tonsil. Luschka's tonsil.

3834 **Rachenwand**, f. pharyngeal wall, etc.

3835 7. **SCHLUCK**, m. 1. draught, gulp, swallow.

3836 **Schluckbewegung**, f. movement of swallowing.

3837 **Schlucken**, n. 2. (from schlucken, to swallow), swallowing.

3838 8. **SCHLUND**, m. 1. pharynx, fauces, throat (see also Rachen for compounds.)

3839 **Schlundarterie**, f. artery of the pharynx.

3840 **Schlundblutader**, f. pharyngeal vein.

3841 **Schlundblutung**, f. hemorrhage from the pharynx.

3842 **Schlundbogen**, m. 2. arch of the fauces.

3843 **Schlundbräune**, f. sore throat, pharyngitis, quinsy.

3844 **Schlunddach**, n. 1. roof of the pharynx.

3845 **Schlunddrüse**, f. pharyngeal gland.

3846 **Schlunderweiterung**, f. dilatation of the pharynx.

3847 **Schlundgaumenbogen**, m. 2. pharyngo-palatine arch.

3848 **Schlundgaumenmuskel**, n. 2. palato-pharyngeus muscle.

3849 **Schlundgefäsz**, n. 1. pharyngeal vessel.

3850 **Schlundgrube**, f. blinde, cul de sac of pharynx.

3851 **Schlundhöhle**, f. pharyngeal cavity.

3852 **Schlundkopf**, m. 1. upper part of pharynx.

3853 **Schlundkopfblutader**, f. pharyngeal vein.

3854 **Schlundkopferweichung**, f. softening of the pharynx.

3855 **Schlundkopfgaumenmuskel**, m. 2. palato-pharyngeal muscle.

3856 **Schlundkopfgeflecht**, n. 1. pharyngeal plexus.

3857 **Schlundkopfheber**, m. 2. } stylo-muscle.
3858 **Schlundkopfmuskel**, m. 2. }

3859 **Schlundkopfnerv**, m. 3. pharyngeal nerve.

3860 **Schlundkopfpulsader**, f. } pharyngeal artery.
3861 **Schlundkopfschlagader**, f. }

3862 **Schlundkopfschleimhaut**, f. pharyngeal mucous membrane.

3863 **Schlundkopfspiegel**, m. 2. pharyngeal speculum.

3864 **Schlundkopfwand**, f. } pharyngeal wall.
3865 **Schlundkopfwandung**, f. }

3866 **Schlundmuskel**, m. 2. pharyngeal muscle.

3867 **Schlundnerv**, m. 3. pharyngeal nerve.

3868 **Schlundpforte**, f. opening of oesophagus.
3869 **Schlundplatte**, f. pharyngeal lamina.
3870 **Schlundpulsader**, f. } artery of the pharynx.
3871 **Schlundschlagader**, f. } artery of the pharynx.
3872 **Schlundrohr**, n. 1. } oesophageal tube.
3873 **Schlundröhre**, } oesophageal tube.
3874 **Schlundschleimhaut**, f. oesophageal mucous membrane.
3875 **Schlundschlieszmuskel**, m. 2. constrictor of the pharynx.
3876 **Schlundspalte**, f. pharyngeal cleft.
3877 **Schlundsonde**, f. } pharyngeal probang.
3878 **Schlundstöszer**, m. 2. } pharyngeal probang.
3879 **Schlundvene**, f. pharyngeal vein.
3880 **Schlundverengerung**, f. constrictor of the pharynx.
3881 **Schlundwand**, f. wall of the pharynx.
3882 **Schlundzäpfleinmuskel**, m. 2. palato-pharyngeus muscle, etc.
3883 9. **SPEICHEL**, m. 2. saliva.
3884 **Speichelabgang**, m. 1. discharge of saliva.
3885 **speichelabsondernd**, adj. sialagogic.
3886 **Speichelabsonderung**, f. secretion of saliva.
3887 **speichelartig**, adj. salivary.
3888 **Speicheldrüse**, f. salivary gland.
3889 **Speichelfistel**, f. salivary fistula.
3890 **Speichelflusz**, m. 1. ptyalism, salivation.
3891 **Speichelflüssigkeit**, f. saliva.
3892 **Speichelgang**, m. 1. salivary duct.
3893 **Speichelgangfistel**, f. salivary duct fistula.
3894 **Speichelkörperchen**, n. 2. salivary corpuscle.
3895 **speichelreizend**, adj. causing a flow of saliva.
3896 **Speichelröhre**, f. salivary duct.
3897 **Speichelstein**, m. 1. salivary concretion or calculus.
3898 **Speichelstoff**, m. 1. ptyalin.
3899 **Speichelzelle**, f. salivary corpuscle, etc.
3900 10. a. **SPEISE**, f. aliment, food, nourishment, nutrition.
3901 **Speisebestandteil**, m. 1. constituent part of food.
3902 **Speisebrei**, m. 1. chyme.
3903 **Speisebreibildung**, f. formation of chyme.
3904 **Speisegang**, m. 1. } alimentary canal.
3905 **Speisecanal**, m. 1. } alimentary canal.
3906 **Speiseordnung**, f. regulation of diet, regimen.
3907 b. **SPEISERÖHRE**, f. oesophagus.
3908 **Speiseröhrenarterie**, f. oesophageal artery.
3909 **Speiseröhrenblutader**, f. oesophageal vein.
3910 **Speiseröhrendurchbohrung**, f. perforation of oesophagus.
3911 **Speiseröhreneröffnung**, f. oesophagotomy.
3912 **Speiseröhrenerweichung**, f. softening of oesophagus.
3913 **Speiseröhrenerweiterung**, f. dilatation of oesophagus.
3914 **Speiseröhrengeflecht**, n. 1. oesophageal plexus.
3915 **Speiseröhrenlähmung**, f. paralysis of oesophagus.
3916 **Speiseröhrenmuskel**, m. 2. muscular coat of oesophagus.
3917 **Speiseröhrenpulsader**, f. } oesophageal artery.
3918 **Speiseröhrenschlagader**, f. } oesophageal artery.
3919 **Speiseröhrenschleimhaut**, f. mucous membrane of oesophagus.
3920 **Speiseröhrenschlitz**, m. 1. oesophageal opening (in diaphragm.)
3921 **Speiseröhrenschnitt**, m. 1. oeeophagotomy.
3922 **Speiseröhrenvene**, f. oesophageal vein.
3923 **Speiseröhrenverengerung**, f. constriction or stricture of oesophagus.
3924 **Speiseröhrenverschwärung**, f. ulceration of the oseophagus, etc.
3925 c. **SPEISESAFT**, m. 1. chyle.
3926 **Speisesaftbehältnis**, n. 1. receptaculum chyli.

3927 **Speisesaftbereitung**, f. } formation of chyle.
3928 **Speisesaftbildung**, f. }
3929 **Speisesaftmangel**, m. 2. deficiency or absence of chyle.
3930 **Speisesaftröhre**, f. thoracic duct.
3931 d. **SAFT**, m. 1. juice, sap, humor; syrup;
3932 pl. Säfte, humors (of the body) in compounds:
3933 **Säfteandrang**, m. 1. congestion of fluids, orgasm.
3934 **Säfteanhäufung**, f. accumulation, gathering of fluids.
3935 **Säfteentmischung**, f. decomposition of fluids.
3936 **Säftemasse**, f. mass, bulk, substance of fluids of the body.
3937 **säftereinigend**, adj. purifying the fluids or juices.
3938 **Säfteverderbnis**, f. vitiation of the fluids or juices.
3939 **Säfteverdickung**, f. thickening of the fluids or juices.
3940 **Säftevergiftung**, f. poisoning of the fluids or juices.
3941 **Säfteverlust**, m. 1. (from v. ir. verlieren, to lose) loss of fluids of the body.
3942 **Säftezuflusz**, m. 1. supply of fluids or juices.
3943 **Saftfülle**, f. abundance of fluid or juice.
3944 **Saftgefäsz**, n. 1. chyliferous vessel, lacteal vessel.
3945 **Saftkanal**, m. 1. } lymph canal.
Saftkanälchen, n. 2. }
3946 **saftlos**, adj. achylous, without chyle.
3947 **Saftlücke**, f. lymph space.
3948 **Saftmangel**, m. 2. achilia, deficiency of chyle.
3949 **saftreich**, adj. juicy, succulent.
3950 **Saftschwellung**, f. oedematous swelling.
3951 **Saftspalte**, lymph space (e. g. between prickle cells of epidermis.)
3952 **Saftspaltensystem**, n. 1. system of lymph spaces.
3953 **Saftzelle**, f. lymph cells, etc.
3954 11. **MAGEN**, m. 2. stomach. überladener (fr. v. ir. überladen, to overload, overloaded stomach;)
3955 **Magen**, verdorbener, (from v. ir. verderben, to spoil, to bring in disorder, disordered stomach.)
3956 **Magenabkühlung**, f. (from abkühlen, to cool, to refrigerate), chilling of the stomach, e. g. by iced drinks or by eating ice cream. In compounds gastric:
3957 **Magenader**, f. gastric vein.
3958 **Magenarterie**, f. gastric artery.
3959 **Magenauftreibung**, f. distention of the stomach.
3960 **Magenausgang**, m. 1. pyloric orifice of the stomach.
3961 **Magenausspülung**, f. washing out of the stomach.
3962 **Magenbewegung**, f. movement of the stomach.
3963 **Magenblähung**, f. gastric flatulency.
3964 **Magenblindsack**, m. 1. cul de sac of the stomach.
3965 **Magenbrei**, m. 1. chyme.
3966 **Magenbrennen**, n. 2. heartburn, pyrosis.
3967 **Magenbruch**, m. 1. gastrocele.
3968 **Magendarmkanal**, m. 1. gastro-intestinal canal.
3969 **Magendrücken**, n. 2. (from drücken, to press), pain in the stomach.
3970 **Magendrüse**, f. gastric gland.
3971 **Magendünndarmfistel**, f. gastro-enteric fistula.
3972 **Mageneingang**, m. 1. oesophageal orifice of the stomach.
3973 **Magenflüssigkeit**, f. fluid of the stomach.
3974 **Magengefäsz**, n. 1. gastric vessel.
3975 **Magengeflecht**, n. 1. coronary plexus of the stomach.
3976 **Magengegend**, f. gastric region.
3977 **Magengekröse**, n. 1, mesogaster.
3978 **Magengrimmdarmnetz**, n. 1. gastro-colic omentum.
3979 **Magengrübchen**, n. 2. depressions or little pits on mucous surface of the stomach.
3980 **Magengrube**, f. scrobiculus cordis, stomach-pit.
3981 **Magengrund**, m. 1. fundus of the stomach.

3982 **Magenhaut**, f. coat of the stomach.
3983 **Magenhöhle**, f. cavity of the stomach.
3984 **Mageninfarct**, m. 1. infarct of the stomach.
3985 **Mageninhalt**, m. 1. contents of the stomach.
3986 **Magenkranzarterie**, f. coronary artery of the stomach.
3987 **Magenkranzgeflecht**, n. 1. coronary plexus of the stomach.
3988 **Magenkranzschlagader**, f, coronary artery of the stomach.
3989 **Magenkrümmung**, f. / **Magenverkrümmung**, f. } curvature of the stomach.
3990 **Magenlabdrüse**, f. peptic gland of the stomach.
3991 **Magenlebernetz**, n. 1. gastro-hepatic omentum.
3992 **Magenleberschlagader**, f. gastro-hepatic artery.
3993 **Magenlymphdrüse**, f. gastric lymphatic gland.
3994 **Magenmund**, m. 1. oesophageal orifice of the stomach.
3995 **Magenmuskelhaut**, f. muscular coat of the stomach.
3996 **Magennaht**, f. suture of the stomach.
3997 **Magennerv**, m. 3. gastric nerve.
3998 **Magennervenschwäche**, f. dyspepsia nervosa.
3999 **Magennetzschlagader**, f. gastro-epiploic artery.
4000 **Magennetzvene**, f. gastro-epiploic vein.
4001 **Magenpförtner**, m. 2. pylorus.
4002 **Magenpulsader**, f. gastric artery.
4003 **Magenrand**, m. 1. margin of the stomach.
4004 **Magenreiz**, m. 1. gastric irritation.
4005 **Magensaft**, m. 1. gastric juice.
4006 **Magensaftdrüse**, f. gastric gland.
4007 **Magensaftsäure**, f. acid of gastric juice.
4008 **Magensäure**, f. acidity of the stomach.
4009 **Magenschall**, m. 1. stomach note (e. g. in percussion).
4010 **Magenschärfe**, f. acidity of the stomach.
4011 **Magenschlagader**, f. gastric artery.
4012 **Magenschleim**, m. 1. gastric mucus.
4013 **Magenschleimdrüse**, f. mucous gland of the stomach.
4014 **Magenschleimhaut**, f. mucous membrane of the stomach.
4015 **magenschwach**, adj. dyspeptic.
4016 **Magenschwäche**, f. dyspepsia.
4017 **Magenschwindel**, m. 2. gastric vertigo.
4018 **Magenstein**, m. 1. gastric concretion.
4019 **Magenton**, m. 1. see Magenschall.
4020 **Magenüberladung**, f. (fr. überladen, to overload), surfeit.
4021 **Magenvene**, f. gastric vein.
4022 **Magenverdauung**, f. gastric digestion.
4023 **Magenverdickung**, f. induration or thickening of the stomach.
4024 **Magenverstimmung**, f. gastric disorder, gastric derangement.
4025 **Magenwand**, f. or **wandung**, f. coat or wall of the stomach.
4026 **Magenzelle**, f. peptic cell.
4027 **Magenzwölffingerdarmschlagader**, f. gastro-duodenal artery, etc.
4028 12. a. **DARM**, m. 1. gut, intestine (in compounds intestinal):
4029 **Darm, blinder**, caecum:
4030 —, **dicker**, colon, large intestine.
4031 —, **dünner**, / —, **enger**, } small intestine.
4032 —, **gerader**, rectum.
4033 —, **gewundener** or **langer**, ileum.
4034 —, **leerer**, the jejunum.
4035 **Darmanlage**, f. intestinal germ or rudiment.
4036 **Darmarterie**, f. intestinal artery.
4037 **Darmausleerung**, f. evacuation of the bowels.
4038 **Darmbauchfistel**, f. intestino-abdominal fistula.

4039 **Darmbandwurm**, m. 1. tapeworm.
4040 **Darmbein**, n. 1. ilium.
4041 **Darmbeinaushöhlung**, f. (from aushöhlen, to hollow out) hollow of the ilium.
4042 **Darmbeinbinde**, f. iliac fascia.
4043 **Darmbeinfläche**, f. surface of ilium.
4044 **Darmbeingrube**.f. iliac fossa.
4045 **Darmbeinhöcker**, m. 2. crest of ilium.
4046 **Darmbeinhöhlung**, f. hollow of ilium.
4047 **Darmbeinkamm**, m. 1. crest of ilium.
4048 **Darmbeinkrümmung**.f.(from krümmen, to make crooked. to bend) sigmoid flexure.
4049 **Darmbeinlefze**, f. lip of the crest of ilium.
4050 **Darmbeinmuskel**, m. 2. iliac muscle.
4051 **Darmbeinpulsader**, f. iliac artery.
4052 **Darmbeinschlagader**, f. iliac artery.
4053 **Darmbeinstachel**. m. 2. iliac spine.
4054 **Darmbewegung**, f. peristaltic movement of intestine.
4055 **Darmblatt**, n. 1. intestine plate or fold, hypoblast.
4056 **Darmblutader**. f. intestinal vein.
4057 **Darmblutflusz**, m. 1. } intestinal hemor-
4058 **Darmblutung**, f. } rhage.
4059 **Darmbruch**, m. 1. rupture, enterocele.
4060 **Darmdrüse**, f. intestinal gland.
4061 **Darmdrüsenblatt**, n. 1. intestinal gland-layer.
4062 **Darmdurchbohrung**, f. (from
4063 **bohren**, to perforate) perforation of the intestines.
4064 **Darmeinklemmung**, f. strangulation or constriction of the intestine.
4065 **Darmentleerung**, f. evacuation of the bowels.
4066 **Darmfell**, n. 1. peritoneum.
4067 **Darmfläche**, f. intestinal surface.
4068 **Darmflusz**, m. 1. intestinal discharge.
4069 **Darmflüssigkeit**, f. intestinal fluid.
4070 **Darmfollikel**. m. and n. 2. intestinal follicular gland.
4071 **Darmfurche**, f. intestinal furrow.
4072 **Darmgang**, m. 1. intestinal canal.
4073 **Darmgas**, n. 1. intestinal gas.
4074 **Darmgefäsz**, n. 1. intestinal vessel.
4075 **Darmgegend**, f. intestinal region.
4076 **Darmgeräusch**, n. 1. intestinal sound.
4077 **Darmhaut**, f. intestinal coat.
4078 **Darmhöhle**, f. intestinal cavity.
4079 **Darminhalt**, m. 1. intestinal contents.
4080 **Darmkanal**, m. 1. intestinal canal.
4081 **Darmklappe**, f. intestinal valve.
4082 **Darmklemme**, f. intestinal clamp.
4083 **Darmknochen**. m. 2. ilium.
4084 **Darmmündung**, f. intestinal aperture.
4085 **Darmmuskel**, m. 2. iliac muscle.
4086 **Darmmuskelhaut**, f. muscular coat of the intestine.
4087 **Darmmuskelwand**, f. wall formed by the iliac muscle.
4088 **Darmnaht**, f. intestinal suture.
4089 **Darmnerv**, m. 3. intestinal nerve.
4090 **Darmnervengeflecht**, n. 1. mesenteric plexus, intestinal nerve-plexus.
4091 **Darmnetz**, n. 1. omentum, epiploon.
4092 **Darmpulsader**, f. intestinal artery.
4093 **Darmreizung**, f. intestinal irritation.
4094 **Darmrinne**, f. intestinal furrow.
4095 **Darmrisz**, m. 1. intestinal tear or laceration.
4096 **Darmrohr**, n. 1. } intestinal
Darmröhre, f. } tube.
4097 **Darmsaft**, m. 1. intestinal juice.
4098 **Darmsaftdrüse**, f. intestinal gland.
4099 **Darmsaugader**, f. intestinal absorbent vessel.
4100 **Darmverdauung**, f. intestinal digestion.

4101-4102 **Darmverschlieszung**, f. (from v. ir. verschlieszen, to shut) intestinal obstruction, occlusion of intestine.

4103 **Darmverstopfung**, f. constipation, obstruction of the intestine.

4104 **Darmvorfall**, m. 1. prolapse, protrusion of intestine.

4105 **Darmwand**, f. } intestinal
Darmwandung f. } wall.

4106 **Darmweiche**, f. iliac region.

4107 **Darmwindung**, f. intestinal convolution.

4108 **Darmzerreiszung**, f. rupture of the intestine.

4109 **Darmzotte**, f. intestinal villus.

4110 **Darmzwang**, m. 1. constipation, twisting of intestine, etc.

4111 **AFTERDARM**, m. 1. (from after, anus, rectum.)

4112 **BLINDDARM**, m. 1. (from blind, sightless) caecum.

4113 **blinddarmähnlich**, adj. resembling the caecum, caecal.

4114 **Blinddarmanhang**, m. 1. vermiform appendix.

4115 **Blinddarmgekröse**, n. 1. meso-caecum.

4116 **Blinddarmklappe**, f. ileo-caecal valve.

4117 **Blinddarmsaft**, m. 1. caecum secretion.

4118 **DICKDARM**, m. 1. (from dick, thick), colon, large intestine.

4119 **Dickdarmausstülpung**, f. colon pouch.

4120 **Dickdarmblasenfistel**, f. intestino-vesical fistula (colon.)

4121 **Dickdarmfalte**, f. colon-fold.

4122 **Dickdarmklappe**, f. ileo-colic-valve.

4123 **Dickdarmschleimhaut**, f. mucous membrane of colon.

4124 **DÜNNDARM**, m. 1. (from dünn, thin, slight), small intestine.

4125 **Dünndarmblutader**, f. mesenteric vein.

4126 **Dünndarmdrüsen**, f. pl. small intestine glands.

4127 **Dünndarmgekröse**, n. 1. mesentery.

4128 **Dünndarmpillen**, f. pl. pills acting only on small intestines.

4129 **Dünndarmsaft**, m. 1. succus entericus.

4130 **Dünndarmschlinge**, f. small intestine loop.

4131-4132 **GRIMMDARM**, m. 1. (from grimmen, to gripe, to be griped)—hence Grimmen, n. 2. colic—), colon.

4133 **Grimmdarmband**, n. 1. colic ligament.

4134 **Grimmdarmblutader**, f. colic vein.

4135 **Grimmdarmgegend**, f. colic region.

4136 **Grimmdarmgekrösdrüse**, f. gland in meso-colon.

4137 **Grimmdarmgekröse**, n. 1. meso-colon.

4138 **Grimmdarmklappe**, f. valvula coli.

4139 **Grimmdarmschlagader**, f. } colic
4140 **Krummdarmschlagader**, f. } artery.

4141 **Krummdarmschlinge**, f. loop of ileum.

4142 **MASTDARM**, m. 1. (from masten or mästen, to fatten) rectum.

4143 **Mastdarmarterie**, f. haemorrhoidal artery.

4144 **Mastdarmblutader**, f. haemorrhoidal vein.

4145 **Mastdarmblutadergeflecht**, n. 1. haemorrhoidal venous plexus.

4146 **Mastdarmblutflusz**, m. 1. haemorrhoids.

4147 **Mastdarmblutgefäsz**, n. 1. haemorrhoidal vessel.

4148 **Mastdarmblutung**, f. hemorrhage from rectum, haemorrhoids.

4149 **Mastdarmgekröse**, n. 1. meso-rectum.

4150 **Mastdarmgeschwür**, n. 1. ulcer of rectum.

4151 **Mastdarmharnblasenmutterscheidenfistel**, f. recto-vesico-vaginal fistula.

4152 **Mastdarmharnröhrenfistel**, f. recto-urethral fistula.

4153 **Marstdarmhäute**, f. pl. coats of rectum.

4154 **Mastdarmheber**, m. 2. levator ani.

4155 **Mastdarmknoten**, m. 2. haemorrhoids, piles.

4156 **Mastdarmnaht**, f. rectal suture.
4157 **Mastdarmnerv**, m. 3. haemorrhoidal nerve.
4158 **Mastdarmöffnung**, f. anus.
4159 **Mastdarmpolyp**, m. 1. rectal polyp.
4160 **Mastdarmpulsader**, f. haemorrhoidal artery.
4161 **M a s t d a rmscheidenbruch**, m. 1. recto-vaginal hernia.
4162 **Mastdarmscheidenwand**, f. recto-vaginal septum.
4163 **M a s t darmumstülpung**, f. (from
4164 umstülpen, to invert) rectum inversion.
4165 **Mastdarmvene**, f. haemorrhoidal vein.
4166 **Mastdarmverengung**, f. rectum stenosis or stricture.
4167 **Mastdarmverschlusz**, m. 1. rectum or anus atresia.
4168 **Mastdarmvorfall**, m. 1. rectum prolapse.
4169 **ZWÖLFFINGERDARM**, m. 1. duodenum.
4170 **Zwölffingerdarmarterie**, f, duodenal artery.
4171 **Z w ö l ffi n g e rdarmentzündung**, f. duodenum inflammation.
4172 **Gedärm**, n. 1. the bowels, entrails, intestines, etc.
4173 b. **Gekröse**, n. 1. mesentery, in compounds :
4174 **Gekrösader**, f. mesenteric vein.
4175 **Gekrösarterie**, f. mesenteric artery.
4176 **gekrösartig**, adj. mesenteric.
4177 **Gekrösblatt**, m. 1. layer of the mesentery.
4178 **Gekrösblutader**, f. mesenteric vein.
4179 **Gekrösbruch**, m. 1. mesenteric hernia.
4180 **Gekrösdärme**, pl. m. 1. jejunum and ileum.
4181 **Gekrösdrüse**, f. mesenteric gland.
4182 **Gekrösdrüsengang**, m. 1. } pancreatic duct.
4183 **Gekrösgang**, m. 1. } pancreatic duct.
4184 **Gekrösgefäsz**, n. 1. mesenteric vessel.
4185 **Gekröshaut**, f. the scum obtained from saccharomyces mesentericus.
4186 **Gekrösplatte**, f. mesenteric layer.
4187 **Gekröspulsader**, f. mesenteric artery.
4188 **Gekrösrand**, m. 1. mesenteric border.
4189 **Gekrösschlagader**, f. mesenteric artery.
4190 **Gekrösvene**, f. mesenteric vein.
4191 **Gekröswurzel**, f. root of the mesentery, etc.
4192 c. **Netz**, n. 1. net, rete, reticulum, plexus; omentum, epiploon, retina. In compounds :
4193 **Netzader**, f. epiploic vein.
4194 **netzähnlich**, adj. } reticular, plexiform, alveolar.
4195 **netzartig**, adj. } reticular, plexiform, alveolar.
4196 **Netzarterie**, f. omental or epiploic artery.
4197 **Netzbeutel**, m. 2. sac of the omentum.
4198 **Netzblatt**, n. 1. layer of the omentum.
4199 **Netzblutader**, f. omental vein.
4200 **Netzbruch**, m. 1. omental hernia, epiplocele.
4201 **Netzchen**, n. 2. reticulum, a small network.
4202 **Netzdarmbruch**, m. 1. entero-epiplocele.
4203 **Netzentzündung**, f. inflammation of omentum, epiploïtis.
4204 **netzförmig**, adj. retiform, reticular, alveolar.
4205 **Netzgefäsz**, n. 1. omental vessel.
4206 **Netzgerüst**, n. 1. reticular framework.
4207 **Netzhaut**, f. retina.
4208 **Netzhaut der Gedärme**, omentum.
4209 **Netzhaut des Ohres**, reticular membrane of Corti's organ (ear).
4210 **Netzhautabhebung**, f. **Netzhautablösung**, f. } detachment of retina.
4211 **Netzhautblutung**, f. retinal hemorrhage.
4212 **Netzhautentzündung**, f. inflammation of retina, retinitis.
4213 **Netzhauterweichung**, f. softening of retina.

4214 **Netzhautgefäsz**, n. 1. retinal vessel.
4215 **Netzhautpulsader**, f. retinal artery, central artery of retina.
4216 **Netzhautschicht**, f. retinal layer.
4217 **Netzhautschlagader**, f. retinal artery, central artery of retina.
4318 **Netzhautschwund**, m. 1. atrophy of retina.
4219 **Netzhautspalte**, f. / **Netzhautspaltung**, f. } coloboma retinae, cleft in retina.
4220 **Netzhautvene**, f. / **Netzhautblutader**, f. } retinal vein.
4221 **Netzknorpel**, m. 2. reticular cartilage.
4222 **Netzleistenbruch**, m. 1. inguinal epiplocele.
4223 **Netznabelbruch**, m. 1. omental umbilical hernia.
4224 **Netznerv**, m. 3. nerve of the omentum.
4225 **Netzpulsader**, f. omental or epiploïc artery.
4226 **Netzschenkelbruch**, m. 1. femoral epiplocele.
4227 **Netzschlagader**, f. omental, or epiploïc artery.
4228 **Netzsehen**, n. 2. obscured vision.
4229 **Netzstrang**, m. 1. omental cord.
4230 **Netzvene**, f. omental vein.
4231 **Netzvorfall**, m. 1. escape of the omentum, epiplocele.
4232 **Netzwerk**, n. 1. network.
4233 **Netzzelle**, f. reticular cell.
4234 **Netzzellensarkom**, n. 1. reticular sarcoma. etc.
4235 13. **GALLAPFEL**, m. 1. (from the Latin *galla*, Gallapfel, pl. Galläpfel), gallapple.
4236 **Galläpfelgerbsäure**, f. (from
4237 **gerben**, to tan and
4238 **Säure**, acid), tannic acid.
4239 **Galläpfeltinktur**, f. tincture of galls.
4240 **GALLE**, f. bile, gall, in compounds:
4241 **Gallen-absonderung**, f. secretion of bile.
4242 **Gallenader**, f. cystic vein.
4243 **gallenartig**, adj. bile-like, bilious.
4244 **Gallenausführungsgang**, m. 1. excretory bile-duct.
4245 **Gallenbehältnis**, n. 1. / 4246 **Gallenblase**, f. } gall-bladder.
4247 **gallenbitter**, adj. bitter as gall.
4248 (**Gallenblasen** is cystic in compounds:)
4249 **Gallenblasenarterie**, f. cystic artery.
4250 **Gallenblasenbauchfistel**, f. abdominal biliary fistula.
4251 **Gallenblasenblutader**, f. cystic vein.
4252 **Gallenblasendarmfistel**, f. biliary intestinal fistula.
4253 **Gallenblasenempyem**, n. 1. suppuration of the gall-bladder.
4254 **Gallenblasengang**, m. 1. cystic duct.
4255 **Gallenblasengrube**, f. fissure or fossa for the gall-bladder.
4256 **Gallenblasenhals**, m. 1. neck of the gall-bladder.
4257 **Gallenblasenhaut**, f. mucous membrane of the gall-bladder.
4258 **Gallenblasenstein**, m. 1. gall-stone.
4259 **Gallendarm**, m. 1. duodenum.
4260 **Gallendrüse**, f. gland of the bile-duct.
4261 **Gallenergieszung**, f. / 4262 **Gallenergusz**, m. 1. } discharge or evacuation of bile.
4263 **Gallenfarbstoff**, m. 1. biliary pigment.
4264 **Gallenpulsader**, f. / **Gallenschlagader**, f. } biliary artery.
4265 **gallenreich**, adj. rich in bile.
4266 **Gallenstauung**, f. biliary engorgement.
4267 **Gallen** or **Gallensteinfett**, n. 1. / 4268 **Gallentalg**, m. 1. } cholesterine.
4269 **gallensüchtig**, adj. bilious, choleric.
4270 **Gallenweg**, m. 1. biliary passage.
4271 **Gallenzufuhr**, f. supply of bile.
4272 **gallicht**, adj. / **gallig**, adj. } bilious, etc.
4273 14. **LEBER**, f. liver, in compounds mostly *hepatic*:
4274 **Leberabscesz**, m. 1. hepatic abscess.
4275 **Leberader**, f. hepatic vein.
4276 **leberähnlich**, adj. hepatic.

4277 **Leberanämie**, f. hepatic anaemia.
4278 **Leberanschoppung**, f. hepatic infarct.
4279 **Leberarterie**, f. hepatic artery.
4280 **leberartig**, adj. hepatic.
4281 **Leberatrophie**, f. atrophy of the liver.
4282 **Leberband**, n. 1. hepatic ligament.
4283 **Leberblasengang**, m. 1. } bile duct, cystic duct.
4284 **Leberblasenkanal**, m. 1. }
4285 **Leberblutader**, hepatic vein.
4286 **Leberblutgeschwulst**, f. blood cyst of the liver.
4287 **Leberblutung**, f. hemorrhage from or into the liver.
4288 **leberbraun**, adj. liverbrown.
4289 **Leberbruch**, m. 1. hepatocele.
4290 **Leberdrüse**, f. hepatic gland.
4291 **Lebereinschnitt**, m. 1. fissure of the liver, hepatic notch.
4292 **Lebereiter**, m. 2. liver-pus.
4293 **Leberentartung**, f. liver induration.
4294 **Leberfurche**, f. fissure of the liver.
4295 **Lebergalle**, f. hepatic bile.
4296 **Lebergallenblasengang**, m. 1. cystic duct.
4297 **Lebergallengang**, m. 1. } hepatic duct.
4298 **Lebergang**, m. 1. }
4299 **Lebergeflecht**, n. 1. hepatic plexus.
4300 **Lebergegend**, f. hepatic region.
4301 **Lebergewebe**, n. 1. hepatic tissue.
4302 **Lebergrube**, f. fossa of the liver.
4303 **Leberhaut**, f. } Glisson's capsule.
4304 **Leberhülle**, f. }
4305 **Leberhülse**, f. }
4306 **Leberinsel**, f. **Leberinselchen**, n. 2. } hepatic lobule.
4307 **Leberläppchen**, n. 2. hepatic lobule.
Leberlappen, m. 2. lobe of the liver.
——, hinterer, Spigelian lobe of the liver.
4308 **Lebernerv**, m. 3. hepatic nerve.
4309 **Leberpforte**, f. porta of the liver.
4310 **Leberprobe**, f. the liver test.
4311 **Leberpulsader**, f. hepatic artery.
4312 **Leberquerfurche**, f. transverse fissure of the liver.
4313 **Leberrinne**, f. fissure of the liver.
4314 **Leberschall**, m. 1. hepatic sound.
4315 **Leberschlagader**, f. hepatic artery.
4316 **Leberschwund**, m. 1. atrophy of the liver.
4317 **Leberstein**, m. 1. gall-stone.
4318 **Leberthran**, m. 1. cod-liver oil.
4319 **Leberumhüllung**, f. capsule of the liver.
4320 **Lebervene**, f. hepatic vein.
4321 **Lebervenenblut**, n. 1. hepatic vein-blood.
4322 **Lebervergröszerung**, f. liver enlargement.
4323 **Leberverhärtung**, f. liver induration.
4324 **Leberverkleinerung**, f. atrophy or shrinking of the liver.
4325 **Leberverletzung**, f. injury to the liver.
4326 **Leberverstopfung**, f. hepatic obstruction.
4327 **Leberzelle**, f. liver cell.
4328 **Leberzellenbälkchen**, n. 2. } liver cell trabeculum.
4329 **Leberzellenbalken**, m. 2. }
4330 **Leberzellennetz**, n. 1. network of liver cells.
4331 **Leberzellenschlauch**, m. 1. canal formed by hepatic cells, etc.
4332 15. **MILZ**, f. spleen, in compounds mostly *splenic:*
4333 **Milzabscesz**, m. 1. splenic abscess.
4334 **Milzader**, f. splenic vein.
4335 **Milzanschoppung**, f. congestion of the spleen.
4336 **Milzanschwellung**, f. enlargement of the spleen.
4337 **Milzarterie**, f. splenic artery.
4338 **Milzbalken**, m. 2. spleen-trabeculum.
4339 **Milzband**, n. 1. splenic ligament or omentum.
4340 **Milzbläschen**, n. 2. Malphigian spleen corpuscle.

4341 **Milzblatter**, f. anthrax pustule.

4342 **Milzblutader**, f. splenic vein.

4343 **Milzblutflusz**, m. 1. } splenic hemorrhage.

4344 **Milzblutung**, f. } splenic hemorrhage.

4345 **Milzbrand**, m. 1. anthrax, charbon, malignant postule, splenic fever.

4346 **Milzbrandkeim**, m. 1. germ of anthrax.

4347 **Milzbruch**, m. 1. splenocele.

4348 **Milzdämpfung**, f. splenic dulness.

4349 **Milzdrüse**, f. spleen.

4350 **Milzgefäsz**, n. 1. splenic vessel.

4351 **Milzgefäszrinne**, f. groove for splenic vessels.

4352 **Milzgeflecht**, n. 1. splenic plexus.

4353 **Milzgegend**, f. splenic region.

4354 **Milzgeschwulst**, f. tumor of the spleen.

4355 **Milzgewebe**, n. 1. splenic tissue.

4356 **Milzinfarkt**, m. 1. splenic infarct.

4357 **Milzkapsel**, f. capsule of the spleen.

4358 **Milzknoten**, m. 2. splenic nodule.

4359 **Milznerv**, m. 3. splenic nerve.

4360 **Milzpocke**, f. anthrax pustule.

4361 **Milzpulpa**, f. splenic pulp.

4362 **Milzpulsader**, f. splenic artery.

4363 **Milzpustel**, f. anthrax pustule.

4364 **Milzschall**, m. 1. splenic note (in percussion).

4365 **Milzschlagader**, f. splenic artery.

4366 **Milzstechen**, n. 2. stitch in the side.

4367 **milzsüchtig**, adj. hypochondriacal.

4368 **Milzvene**, f. splenic vein.

4369 **Milzvergröszerung**, f. spleen enlargement.

4370 **Milzverhärtung**, f. spleen induration.

4371 **Milzverstopfung**, f. spleen engorgement.

4372 **Milzzelle**, f. splenic cell.

4373 **Milzzerreiszung**, f. laceration or rupture of the spleen, etc.

4374 16. **PANKREAS**, n. 1. pancreas (see also Bauchspeicheldrüse for compounds), in compounds;

4375 **Pankreassaft**, m. 1. pancreatic juice.

4376 **Pankreasstein**, m. 1. pancreatic concretion.

4377 **Pankreasverdauung**, f. pancreatic digestion.

4378 **pankreatisch**, adj. pancreatic, etc.

4379 17. **STUHL**, m. 1. stool, night-chair, evacuation of the bowels, in compounds;

4380 **Stuhlabgang**, m. 1. escape of faeces.

4381 **Stuhlausleerung**, f. evacuation of the bowels.

4382 **stuhlbefördernd**, adj. } aperient.

4383 **stuhlbeschleunigend**, adj. } aperient.

4384 **Stuhlbeförderung**, f. } promoting or furthering action of the bowels.

4385 **Stuhlbeschleunigung**, f. } promoting or furthering action of the bowels.

4386 **Stuhlbeschwerden**, f. pl. troubles of defaecation.

4387 **Stuhldrang**, m. 1. tenesmus.

4388 **Stuhlentleerung**, f. } evacuation of the bowels.

4389 **Stuhlgang**, m. 1. } evacuation of the bowels.

4390 **Stuhlmangel**, m. 2. constipation.

4391 **Stuhlträgheit**, f. sluggishness of the bowels.

4392 **Stuhlverhaltung**, f. retention of faeces.

4393 **Stuhlverstopfung**, f. constipation.

4394 **Stuhlzwang**, m. 1. tenesmus.

4395 **Reiswasserstuhl**, m. 1. rice-water stool, fig., referring to the rice-water-like discharges from the bowels, etc.

4396 18. **VERDAUUNG**, f. (from verdauen, to digest) digestion.

4397 **verdaulich**, adj. digestible.

4398 **Verdaulichkeit**, f. digestibility.

4399 **verdauungsbefördernd**, adj. digestive, peptic (lit. helping digestion). In compounds:

4400 **Verdauungsakt**, m. 1. act of digestion.

4401 **Verdauungsapparat**, m. 1. digestive apparatus.

4402 **Verdauungsblut**, n. 1. the blood from or during digestion.

4403 **Verdauungsdrüse**, f. alimentary gland (e. g. salivary
4404 gland, Bauchspeicheldrüse, etc.).
4405 **Verdauungsflüssigkeit**, f. digestive fluid or juice.
4406 **verdauungsfördernd**, adj. digestive, peptic.
4407 **Verdauungsgeschäft**, n. 1. digestive process.
4408 **Verdauungskanal**, m. 1. digestive canal.
4409 **Verdauungskraft**, f. digestive power.
4410 **Verdauungsorgan**, n. 1. digestive organ (organ of digestion).
4411 **Verdauungssaft**, m. 1. digestive fluid or juice.
4412 **Verdauungsschleimhaut**, f. digestive mucous membrane.
4413 **Verdauungsschwäche**, f. dyspepsia, weakness of digestion.
4414 **Verdauungssekret**, n. 1. digestive fluid or secretion.
4415 **Verdauungsstörung**, f. disturbance of digestion.
4416 **Verdauungstraktus**, m. 1. digestive tract.
4417 **Verduungsverlauf**, m. 1. course of digestion.
4418 **Verdauungsvorgang**, m. 1. process of digestion.
4419 **Verdauungsweg**, m. 1. digestive tract.
4420 **Verdauungswerk**, n. 1. digestive process.
4421 **Verdauungswerkzeug**, n. 1. digestive apparatusor organ, etc.
4422 19. **ZWERGFELL**, m. 1. diaphragm, in compounds:
4423 **Zwergfellader**, f. vein of the diaphragm.
4424 **Zwergfellarterie**. f. artery of the diaphragm.
4425 **Zwergfellatmung**, f. diaphragmatic respiration.
4426 **Zwergfellband**, n. 1. crus or ligament of the diaphragm.
4427 **Zwergfellbruch**, m. 1. diaphragmatic hernia.
4428 **Zwergfellkrampf**, m. 1. spasm of the diaphragm.
4429 **Zwergfellkuppe**, f. } dome of the diaphragm.
4430 **Zwergfellkuppel**, f. }
4431 **Zwergfellleiden**, n. 2. diaphragmatic pain.
4432 **Zwergfellmagenband**, n. 1. gastro-phrenic ligament.
4433 **Zwergfellverdrängung**, f. displacement of the diaphragm.
4434 **Zwergfellverletzung**, f. injury to the diaphragm.
4435 **Zwergfellwölbung**, f. (from
4436 wölben, to vault) dome of the diaphragm.
4437 **Zwergfellzacke**, f. crus of the diaphragm, etc.
4438 §14. **Die Geschlechtsorgane**, The Sexual Organs. In compounds:
4439 1. **GESCHLECHT**, n. 1. sex, species, genus, kind, race.
4440 **geschlechtlich**, adj. generic, sexual.
4441 **geschlechtlos**, adj. sexless.
4442 **Geschlechtsabneigung**, f. sexual disinclination, anaphrodisia.
4443 **Geschlechtsapparat**, m. 1. sexual apparatus.
4444 **Geschlechtsart**, f. genus, species, kind, race.
4445 **Geschlechtsausschweifung**, f. sexual excess, excessive venery.
4446 **Geschlechtsdrüse**, f. genital gland, ovary.
4447 **Geschlechtseigentümlichkeit**, f. sexual peculiarity.
4448 **Geschlechtsempfindung**, f. sexual feeling, sensibility.
4449 **Geschlechtsentwickelung**, f. sexual development.
4450 **Geschlechtsfalte**, f. genital fold.
4451 **Geschlechtsgang**, m. 1. genital duct, passage or canal.
4452 **——Müller's duct.**
4453 **Geschlechtsgenusz**, m. 1. sexual intercourse, sexual pleasure.
4454 **Geschlechtsglied**, n. 1. sexual organ, pl. genitals.
4455 **Geschlechtshöcker**, m. 2. genital eminence or protuberance.
4456 **Geschlechtsleben**, n. 2. sexual condition or habit.
4457 **Geschlechtslust**, f. sexual appetite.
4458 **Geschlechtsneigung**, f. sexual impulse or instinct.

6

4459 **Geschlechtsorgan**, n. 1. sexual organ.
4460 **geschlechtsreif**, adj. being ripe in puberty.
4461 **Geschlechtsreife**, f. puberty.
4462 **Geschlechtsreiz**, m. 1. sexual impulse or instinct.
4463 **geschlechtsreizend**, adj. aphrodisiac.
4464 **Geschlechtsteile**, m. 1. pl. genitals, the sexual organs.
4465 **Geschlechtstrieb**, m. 1. sexual impulse or instinct.
4466 **Geschlechtsverbindung**, f. } coition, sexual intercourse.
4467 **Geschlechtsverrichtung**, f. } coition, sexual intercourse.
4468 **Geschlechtsweg**, m. 1. genital passage.
4469 **Geschlechtswerkzeug**, n. 1. sexual apparatus.
4470 **Geschlechtszeichen**, n. 2. genitals.
4471 2. **BEGATTUNG**, f. (from begatten, to copulate), coition, copulation.
4472 **Begattungsorgan**, n. 1. generative organ.
4473 **Begattungstrieb**, m. 1. sexual impulse or instinct, etc.
4474 § 15. **SCHAMTEILE**, männliche, m. 1. pl. pudenda, male; (for compounds see also *Scham*) in compounds:
4475 1. **GLIED**, männliche, n. 1. } penis.
4476 **Penis**, m. 1. } penis.
4477 **Rute**, f. (rod, yard.) } penis.
4478 2. **EICHEL** (der Rute), f. glans penis.
4479 **Eichelband**, n. 1. fraenum of the penis.
4480 **eichelförmig**, adj. acorn-shaped.
4481 **Eichelharnröhre**, f. (the part of the) urethra in the glans penis.
4482 **Eichelkrone**, f. corona glandis.
4483 **Eichelkronenfurche**, f. groove of corona glandis.
4484 **Eichelstein**, m. 1. preputial concretion.
4485 3. **VORHAUT**, f. prepuce.
4486 **Vorhautband**, n. 1. } fraenum of the prepuce.
Vorhautbändchen, n. 2. } fraenum of the prepuce.
4487 **Vorhautdrüse**, f. preputial gland.
4488 **Vorhautplatte**, f. preputial membrane or fold.
4489 **Vorhautstein**, m. 1. preputial calculus.
4490 4. **HODE**, f. } testicle (s)
HODEN, m. 2. } testicle (s)
4491 **Hodenanschwellung**, f. swelling of the testicle.
4492 **Hodenarterie**, f. artery of the testicle.
4493 **Hodenatrophie**, f. atrophy of the testicle.
4494 **Hodenaufhebermuskel**, m. 2. (from heben, to lift), cremaster muscle.
4495 **Hodenausrottung**, f. castration.
4496 **Hodenbruch**, m. 1. scrotal hernia.
4497 **Hodendrüse**, f. testicle.
4498 **Hodenextirpation**, f. castration.
4499 **Hodenfleischhaut**, f. dartos of the scrotum.
4500 **Hodengefäsz**, n. 1. vessel of the testicle.
4501 **Hodengeschwulst**, f. swelling or tumor of the testicle.
4502 **Hodengewebe**, n. 1. parenchyma of the testicle.
4503 **Hodenhaut**, f. covering of the testicle.
4504 **Hodenherabsteigung**, f. descent of the testicle.
4505 **Hodenkanälchen**, n. 2. seminal duct or tube.
4506 **Hodenkopf**, m. 1. epididymis, globus major.
4507 **Hodenläppchen**, n. 2. lobule of the testicle.
4508 **hodenlos**, adj. without testicles.
4509 **Hodenmuskel**, m. 2. cremaster.
4510 **Hodenmuskelhaut**, f. sheath of cremaster.
4511 **Hodennerv**, m. 3. spermatic nerve.
4512 **Hodennetz**, n. 1. rete testis.
4513 **Hodenpulsader**, f. artery of the testicle.
4514 **Hodenröhrchen**, n. 2. seminal duct or tube.
4515 **Hodensack**, m. 1. scrotum.
4516 **Hodensacknaht**, f. raphe of the scrotum.
4517 **Hodensacknerv**, m. 3. scrotal nerve.

4518 **Hodensackpulsader**, f. scrotal artery.
4519 **Hodenwassersucht**, f. hydrocele.
4520 **Hodenzellhaut**, f. dartos.
4521 **Hodenzurückhaltung**, f. retained testicle, etc.
4522 5. **SAME**, m. 2. } seed,
SAMEN, m. 2. } semen.
4523 **Samenabflusz**, m. 1. spermatorrhœa.
4524 **Samenabführungsgang**, m. 1. spermatic duct, vas deferens.
4525 **Samenabgang**, m. 1. discharge of semen.
4526 **——, unbemerklicher**, imperceptible discharge of semen.
4527 **Samenader**, f. spermatic vein.
4528 **Samenadergeflecht**, n. 1. spermatic venous plexus.
4529 **Samenaderschnur**, f. spermatic cord.
4530 **Samenbläschen**, n. 2. seminal vesicle.
4531 **Samendrüse**, f. spermatic gland, prostate gland.
4532 **Samenkanälchen**, n. 2. seminal tubule.
4533 **Samenkeim**, m. 1. embryo, germ, spore.
4534 **Samenkern**, m. 1. sperm cell.
4535 **Samenplethora**, f. plethora of semen.
4536 **Samenpulsader**, f. spermatic artery.
4537 **Samenröhrchen**, n. 2. } seminal
Samenröhre, f. } tubule.
4538 **Samensaft**, m. 1. seminal fluid.
4539 **Samenschneller**, m. 2. ejaculator (seminalis) urinæ.
4540 **Samenschwäche**, f. seminal debility.
4541 **Samenstrang**, m. 1. spermatic cord.
4542 **Samentasche**, f. vesicula seminalis.
4543 **Samentier**, n. 1. spermatozoon.
4544 **Samenverhaltung**, f. retention of semen.
4545 **Samenverlust**, m. 1. loss of semen.
4546 **Samenweg**, m. 1. seminal passage.
4547 **Samenwerkzeug**, n. 1. seminal organ or apparatus.
4548 **Samenzelle**, f. seminal cell.
4549-4550 6. **ZEUGUNG**, f. (from zeugen (erzeugen) to beget, to generate) begetting, generation, procreation.
4551 **Zeugungsakt**, m. 1. act of begetting.
4552 **Zeugungsdrüse**, f. genital gland (testicle or ovary.)
4553 **zeugungsfähig**, adj. capable of begetting (of male or female.)
4554 **Zeugungsfaktor**, m. 1. the impregnating spermatozoon.
4555 **Zeugungsflüssigkeit**, f. semen.
4556 **Zeugungsgeschäft**, n. 1. act of begetting, copulation.
4557 **Zeugungsglied**, n. 1. genitals.
4558 **Zeugungskraft**, f. generative capacity or power.
4559 **Zeugungsorgan**, n. 1. generative organ.
4560 **zeugungsreif**, adj. } of age to beget, pube-
mannbar, adj. } scent, virile.
4561 **Zeugungsreife**, f. } puberty,
Mannbarkeit, f. } virility.
Mannheit, f. }
4562 **Zeugungsteile**, m. 1. pl. genitals.
4563 **Zeugungstrieb**, m. 1. generative or procreative impulse or instinct.
4564 **zeugungsunfähig**, adj. impotent (male), sterile (female).
4565 **Zeugungsunfähigkeit**, f. } impotence (male)
4566 **Zeugungsunvermögen**, n. 2. } sterility, (female).
4567 **Zeugungsvermögen**, n. 2. capability of begetting (of male or female), etc.
4568 § 16. **SCHAMTEILE**, weibliche, pl. m. 1. pudenda female. (See also Scham § 8, 21.) In compounds:
4569 1. **SCHEIDE**, f. sheath, vagina.
4570 { **Scheidehaut**, f. } tunica
{ **Scheidehäutchen**, n. 2. } vaginalis.
4571 **Scheidenabscesz**, m. 1. thecal abscess.
4572 **Scheidenachse**, f. vaginal axis.
4573 **Scheidenader**, f. vaginal vein.
4574 **scheidenähnlich**, adj. } sheath-
4575 **scheidenartig**, adj. } like.

4576 **Scheidenansatz**, m. 1. vaginal insertion.
4577 **Scheidenarterie**, f. vaginal artery.
4578 **Scheidenausflusz**, m. 1. vaginal discharge.
4579 **Scheidenausstülpung**, f. extro-version of the vagina.
4580 **Scheidenband**, n. 1. vaginal ligament.
4581 **Scheidenblindsack**, m. 1. vaginal cul-de-sac.
4582 **Scheidenblutader**, f. vaginal vein.
4583 **Scheidenblutadergeflecht**, n. 1. vaginal venous plexus.
4584 **Scheidenbrand**, m. 1. gangrene of the vagina.
4585 **Scheidenbruch**, m. 1. vaginal hernia.
4586 **Scheidenbruchsack**, m. 1. sac of vaginal hernia.
4587 **Scheidendammfistel**, f. perineal fistula.
4588 **Scheidendammrisz**, m. 1. perineo-vaginal rupture.
4589 **Scheidendarmbruch**, m. 1. intestino-vaginal hernia.
4590 **Scheidendünndarmfistel**, f. exterico-vaginal fistula.
4591 **Scheideneingang**, m. 1.
4592 **Scheidenmündung**, f.
4593 **Scheidenmund**, m. 1.
} orifice of vagina.
4594 **Scheidennaht**, f. vaginal suture; elytrorrhaphy.
4595 **Scheidenpolyp**, m. 1. vaginal polyp.
4596 **Scheidenpuls**, m. 1. vaginal pulse.
4597 **Scheidenraum**, m. 1. vaginal space.
4598 **Scheidenrisz**, m. 1. laceration of vagina.
4599 **Scheidenrohr**, n. 1. vaginal canal.
4600 **Scheidenrunzel**, f. vaginal fold or ruga.
4601 **Scheidenschleim**, m. 1. vaginal mucus.
4602 **Scheidenschleimflusz**, m. 1. vaginal leucorrhœa.
4603 **Scheidenschmerz**, m. 1. vaginal pain.
4604 **Scheidenschnürer**, m. 2. sphinxter vaginae.
4605 **Scheidenvorfall**, m. 1. prolapse of vagina.
4606 **Scheidenvorhof**, m. 1. vestibulum vaginae.
4607 **Scheidenwand**, f. vaginal wall.
4608 **Scheidenwulst**, f. vaginal ruga or fold, etc.
4609 2. **MUTTER**, f. mother, uterus, womb (see also Gebärmutter). In compounds:
4610 **Mutterader**, f. uterine vein.
4611 **Mutterast**, m. 1. uterine branch.
4612 **Mutterband**, n. 1. uterine ligament.
4613 **Mutterbett**, n. 1. childbed.
4614 **Mutterblutflusz**, m. 1. flooding.
4615 **Mutterdrüse**, f. uterine cotyledon.
4616 **Mutterende**, n. 1. fundus uteri, extremity of uterus.
4617 **Muttergang**, m. 1. uterine passage, vagina.
4618 **Muttergewebe**, n. 1. uterine tissue, mother tissue.
4619 **Muttergrund**, m. 1. fundus uteri.
4620 **Mutterhals**, m. 1. cervix uteri.
4621 **Mutterhalskanal**, m. 1.
4622 **Mutterhalsrinne**, f.
} canal of cervix uteri.
4623 **Mutterhalter**, m. 2. hysterophore, uterine pessary.
4624 **Mutterhorn**, n. 1. cornu uteri.
4625 **Mutterkörper**, m. 2. corpus uteri, uterus body.
4626 **Mutterkranz**, m. 1. pessary.
4627 **Mutterkuchen**, m. 2. placenta.
4628 **Mutterkuchenblutkreislauf** m. 1. placental circulation.
4629 **Mutterkyste**, f. cyst of the uterus.
4630 **Mutterleib**, m. 1. uterus, womb.
4631 **mütterlich**, adj. maternal, uterine.
4632 **Mutterlippe**, f. uterine lip.
4633 **Muttermasse**, f. uterus, womb.
4634 **Muttermilch**, f. mother's milk.
4635 **Muttermund**, m. 1. os uteri.
4636 **Muttermundlippe**, f. lip of os uteri.

4637 **Muttermundöffnung**, f. } os uteri.
4638 **Muttermundring**, m. 1. }
4639 **Muttermundsaum**, m. 1. lip of os uteri.
4640 **Mutterring**, m. 1. uterine pessary.
4641 **Mutterrohr**, n. 1. uterine tube, vaginal pipe of douche, Fallopian tube.
4642 **Mutterschaft**, f. maternity.
4643 **Mutterschaftszeichen**, n. 2. sign of maternity.
4644 **Mutterscheide**, f. vagina.
4645 **Mutterscheidengrübchen**, n. 2. fossa navicularis, vaginal dimple.
4646 **Mutterscheidenteil**, m. 1. vaginal portion of uterus.
4647 **Muttersenkung**, f. dexensus uteri, uterine descent before labor.
4648 **Muttersonde**, f. uterine sound.
4649 **Mutterspiegel**, m. 2. vaginal speculum.
4650 **Mutterspritze**, f. uterine syringe.
4651 **Mutterträger**, m. 2. uterine support.
4652 **Muttertrompete**, f. Fallopian tube.
4653 **Muttertrompetenschwangerschaft**, f. tubal pregnancy.
4654 **Muttervorfall**, m. 1. uterus prolapse.
4655 **Mutterweh**, n. 1. } uterine pain,
4656 **Mutterwehen**, pl. } labor pains.
4657 **Mutterzäpfchen**, n. 2. } cone-shaped
Mutterzapfen, m. 2. } pessary, etc.

(Appendix), compounds pertaining to menstruation.

4658 **Menstrualausschlag**, m. 1. menstrual eruption.
4659 **Menstrualblut**, n. 1. menstrual blood.
4660 **Menstrualflüssigkeit**, f. menstrual discharge.
4661 **Menstrualkolik**, f. dysmenorrhoea.
4662 **Menstrualschweisz**, m. 1. perspiration during the menstrual period.
4663 **Menstruation**, f. } menstruation,
4664 **Monatliche Reinigung**, f. } monthly purification.
4665 **Menstruationsstörung**, f. disturbance in menstruation.
4666 **menstruieren**, to menstruate, etc.
4667 **GEBÄRENDE**, f. } (from:
4668 **Gebärerin**, f. }
4669 **gebären**, to bring forth. to bear a child), a woman in labor.
4670 **Gebären**, n. 1. childbirth, parturition,
4671 **Gebärachse**, f. axis of parturition.
4672 **Gebäranstalt**, f. lying-in institution.
4673 **gebärfähig**, adj. capable of bringing forth or of bearing children.
4674 **Gebärfähigkeit**, f. capability of bringing forth children.
4675 **Gebärhaus or Hospital**, n. 1. lying-in hospital.
4676 3. **GEBÄRMUTTER**, f. uterus, womb (see also Mutter, uterus, womb), in compounds:
4677 **Gebärmutterabscesz**, m. 1. uterus abscess.
4678 **Gebärmutterband**, n. 1. ligamentum uteri.
4679 **Gebärmutterbeugung**, f. flexion of uterus.
4680 **Gebärmutterblutader**, f. uterine vein.
4681 **Gebärmutterblutadergeflecht**, n. 1. uterine venous plexus.
4682 **Gebärmuttergeflecht**, n. 1. uterine plexus.
4683 **Gebärmuttergeräusch**, n. 1. uterine murmur or souffle.
4684 **Gebärmuttergewebe**, n. 1. uterine tissue.
4685 **Gebärmuttergrund**, m. 1. fundus uteri.
4686 **Gebärmutterhals**, m. 1. neck of uterus, cervix uteri.
4687 **Gebärmutterhöhle**, f. uterine cavity.
4688 **Gebärmutterhorn**, m. 1. cornu or horn of uterus.
4689 **Gebärmutterknickung**, f. uterine flexion.
4690 **Gebärmutterkörper**, m. 2. body of uterus.
4691 **Gebärmutterkranz**, m. 1. pessary.

4692 **Gebärmutterkuppe**, f. dome-shaped portion of uterus, fundus uteri.
4693 **Gebärmuttermund**, m. 1. mouth of uterus.
4694 **Gebärmutternaht**, f. uterine suture.
4695 **Gebärmutterneigung**, f, version of uterus.
4696 **Gebärmutternerv**, m. 3. uterine nerve.
4697 **Gebärmutterpulsader**, f. uterine artery.
4698 **Gebärmutterrisz**, m. 1. laceration of uterus.
4699 **Gebärmutterscheidenteil**, m. 1. vaginal part of uterus.
4700 **Gebärmutterschlagader**, f. uterine artery.
4701 **Gebärmutterschleimhaut**, f. uterine mucous membrane.
4702 **Gebärmuttervene**, f. uterine vein.
4703 **Gebärmuttervollblütigkeit**, f. congestion of uterus.
4704 **Gebärmutterwand**, f. uterine wall.
4705 **Gebärmutterzerreiszung**, f. laceration or rupture of uterus.
4706 **Gebärmutterzusammenziehung**, f. contraction of uterus.
4707 **Gebärorgan**. n. 1. uterus.
4708 **gebärunfähig**, adj. incapable of bringing forth children.
4709 **Gebärunfähigkeit**, f. incapability of bringing forth children.
4710 **Gebärunmöglichkeit**, f. impossibility of delivery or parturition.
4711 **Gebärwehen**, labor pains.
4712 **Gebärzeit**, f. period or time of delivery, etc.
4713 4. **EI**, n. 1. egg, ovum, ovule; in compounds:
4714 **Eiachse**, f. axis of ovum.
4715 **Eiaustritt**, m. 1. exit of ovum.
4716 **Eiballen**, m. 2. ovarian vesicle.
4717 **Eiballenzone**, f. nest of ovarian vesicle.
4718 **Eidotter**, m. 2. yolk, vitellus.
4719 **Eidotterfett**. n. 1. lecithine.
4720 **Eientwickelung**, f. egg—development.
4721 **Eieralbumin**, n. 1. white of an egg.
4722 **Eiergang**, m. 1. oviduct.
4723 **Eiersack**, m. 1. ovarian follicle, etc.
4724 5. **EIERSTOCK**, m. 1. ovary.
4725 **Eierstocksanschwellung**, f. enlargement of the ovary.
4726 **Eierstocksarterie**, f. ovarian artery.
4727 **Eierstocksausrottung**, f. extirpation of the ovary.
4728 **Eierstocksband**, n. 1. ovarian ligament.
4729 **Eierstocksbruch**, m. 1. ovarian hernia.
4730 **Eierstockscyste**, f. ovarian cyst.
4731 **Eierstockseiterung**, f. suppuration of the ovary.
4732 **Eierstocksgefäsz**, n. 1. ovarian vessel.
4733 **Eierstocksgekröse**, n. 1. meso-ovarium.
4734 **Eierstocksgeschwulst**, f. ovarian tumor.
4735 **Eierstocksnerv**, m. 3. ovarian nerve.
4736 **Eierstockspulsader**, f. ovarian artery.
4737 **Eierstocksschwangerschaft**, f. ovarian pregnancy.
4738 **Eierstocksschwund**, m. 1. ovarian atrophy.
4739 **Eierstocksvene**, f. ovarian vein.
4740 **Eierstocksverhärtung**, f. ovary-induration.
4741 **Eierstocksvorfall**, m. 1. ovary-prolapse.
4742 **Eierweisz**, n. 1. white of an egg.
4743 **Eierzelle**, f. ovum.
4744 **Eihaftung**, f. (from haften, to adhere) adherance of ovum.
4745 **Eihaut**, f. membrane of ovum, amniotic membrane, chorion.
4746 **Eihautschlagader**, f. capsular ovarian artery.
4747 **Eihöhle**, f. egg-cavity.
4748 **Eihülle**, f. tunic of the ovum, decidua.
4749 **Eikapsel**, f. Gräfian follicle.
4750 **Eikeim**, m. 1. egg-germ.
4751 **Eikern**, m. 1. nucleus of ovum, germinal ossicle.
4752 **Eileiter**, m. 2. Fallopian tube, oviduct.
4753 **Eileiterkanal**, m. 1. canal of Fallopian tube.

4754 **Eileitermündung**, f. ostium of Fallopian tube.
4755 **Eileiterschwangerschaft**, f. tubal pregnancy, etc.
4756 6. **FRUCHT**, f. fruit, embryo, foetus;
4757 ——, **falsche**, mole.
In compounds :
4758 **fruchtabtreibend**, adj. ecbolic, abortierend, adj. abortive, (from abortieren, to abort)
4759 **Fruchtabtreibung**, f. abortion ; (from v. ir.
4760 **abtreiben**, to drive off, to abort, to miscarry.)
4761 **Fruchtabtreibungsmittel**, n. 2. an abortive.
4762 **Fruchtachse**, f. axis of the embryo.
4763 **Fruchtachsendruck**, m. 1. foetal axis pressure.
4764 **Fruchtanhang**, m. 1. embryonic appendage.
4765 **Fruchtauge**, n. 1. germ, bud.
4766 **fruchtbar**, adj. fruitful, fertile, productive.
4767 **Fruchtbarkeit**, f. fecundity, fertility, productiveness.
4768 **Fruchtbewegung**, f. foetal movement.
4769 { **Fruchtbildung**, f. fructification. **Befruchtung**, f. (from befruchten, to fructify.) }
4770 **Fruchtblase**, f. amnion sac.
4771 **Fruchtblasensprung**, m. 1. rupture of the amnion sac.
4772 **Fruchtblasenvorfall**, m. 1. prolapse of the amnion.
4773 **Fruchthalter**, m. 2. uterus.
4774 **Fruchthalterhöhle**, f. cavity of the uterus.
4775 **Fruchthaut**, f. } amnion,
4776 **Fruchthäutchen**, n. 2. } chorion.
4777 **Fruchthautzotte**, f. villus of the chorion.
4778 **Fruchthof**, m. 1. area of germination.
4779 **Fruchthyphen**, n. 1. zygospore, germinal hypha.
4780 **Fruchtkeim**, m. 1.
4781 { **Fruchtknospe**, f. | germ, **Fruchtknoten**, m. 2. | embryo. }
4782 **Fruchtknotenwulst**, m. 1. & f. embryonic prominence.
4783 **Fruchtkopf**, m. 1. foetal head.
4784 **Fruchtkuchen**, m. 2. foetal placenta.
4785 **Fruchtlager**, m. 2. sporangium.
4786 **Fruchtleben**, n. 2. foetal life.
4787 **fruchtlos**, adj. barren, sterile.
4788 **unfruchtbar**, adj. unproductive.
4789 **Fruchtlosigkeit**, f. } barrenness,
4790 **Unfruchtbarkeit**, f. } sterility,
4791 **Fruchtsack**, m. 1. foetal sac, ovi-sack, egg-sack.
4792 **Fruchtschleim**, m. 1. } vernix
4793 **Fruchtschmiere**, f. } caseosa.
4794 **Fruchtstand**, m. 1. germinal hypha.
4795 **Fruchttod**, m. 1. foetal death.
4796 **Fruchtträger**, m. 2. germinal hypha, zygospore.
4797 **Fruchtwasser**, n. 2. liquor amnii.
4798 **Fruchtwasserabsonderung**, f. secretion of amniotic fluid.
4799 **Fruchtwasserbildung**, f. formation of amniotic fluid.

APPENDIX regarding compounds pertaining to age, puberty, etc., e. g.:

4800 **heiratsfähig**, adj. marriageable.
4801 **Heirat**, f. marriage (from heiraten, to marry).
4802 **Jungfer**, f. } maiden,
4803 **Jungfrau**, f. } virgin.
4804 **Jungfernfieber**, n. 1. chlorosis.
4805 **Jungfernhäutchen**, n. 2. hymen.
4806 **Jungfernschaft**, f. maidenhood, virginity.
4807 **Jungfernsucht**, f. }
4808 **Jungfernkrankheit**, f. } chlorosis.
4809 **Jungfernbleichsucht**, f. }
4810 **Jungfernzeugung**, f. parthenogenesis.
4811 **Jungfrauenalter**, n. 2. woman between 14 and 18.
4812 **jungfräulich**, adj. virgin.
4813 **Jungfräulichkeit**, f. } maiden-
4814 **Jungfrauschaft** f. } hood, virginity.
4815 **Jüngling**, m. 1. youth, young man.

4816 **Jünglingsalter**, m. 2. youth between 14 and 20.
4817 7. **MILCH**, f. milch, in compounds:
4818 **milchähnlich**, adj. } milky,
4819 **milchartig**, adj. } lacteal.
4820 **Milchbackenzahn**, m. 1. deciduous molar tooth.
4821 **Milchbehälter**, m. 2. acinus of the breast.
4822 **Milchbereitung**, f. } milk for-
4823 **Milchbildung**, f. } mation.
4824 **Milchblattern**, f. pl. cow-pox.
4825 **Milchborke**, f. crusta lactea, porrigo.
4826 **Milchbruch**, m. 1. galactocele, milk-cyst.
4827 **Milchbrustgang**, m. 1. thoracic duct.
4828 **Milchcyste**, f. milk-cyst, galactocele.
4829 **Milchdiät**, f. milk diet.
4830 **Milchdrüse**, f. lacteal or mammary gland.
4831 **Milchdrüsengang**, m. 2. milk-duct.
4832 **Milchdrüsenläppchen**, n. 2. lobule of mammary gland.
4833 **Milchdrüsenschlagader**, f. artery of the mamma.
4834 **milchenthaltend**, adj. milk containing, lactiferous.
4835 **Milchfistel**, f. lacteal or mammary fistula.
4836 **Milchflusz**, m. 1. galactorrhœa.
4837 **Milchgang**, m. 1. lactiferous duct.
4838 **milchgebend**, adj. milk yielding.
4839 **Milchgebisz**, n. 1. milk teeth.
4840 **Milchgefäsz**, n. 1. lacteal vessel.
4841 **Milchgeschwulst**, f. milk tumor.
4842 **Milchglas**, n. 1. breast pump, breast glass.
4843 **Milchhaare**, n. 1. pl. down.
4844 **Milchharn**, m. 1. chylous urine.
4845 **Milchharnen**, n. 2. } chy-
4846 **Milchharnflusz**, m. 1. } luria.
4847 **milchicht**, adj. } milky, lac-
milchig, adj. } teal.
4848 **Milchkanal**, m. 1. } lactifer-
Milchkanälchen, n. 2. } ous duct.
4849 **Milchknoten**, m. 2. milk tumor (from retained milk in the breast).
4850 **Milchkügelchen**, n. 2. milk globule.
4851 **Milchleiter**, m. 2. lactiferous duct.
4852 **Milchnahrung**, f. milk diet.
4853 **Milchprüfung**, f. testing of milk.
4854 **Milchpumpe**, f. breast pump.
4855 **Milchröhrchen**, n. 2. lactiferous tube.
4856 **Milchsäckchen**, n. 2. sinus lactiferous.
4857 **Milchsaft**, m. 1. chyle.
4858 **Milchsaftgang**, m. 1. thoracic duct.
4859 **Milchsaftgefäsz**, n. 1. lacteal vessel.
4860 **Milchsäure**, f. lactic acid.
4861 **Milchschneidezahn**, m. 1. deciduous or milk incisor teeth.
4862 **Milchserum**, n. 1. serum lactis, whey.
4863 **Milchspeise**, f. milk diet.
4864 **Milchstar**, m. 1. milky cataract.
4865 **Milchstauung**, f. retention of milk.
4866 **Milchstockung**, f. arrest of milk secretion.
4867 **milchtreibend**, adj. } galactagogic, acceler-
4868 **milchfördernd**, adj. } ating milk-flow.
4869 **Milchüberflusz**, m. 1. milk-superabundance.
4870 **Milchverfälschung**, f. milk adulteration.
4871 **Milchverhaltung**, f. retention of milk.
4872 **Milchverlust**, m. 1. loss of milk.
4873 **Milchwage**, f. lactometer.
4874 **Milchwasser**, n. 2. whey.
4875 **Milchwein**, m. 1. koumiss, kephir.
4876 **Milchzahn**, m. 1. milk tooth.
4877 **Milchzahnperiode**, f. time from 1st to 7th year in life.
4878 **Milchzieher**, m. 2. breast-pump.
4879 **Milchzisterne**, f. milk duct, etc.
4880 8. **SCHWANGERSCHAFT**, f. pregnancy, (from
4881 **schwängern**, to impregnate, saturate).
4882 **schwanger**, adj. pregnant.

4883 **enceinte**; in andern or gesegneten Umständen sein, or sich befinden, to be in other or blessed circumstances, to be with child.
4884 **schwängerbar**, adj. capable of being impregnated.
4885 **Schwängerer**, m. 2. the male who impregnated a woman.
4886 **Schwängerung**, f. impregnation.
4887 **Schwangerschaftsbeginn**, m. 1. beginning of pregnancy.
4888 **Schwangerschaftsblutung**, f. hemorrhage of pregnancy.
4889 **Schwangerschaftsdauer**, f. duration of pregnancy, (neun Monate oder 274 Tage, nine months or 274 days).
4890 **Schwangerschaftserscheinung**, f. sign or phenomenon of pregnancy.
4891 **Schwangerschaftsmonat**, m. 1. month of pregnancy.
4892 **Schwangerschaftsnarbe**, f.
4893 **Schwangerschaftsstreifen**, m. 2. pl.
} white lines on the abdomen after pregnancy.
4894 **Schwangerschaftsvorgang**, m. 1. process of pregnancy.
4895 **Schwangerschaftswachstum**, n. 1. progress of pregnancy.
4896 **Schwangerschaftswahn**, m. 1. delusion of being pregnant.
4897 **Schwangerschaftswehen**, pl. n. 1. pregnancy pains.
4898 **Schwangerschaftswoche**, f. week of pregnancy;
4899 **in Wochen sein**, to be in childbed, lying-in.
4900 **Schwangerschaftszeit**, f. time or period of pregnancy, etc.
4901 9. **GEBURT**, f. (from v. ir.
4902 **gebären**, to bring forth, to bear a child), birth, labor (of women), parturition; delivery, child-birth.
4903 **Geburtenzahl**, f. the number of births.
4904 **gebürtig**, adj. born, native.
4905 **Geburtsachse**, f. axis of delivery.
4906 **Geburtsarbeit**, f. labor.
4907 **geburtsfördernd**, adj. assisting labor, ecbolic.
4908 **Geburtsdauer**, f. duration of labor.
4909 **Geburtsfehler**, m. 2. congenital defect.
4910 **Geburtsglieder**, n. 1. pl. genitals.
4911 **Geburtshelfer**, m. 2. accoucheur, obstetrician.
4912 **Geburtshelferin**, f. midwife.
4913 **Geburtshergang**, m. 1. procedure or process of labor.
4914 **Geburtsschein**, m. 1. certificate of birth.
4915 **Geburtsteile**, m. 1. pl. female genital organs.
4916 **Geburtsweg**, m. 1.
4917 **Geburtspassage**, f.
} generative passage.
4918 **Geburtswehen**, n. 1. pl. labor pains.
4919 **Geburtszange**, f. obstetrical forceps.
4920 **Geburtszeit**, f. term or time of delivery, etc.
4921 **Frühgebären**, n. 2.
} immature birth.
4922 **Frühgeburt**, f.
4923 **unzeitige Geburt**, f.
} premature birth (after 28 weeks).
4924 **Kaisergeburt**, f. delivery by Caesarean section.
4925 **Kaiserschnitt**, m. 1. (from v. ir.
4926 **schneiden**, to cut), Caesarean section, hysterotomy.
4927 **Miszgeburt**, f. abortion, miscarriage, monster.
4928 **Nachgeburt**, f. placenta, afterbirth.
4929 **Nachgeburtsblutung**, f. postpartum hemorrhage.
4930 **Nachgeburtsperiode**, f. third stage of labor.
4931 **Nachgeburtsvorfall**, m. 1. placenta prolapse.
4932 **Nachgeburtswehen**, n. 1. pl.
Nachwehen,
} after-pains.
4933 **Nachgeburtszange**, f. placental forceps.
4934 **Zangengeburt**, f. delivery by forceps, etc.
4935 **Zwilling**, m. 1. twin, etc.
4936 **Geschwister**, pl. brothers and sisters.
4937 10. **ENTBINDUNG**, f. (from v. ir.
4938 **entbinden**, to deliver), delivery, confinement.
4939 **Entbindungsakt**, m. 1. act of delivery.

4940 **Entbindungsanstalt**, f. } lying-in hospital.
4941 **Entbindungshaus**, n. 1. }
4942 **Entbindungsklinik**, f. obstetric department.
4943 **Entbindungsverfahren**, n. 2. method of delivery.
4944 **Entbindungswerkzeug**, n. 1. obstetric instrument, etc.
4945 11. **NIEDERKUNFT**, f. (from v. ir.
4946 **niederkommen**, to be delivered, to lie in), accouchement, delivery, labor.
4947 **Neuentbundene**, f. newly delivered woman.
4948 **Neugeborne**, n. 3. the new born infant.
4949 **neugeboren**, adj. newly born (from neonatus, newly born).
4950 **vorzeitige Niederkunft**, f. premature accouchement, etc.
4951 12. **WEHEN**, n. 1. pl. labor pains.
4952 **Weh or Wehe**, n. 1. is not much used (from
4953 **weh thun**, to ache, hurt, used with dative, e. g.
4954 **Die Brust thut mir weh**, my breast aches; dem
4955 **Kinde weh thun**, to hurt the child.
4956 **weh or wehe**, adj. e. g. sein weher
4957 **Hals**. his sore throat, etc.
4958 **Wehen haben, in Kindesnöten sein**, } to be in labor.
4959 **wehenähnlich**, adj. } labor pain-like.
4960 **wehenartig**, adj. }
4961 **Wehendruck**, m. 1. pressure during labor pains.
4962 **Weheneintritt**, m. 1. beginning of labor pains.
4963 **Wehenpause**, f. pause between labor pains.
4964 **Wehenthätigkeit**, f. activity of labor pains.
4965 **Wehfrau**, f. **Hebamme**, f. } midwife.
4966 **Wehmutter**, f. }
4967 **Amme**, f. nurse, wet-nurse.
4968 **Ammenmilch**. f. wet-nurse's milk, (from nässen, to wet, to moisten).
4969 **Ammenstube**, f. } nursery.
4970 **Ammenzimmer**, n. 2. }
4971 **Säugamme**. f. wet-nurse. (from
4972 **säugen**, to suckle, give suck, to nurse).
4973 **Saugflasche**. f. } (from v. ir. saugen, to suck, absorb, bottle or glass from which the child sucks or drinks).
4974 **Saugglas**, n. 1. }
4975 **mit der Flasche aufziehen**, v. ir. to bring up a child by hand, to nurse a child from the bottle or glass.
4976 **abgewöhnen**, to disaccustom, to wean.
4977 **Entwöhnung**, f. (from
4978 **entwöhnen**, to wean a child from the milk or from the breast of the mother), weaning, ablactation.
4979 **Weibergelüste**, f. pl. (from
4980 **gelüsten**, to lust), lusts of women, (as here applied, it has reference to the peculiar appetite of pregnant women).
4981 13. **WOCHE**, f. week. pl. Wochen. In compounds.
4982 **Wochen**, f. pl. die Wochen halten, } to be confined, to lie in.
4983 —, in die Wochen kommen, }
4984 —, in den Wochen sein, etc. }
4985 **Wochenbett**, n. 1. childbed.
4986 **Wochenbettkrankheit**, f. puerperal disease.
4987 **Wochenbettpflege**, f. care of lying-in woman.
4988 **Wochenbettwehen**, n. 1. pl. pains of lying-in.
4989 **Wochenbinde**, f. obstetric binder.
4990 **Wochenfieber**, n. 2. puerperal fever.
4991 **Wochenflusz**, m. 1. lochia.
4992 **Wochenkind**, n. 1. fresh born or new born child.
4993 **Wochenkost**, f. diet of lying-in woman.
4994 **Wochenlager**, n. 2. lying-in couch.
4995 **Wochenreinigung**, f. lochia.
4996 **Wochenschweisz**, m. 1. perspiration of the lying-in woman.
4997 **Wochenstube**, f. } lying-in room.
4998 **Wochenzimmer**, n. 2. }

4999 **Wochenzeit,** f. lying-in period.
5000 **Wöchnerin,** f. lying-in woman.
5001 **Wöchnerinnenfieber,** n. 2. puerperal fever.
5002 **Wöchnerinnen-friesel,** m. 2. military rash during the puerperal period, etc.
5003 §17. **DIE HARNWERKZEUGE,** the Urinary Organs, in compounds:
5004 1. **HARN,** m. 1. urine.
5005 **URIN,** m. 1. urine.
5006 **Harnabflusz,** m. 1. passing or escape of urine.
5007 **Harnabgang,** m. 1. passing or escape of urine.
5008 **Harnabsonderung.** f. excretion or secretion of urine.
5009 **Harnabträufeln,** n. 2. incontinence of urine.
5010 **harnähnlich.** adj. urin-like, urinous.
5011 **harnartig.** adj. urin-like, urinous.
5012 **Harnapparat,** m. 1. urinary apparatus.
5013 **Harnausleerung,** f. evacuation of urine. diuresis.
5014 **Harnauspressor,** m. 2. detrusor urinae muscle.
5015 **Harnausscheidung,** f. excretion of urine.
5016 **Harnbeschauung,** f. urinoscopy, examination of urine.
5017 **Harnbesichtigung,** f. urinoscopy, examination of urine.
5018 **Harnbestandteil,** m. 1. constituent part of urine.
5019 **Harnbildung,** f. formation of the urine.
5020 **Harnblase,** f. urinary bladder.
5021 **Harnblasenband,** n. 1. vesical ligament.
5022 **Harnblasenblutader,** f. vesical vein.
5023 **Harnblasenblutadergeflecht,** n. 1. vesical venous plexus.
5024 **Harnblasendrang,** m. 1. stranguary.
5025 **Harnblasengang,** m. 1. urethra.
5026 **Harnblasenhals,** m. 1. neck of the bladder.
5027 **Harnblasenhaut,** f. coat of the urinary bladder.
5028 **Harnblasenmuskel,** m. 2. muscular coat of the bladder.
5029 **Harnblasenschlagader,** f. vesical artery.
5030 **Harnblasenschleimhaut,** f. mucous membrane of the bladder.
5031 **Harnblasenwand,** f. bladder-wall.
5032 **harnen,** to pass water, to urinate.
5033 **Harnentleerung,** f. emptying of the bladder.
5034 **Harnfarbstoff,** m. 1. coloring matter of the urine.
5035 **Harnfäulnis,** f. decomposition of the urine.
5036 **Harnflusz,** m. 1. discharge or flow of the urine.
5037 **Harnflusz, unwillkürlicher,** incontinence of urine, enuresis.
5038 **Harngang,** m. 1. urinary passage.
5039 **Harngährung,** f. fermentation or decomposition of urine.
5040 **Harngefäsze,** n. 1. pl. urinary vessels.
5041 **Harngenitalfistel,** f. urinogenital fistula.
5042 **Harnleiter,** m. 2. ureter, catheter.
5043 **Harnleiterfistel,** f. fistula of the ureter.
5044 **Harnleitermündung,** f. orifice of ureter.
5045 **Harnleiterschlitz,** m. 1. orifice of ureter.
5046 **Harnorgan,** n. 1. urinary organ.
5047 **Harnröhre,** f. urethra.
5048 **Harnröhrenband,** n. 1. triangular ligament of the urethra.
5049 **Harnröhrendrüse,** f. urethral gland.
5050 **Harnröhrennaht,** f. suture of the urethra.
5051 **Harnröhrenöffnung,** f. meatus urinarius.
5052 **Harnröhrenschanker,** m. 2. urethral chancre.
5053 **Harnröhrenschleimhaut,** f. mucous membrane of the urethra.
5054 **Harnsand,** m. 1. gravel.
5055 **Harnsäure,** f. uric acid.
5056 **Harnsediment,** n. 1. urinary deposit.
5057 **Harnstoff,** m. 1. urea.

5058 **harnstoffhaltig**, adj. containing urea.
5059 **Harnstoffvergiftung**, f. uraemia.
5060 **Harnstrang**, m. 1. urachus.
5061 **Harnträufeln**, n. 2. dribbling of urine.
5062 **harntreibend**, adj. } diuretic.
diuretisch, adj. }
5063 **Harnunterdrückung**, f. suppression of urine.
5064 **Harnverhaltung**, f. retention of urine.
5065 **Harnweg**, m. 1. urinary passage.
5066 **Harnwerkzeug**, n. 1. urinary apparatus.
5067 **Harnwolke**, f. urinary nebula, cloudy urine.
5068 **Harnzapfer**, m. 2. catheter.
5069 **Harnzersetzung**, f. decomposition of urine.
5070 **Harnzucker**, m. 2. sugar in the urine (in diabetes).
5071 **Harnzwang**, m. 1. stranguary, dysuria, etc.
5072 2. **URIN**, n. 1. Urin (see also Harn for compounds).
5073 **Urinabgang**, m. 1. see Harnabgang.
5074 **Urinabscesz**, m. 1. urinary abscess.
5075 **Urinbeschwerde**, f. urinary affection or difficulty.
5076 **Urinblase**, f. urinary bladder.
5077 **Urincyste**, f. urinary cyst.
5078 **Urindrang**, m. 1. stranguary, dysuria.
5079 **urinieren**, to urinate.
5080 **Urinröhrchen**, n. 2. catheter.
5081 **Urinsäure**, f. uric acid.
5082 **Urinschau**, .f examination of the urine.
5083 **Urinstein**, m. 1. urinary calculus.
5084 **urintreibend**, adj. diuretic.
5085 **Urinverhaltung**, f. retention of urine.
5086 *Note* 1. **Die Farbe des Urins mag sein**. the color of the urine may be :
5087 **blasz**, pale.
5088 **braun**, brown.
5089 **braun schäumend**, brownish foaming.
5090 **dunkel,(schwarz)**, of a dark hue.
5091 **dick und trübe**, thick and dark.
5092 **grünisch gelb**, greenish yellow.
5093 **hellgelb**, bright yellow.
5094 **hell, sehr hell**, bright, very bright.
5095 **hochgestellt** (high placed), high colored.
5096 **rauchig**, smoky.
5097 **seifenartig**. soapy, soap-like.
5098 **wolkig**, cloudy, etc.
5099 *Note* 2. **Das spezifische Gewicht des Urins mag sein**, the specific weight (gravity)of the urine may be:
5100 **Im Urin mag vorhanden oder gegenwärtig sein**, In the Urine may be present:
5101 **excessif**, excessive
5102 **Azoturie**, f. too much excretion of urea.
5103 **Das Urinieren**, the urinating may be :
5104 **häufig**, } frequent.
frequent, }
5105 **langsam**, slowly.
5106 **schmerzhaft**, } painful.
schmerzlich, }
5107 **sparsam**, } scanty.
sparsamlich, }
5108 **tropfenweise**, drop by drop.
5109 **ununterbrochen**, (from v. ir. brechen, to break), continuous, when flowing.
5110 **unwillkürlich**, involuntary, spontaneously, etc.
5111 3. **NIERE**, f. pl. Nieren, kidney, in compounds *renal:*
5112 **Nierenabscesz**, m. 1. renal abscess.
5113 **Nierenabsonderung**, f. renal excretion.
5114 **Nierenader**, f. renal vein.
5115 **Nierenarterie**, f. renal artery.
5116 **nierenartig**, adj. renal, reniform.
5117 **Nierenbecher**, m. 2. } calyx of kidney.
5118 **Nierenkelch**, m. 1. }
5119 **Nierenbecken**, n. 2. pelvis of kidney.
5120 **Nierenblutader**, f. renal vein.
5121 **Nierendrüse**, f. renal gland.
5122 **Nierenfett**, n. 1. fat around the kidney, peri-renal fat.
5123 **nierenförmig**, adj. reniform, kidney-shaped.
5124 **Nierengefäsz**, n. 1. renal vessel.

5125 **Nierengeflecht**, n. 1. renal plexus.
5126 **Nierengegend**, f. renal region.
5127 **Nierenhaut**, f. capsule of the kidney.
5128 **Nierenkanälchen**, n. 2. uriniferous tubule.
5129 **Nierenkapsel**, f. capsule of the kidney.
5130 **Nierenkegel**, m. 2. pyramid of the kidney.
5131 **Nierenkyste**, f. renal cyst.
5132 **Nierenläppchen**, n. 2. } renal lobule.
Nierenlappen, n. 2. }
5133 **Nierenlappung**, f. renal lobe, renal lobulation.
5134 **Nierenlendenfistel**, f. renal fistula in the loin.
5135 **Nierenmark**, n. 1. medullary or tabular portion of the kidney.
5136 **Nierennerv**, m. 3. renal nerve.
5137 **Nierenpapille**, f. renal papilla.
5138 **Nierenpfortader**, f. vein of hilus of kidney.
5139 **Nierenpfortadersystem**, n. 1. renal portal system.
5140 **Nierenpforte**, f. hilus of the kidney.
5141 **Nierenpulsader**, f. renal artery.
5142 **Nierenpyramide**, f. renal pyramid.
5143 **Nierenrinde**, f. cortex of kidney.
5144 **Nierensand**, m. 1. gravel.
5145 **Nierenschlagader**, f. renal artery.
5146 **Nierensubstanz**, f. substance of the kidney.
5147 **Nierenthätigkeit**, f. action of the kidney.
5148 **Nierenvene**, f. renal vein.
5149 **Nierenwarze**, f. renal papilla.
5150 **nierenweise**, adj. kidney-like, etc.

5151 § 18. **Die FÜNF SINNE**, m. 1. pl. the five senses, in compounds:

5152 1. **GEFÜHL**, n. 1. (from
5153 **fühlen**, hence **befühlen**, to feel), feeling, touch, sensibility, sensation.
5154 **gefühllos**, adj. insensible, apathetic.
5155 **Gefühllosigkeit**, f. stupor, insensibility.
5156 **Gefühlsabstumpfung**, f. dulling of sensation.
5157 **Gefühlshaar**, n. 1. tactile hair, cilium.
5158 **Gefühlslähmung**, f. paralysis of sensation.
5159 **Gefühlsnerv**, m. 3. sensory nerve.
5160 **Gefühlsnervenstörung**, f. disturbance of sensory nerves.
5161 **Gefühlsorgan**, n. 1. organ of touch.
5162 **Gefühlspapille**, f. tactile papilla.
5163 **Gefühlssinn**, m. 1. sense of feeling or touch.
5164 **Gefühlsvermögen**, n. 2. power of feeling, sensibility.
5165 **Gefühlswärzchen**, n. 2. tactile papilla.
5166 **Gefühlswerkzeug**, n. 1. organ of feeling, etc.
5167 2. **GEHÖR**, n. 1. (from hören, to hear), hearing, ear, audition, in compounds auditory: (see also compounds with Ohr).
5168 **Gehörbläschen**, n. 2. } auditory vesicle.
Gehörblase, f. }
5169 **Gehörfehler**, m. 2. defect of hearing.
5170 **Gehörgang**, m. 1. auditory canal or meatus.
5171 **Gehörgangshaut**, f. lining of the auditory canal.
5172 **Gehörhaar**, n. 1. auditory cilium.
5173 **Gehörhöhle**, f. auditory cavity.
5174 **Gehörknöchelchen**, n. 2. } auditory ossicle.
Gehörknochen, n. 2. }
5175 **Gehörknöchelchenkette**, f. chain of auditory ossicles.
5176 **Gehörleiste**, f. crista acustica.
5177 **Gehörloch**, n. 1. auditory foramen.
5178 **gehörlos**, adj. deaf.
5179 **Gehörlosigkeit**, f. deafness.
5180 **Gehörnerv**, m. 3. auditory nerve.
5181 **Gehörnervenfaser**, f. auditory nerve fibre.
5182 **Gehörorgan**, n. 1. organ of hearing.
5183 **Gehörrohr**, n. 1. ear trumpet.

5184 **Gehörsand**, m. 1. otoconia, otolith.
5185 **Gehörschnecke**, f. cochlea.
5186 **Gehörschwindel**, m. 2. auditory vertigo.
5187 **Gehörsempfindung**, f. an auditory sensation.
5188 ——, entotische, f. an auditory sensation caused in the auditory apparatus.
5189 ——, subjektive, f. an auditory sensation produced outside of the ear.
5190 **Gehörssinn**, m. 1. sense of hearing.
5191 **Gehörstäbchen**, n. 2. auditory rod, bacillum acusticum.
5192 **Gehörsteinchen**, n. 2. otoconia, otolith.
5193 **Gehörstörung**, f. disturbance of hearing.
5194 **Gehörtäuschung**, f. deception or delusion of hearing.
5195 **Gehörtrichter**, m. 2. ear trumpet.
5196 **Gehörtrommel**, f. tympanum.
5197 **Gehörtrompete**, f. Eustachian tube.
5198 **Gehörvermögen**, n. 2. power of hearing.
5199 **Gehörvorhof**, m. 1. vestibule.
5200 **Gehörwasser**, n. 2. fluid of inner ear, liquor cotunnii.
5201 **Gehörweg**, m. 1. auditory meatus or canal.
5202 **Gehörwerkzeug**, n. 1. organ of hearing.
5203 **Gehörzahn**, m. 1. organ of Corti, auditory tooth of Huschke, etc.
5204 3. **GERUCH**, m. 1. (from v. ir. riechen, to smell)—
5205 **Riechen**, n. 2. smelling,—see also
5206 **Nase**, f. nose, for compounds), smell, smelling, odor, scent.
5207 **geruchlos**, adj. inodorous, scentless.
5208 **Geruchlosigkeit**, f. scentlessness.
5209 **Geruchsapparat**, m. 1. the olfactory apparatus.
5210 **Geruchseindruck**, m. 1. olfactory impression or sensation.
5211 **Geruchsempfindung**, f. sensation or appreciation of smelling.
5212 **Geruchsgrübchen**, n. 2. } olfactory fossa.
5213 **Geruchsgrube**, f. }
5214 **Geruchshaut**, f. } olfactory or Schneiderian membrane.
5215 **Riechhaut**, f. }
5216 **Geruchsknochen**, m. 2. ethmoid bone.
5217 **Geruchsnerv**, m. 3. } olfactory nerve.
5218 **Riechnerv**, m. 3. }
5219 **Geruchsorgan**, n. 1. olfactory organ, the nose.
5220 **Geruchsreiz**, m. 1. irritant to the sense of smelling.
5221 **Geruchssinn**, m. 1. the sense of smelling.
5222 **Geruchsvermögen**, n. 2. power of smelling.
5223 **Geruchswerkzeug**, n. 1. olfactory organ.
5224 **Geruchszelle**, f. } olfactory cell, etc.
5225 **Riechzelle**, f. }
5226 4. **GESCHMACK**, m. 1. (from
5227 **schmecken**, to taste), taste, relish, flavor, (see also *Gaumen*, palate, and *Zunge*, tongue, for compounds).
5228 **geschmacklos**, adj. tasteless, insipid.
5229 **Geschmacklosigkeit**, f. tastelessness, insipidity.
5230 **Geschmackreiz**, m. 1. irritant to the sense of taste.
5231 **Geschmacksempfindung**, f. perception of taste.
5232 **Geschmacksinn**, m. 1. sense of taste.
5233 **Geschmacksnerv**, m. 3. gustatory nerve, glosso-pharyngeal nerve.
5234 **Geschmacksorgan**, n. 1. organ of taste.
5235 **Geschmacksstörung**, f. disturbance of the sense of taste.
5236 **Geschmackstäuschung**, f. deception of taste.
5237 **Geschmackswärzchen**, n. 2. } gustatory papilla.
Geschmackswarze, f. }
5238 **Geschmackswerkzeug**, n. 1. organ of taste.
5239 **Geschmackszelle**, f. gustatory cell, etc.

5240 5. *a*. **GESICHT**, n. 1. (from
5241 v. ir. sehen, to see), eyesight, sight, vision, sense or faculty of seeing, (for Gesicht, countenance, face, visage, see § 8, 14.) In compounds visual:

5242 **gesichtlos**, adj. blind, sightless.

5243 **Gesichtlosigkeit**, f. blindness.

5244 **Gesichtsachse**, f. visual axis.

5245 **Gesichtsbetrug**, m. 1. } optical illusion.
5246 **Gesichtstäuschung**, f. }

5247 **Gesichtsblödigkeit**, f. } dimness of vision, amblyopia.
5248 **Gesichtsschwäche**, f. }

5249 **Gesichtsempfindung**, f. perception or sensation of sight.

5250 **Gesichtserscheinung**, f. optical phenomenon.

5251 **Gesichtsfehler**, m. 2. defect of eyesight or vision.

5252 **Gesichtsfeldeinengung**, f. limitation of vision-field.

5253 **Gesichtshügel**, m. 2. optic thalamus.

5254 **Gesichtskreis**, m. 1. range of vision.

5255 **Gesichtsorgan**, n. 1. organ of vision.

5256 **Gesichtsprüfung**, f. testing of vision.

5257 **Gesichtspunkt**, m. 1. visual point of distance.

5258 **Gesichtssinn**, m. 1. sense of vision.

5259 **Gesichtsstörung**, f. (from
5260 **stören**. to disturb), disturbance of vision.

5261 **Gesichtsstrahl**, m. 1. visual ray.

5262 **Gesichtsverdunkelung**, f. } obscuration of vision.
5263 **Gesichtsverdüsterung**, f. }

5264 **Gesichtsvorstellung**, f. visual perception.

5265 **Gesichtsweite**, f. visual distance.

5266 **Gesichtswerkzeug**, n. 1. organ of vision, etc.

5267 b. **SEHEN**, n. 2. from v. ir.
5268 **sehen**, to see, seeing, eyesight, sense or faculty of seeing, in compounds visual:

5269 **Sehachse**, f. axis of vision.

5270 **Sehe**, f. pupil, sight; eye.

5271 **Sehfähigkeit**, f. capability of seeing.

5272 **Sehfehler**, m. 2. defective eyesight.

5273 **Sehfeld**, n. 1. field of vision.

5274 **Sehhügel**, m. 2. optic thalamus.

5275 **Sehkanal**, m. 1. foramen opticum.

5276 **Sehkraft**, f. power or faculty of seeing or vision.

5277 **Sehkreis**, m. 1. } field of vision, horizon;
5278 **Gesichtskreis**, m. 1. } horopter.

5279 **Sehlehre**, f. optics.

5280 **Sehleistung**, f. visual capacity.

5281 **Sehlinie**, f. visual line.

5282 **Sehloch**, n. 1. optic foramen, pupil.

5283 **Sehlochhaut**, f. membrana pupillaris.

5284 **Sehmal.**, n. 1. visual point.

5285 **Sehmesser**, n. 2. optometer.

5286 **Sehnerv**, m. 3. optic nerve.

5287 **Sehnervenfaser**, f. fibre of optic nerve.

5288 **Sehnervenfaserschicht**, f. fibrous layer of optic nerve.

5289 **Sehnervenhügel**, m. 2. colliculus of optic nerve.

5290 **Sehnervenkern**, m. 1. nucleus of optic nerve.

5291 **Sehnervenkopf**, m. 1. optic disc.

5292 **Sehnervenkreuzung**, f. chiasm of the optic nerve.

5293 **Sehnervenöffnung**, f. optic foramen.

5294 **Sehnervenscheibe**, f. optic disc.

5295 **Sehnervenschwund**, m. 1. atrophy of optic nerve.

5296 **Sehnervenverfärbung**, f. discoloration of optic nerve.

5297 **Sehorgan**, n. 1. organ of vision.

5298 **Sehpunkt**, m. 1. visual point.

5299 **Sehschärfe**, f. acuteness of vision.

5300 **Sehschwäche**, f. weakness of vision.

5301 **Sehstörung**, f. disturbance of vision.

5302 **Sehstrahl**, m. 1. visual ray.

5303 **Sehstrahlung**, f. visual radiation.

5304 **Sehstrang**, m. 1. optic tract.

5305 **Sehstrangkreuzung**, f. chiasm of the optic nerves.
5306 **Sehstreifen**, m. 2. optic tract.
5307 **Sehvermögen**, n. 2. faculty of seeing or vision.
5308 **Sehweite**, f. visual range or distance.
5309 **Sehweitemesser**, n. 2. optometer.
5310 **Sehwerkzeug**, n. 1. visual apparatus.
5311 **Sehwinkel**, m. 2. visual angle, etc.

5312 §19. **Die DRÜSEN**, the glands in compounds:

5313 **DRÜSE**, f. } gland, pl. Drüsen,
5314 **Aden**, f. } glands.
5315 **Absonderungsdrüse**, f. secretion gland.
5316 **Achseldrüse**, f. axillary gland.
5317 **Achsellymphdrüse**, f. axillary lymph gland.
5318 **Aden**, f. gland.
5319 **Adenographie**, f. description of glands.
5320 **Augendrüse**, f. lachrymal gland.
5321 **Augenliderdrüse**, f. meibomian gland.
5322 **Balgdrüse**, f. follicular gland.
5323 **Bauchspeicheldrüse**, f. pancreas.
5324 **Beckendrüse**, f. pelvic gland.
5325 **Blutdrüse**, f. vascular gland.
5326 **Bronchialdrüse**, f. bronchical gland.
5327 **Bronchialschleimdrüse**, f. bronchial mucous gland.
5328 **Brustdrüse**, f. thoracic gland, mammary gland, thymus.
5329 **Carotidendrüse**, f. carotid gland.
5330 **Darmdrüse**, f. } intestinal
5331 **Darmsaftdrüse**, f. } gland.
5332 **Dünndarmdrüsen**, f. pl. glands of the small intestines.
5333 **Fettdrüse**, f. sebacious gland.
5334 **Gallendrüse**, f. gland of the bile duct.
5335 **Gallengangdrüse**, f. bile duct gland.
5336 **Gaumendrüse**, f. palatine gland.
5337 **Gefäszdrüse**, f. vascular gland.
5338 **Gekrösdrüse**, f. mesenteric gland.
5339 **Gelenkdrüse**, f. synovial gland.
5340 **Generationsdrüse**, f. generative gland.
5341 **Genickdrüse**, f. cervical gland.
5342 **Geschlechtsdrüse**, f. genital gland, ovary.
5343 **Grimmdarmgekrösdrüse**, f. gland in meso-colon.
5344 **Haarbalgdrüse**, f. gland of the hair follicles or sebaceous gland.
5345 **Haardrüse**, f. gland of hair follicles.
5346 **Halsdrüse**, f. cervical gland; tonsil.
5347 **Harnröhrendrüse**, f. urethral gland.
5348 **Haufendrüse**, f. conglomerate gland, Peyer's patch.
5349 **Hautdrüse**, f. sebaceous gland.
5350 **Hautfettdrüse**, f. skin fat-gland (mammary).
5351 **Hautsalbendrüse**, f. } sebaceous
5352 **Hauttalgdrüse**, f. } gland.
5353 **Herzdrüse**, f. cardiac gland.
5354 **Hodendrüse**, f. testicle.
5355 **Hohldrüse**, f. follicular gland.
5356 **Hopfendrüse**, f. pl. glandulæ lupuli.
5357 **Inguinaldrüse**, f. inguinal gland.
5358 **Kehldeckeldrüse**, f. epiglottis gland.
5359 **Kehlkopfdrüse**, f. laryngeal gland.
5360 **Keimdrüse**, f. germinal gland.
5361 **Kieferdrüse**, f. submaxillary gland.
5362 **Kieferlymphdrüse**, f. submaxillary lymphatic gland.
5363 **Kinnbackendrüse**, f. submaxillary gland.
5364 **Knäueldrüse**, f. sweat gland.
5365 **Kniekehlendrüse**, f. popliteal gland.
5366 **Kropfdrüse**, f. thyroid gland; goitre.
5367 **Labdrüse**, f. peptic gland, digestive gland (from laben, to nourish, refresh.)
5368 **Leberdrüse**, f. hepatic gland.
5369 **Leistendrüse**, f. inguinal gland.
5370 **Lendendrüse**, f. lumbar gland.

5371 **Lippendrüse**, f. labial gland.
5372 **Luftröhrendrüse**, f. bronchial gland.
5373 **Lungendrüse**, f. bronchial gland.
5374 **Lymphdrüse**, f. lymphatic gland.
5375 **Magendrüse**, f. } gastric
5376 **Magensaftdrüse**, f. } gland.
5377 **Magenlabdrüse**, f. peptic gland of the stomach.
5378 **Magenschleimdrüse**, f. mucous gland of the stomach.
5379 **Mandeldrüse**, f. tonsil.
5380 **Mediastinal-drüse**, f. } mediastinal
5381 **Mittelfelldrüse**, f. } gland.
5382 **Mesenterialdrüse**, f. mesenteric gland.
5383 **Metakerastische Drüsen**, pl. f. ductless glands.
5384 **Milchdrüse**, f. lacteal or mammary gland.
5385 **Milzdrüse**, f. spleen.
5386 **Mittelfelldrüse**, f. mediastinal gland.
5387 **Moll'sche Drüsen**, pl. modified sweat-glands at the margin of the eyelid.
5388 **Munddrüse**, f. oral gland.
5389 **Mundhöhlendrüse**, f. buccal gland.
5390 **Mundspeicheldrüse**, f. salivary gland.
5391 **Mutterdrüse**, f. uterine cotyledon.
5392 **Nackendrüse**, f. cervical gland.
5393 **Nackenlymphdrüse**, f. cervical lymph gland.
5394 **Nebenbauchspeicheldrüse**, f. accessory pancreatic gland.
5395 **Nebendrüse**, f. accessory gland.
5396 **Nebenschilddrüse**, f. accessory thyroid gland.
5397 **Nebenspeicheldrüse**, f. accessory salivary gland.
5398 **Nervendrüse**, f. nerve gland (as applied by Remak to supra renal capsule).
5399 **Nierendrüse**, f. renal gland.
5400 **Ohrdrüse**, f. } parotid
Ohrendrüse, f. } gland.
5401 **Ohrschmalz-drüse**, f. } ceruminous
Ohrenschmalz-drüse, f. } gland.
5402 **Ohrspeicheldrüse**, f. parotid gland.
5403 **Pepsindrüse**, f. pepsine or peptic gland.
5404 **Pestdrüse**, f. plague bubo.
5405 **Pinealdrüse**, f. pineal gland.
5406 **Pulmonaldrüse**, f. pulmonary gland.
5407 **Samendrüse**, f. spermatic gland, testicle.
5408 **Saugaderdrüse**, f. lymphatic gland.
5409 **Schamdrüse**, f. inguinal gland.
5410 **Schilddrüse**, f. thyroid gland.
5411 **Schleimdrüse**, f. } mucous
5412 **Schleimhaut-drüse**, f. } gland.
5413 **Schlunddrüse**, f. pharyngeal gland.
5414 **Schweiszdrüschen**, n. 2. }
5415 **Schweiszdrüse**, f. } sweat gland.
5416 **Schweiszknäuel-drüse**, f. }
5417 **Sekretionsdrüse**, f. secreting gland.
5418 **Speicheldrüse**, f. salivary gland.
5419 **Synovialdrüse**, f. synovial gland.
5420 **Thränendrüse**, f. lachrymal gland.
5421 **Trachomdrüse**, f. } trachoma
5422 **Trachomfollikel**, n. 2. } granule.
5423 **Unterkieferdrüse**, f. submaxillary gland.
5424 **Uterindrüse**, f. uterine or utricular gland.
5425 **Vorhautdrüse**, f. preputial gland.
5426 **Weichendrüse**, f. inguinal gland.
5427 **Zeugungsdrüse**, f. genital gland (testicle or ovary).
5428 **Zirbel**, f. } pineal gland.
5429 **Zirbeldrüse**, f. }
5430 **Zungendrüse**, f. lingeal gland. etc.
5431 §20. **DIE FISTEL**. The Fistula, in compounds:
5432 **Fistel**, f. } fistula, in com-
5433 **Hohlgang**, m. 1. } pounds: passage, fistula.
5434 **fistelartig**, adj. fistulous.
5435 **Fistelaufschneiden**, n. 2. slitting of a fistula.
5436 **Fistelbistouri**, n. 1. bistoury for fistula.
5437 **Fistelgang**, m. 1. fistulous tract, sinus.

5438 **Fistelgeschwür**, n. 1. fistulous ulcer.
5439 **Fistelmembran**, f. membrane lining a fistula.
5440 **Fistelöffnung**, f. opening of a fistula.
5441 **Fistelstimme**, f. falsetto voice.
5442 **fistulös**, adj, fistulous, etc.
5443 **Augenfistel**, f. lachrymal fistula.
5444 **Backenfistel**, f. buccal fistula.
5445 **Blasenbauchwandfistel**, f. abdomino-vesical fistula, (from
5446 **Blase**, f. bladder, etc.)
5447 **Blasencervicalfistel**, f. cervico-vesical fistula.
5448 **Blasendarmfistel**, f. vesico-intestinal fistula.
5449 **Blasendünndarmfistel**, f. vesico intestinal fistula of small intestines.
5450 **Blasenfistel**, f. vesical fistula.
5451 **Blasengebärmutterfistel**, utero-vesical fistula.
5452 **Blasengebärmutterscheidenfistel**, f. vesico-utero-vaginal fistula.
5453 **Blasenmastdarmfistel**, f. recto-vesical fistula.
5454 **Blasenmutterfistel**, f. vesico-uterine fistula.
5455 **Blasenscheidengebärmutterfistel**, f. vesico-vagino-uterine fistula.
5456 **Blasenscheidenmastdarmfistel**, f. recto-vesico-vaginal fistula.
5457 **Brustfellfistel**, f. fistulous opening in the pleura.
5458 **Brustfistel**, f. thoracic fistula (after empyema.)
5459 **Darmfistel**, f. intestinal fistula.
5460 **Darmscheidenfistel**, f. intestino-vaginal fistula.
5461 **Dünndarmblasenfistel**, f. intestino-vesical fistula (of small intestines.)
5462 **Gallenblasenbauchfistel**, f. abdominal biliary fistula.
5463 **Gallenblasendarmfistel**, f. biliary intestinal fistula.
5464 **Gallenbronchialfistel**, f. biliary bronchial fistula.
5465 **Gallenfistel**, f. } biliary fistula.
5466 **Gallengefäszfistel**, f. } biliary fistula.
5467 **Gallenpleurafistel**, f. pleuro-biliary fistula.
5468 **Gebärmutterdarmfistel**, f. utero-intestinal fistula.
5469 **Gefäszgallenfistel**, f. circulatory biliary fistula.
5470 **Gefäszfistel**, f. fistula in gluteal region.
5471 **Halsfistel**, f. cervical fistula.
5472 **Harnblasendarmfistel**, f. vesico - intestinal fistula, (from
5473 **Harnblase**, f. urinary bladder.)
5474 **Harnblasenfistel**, f. urinary fistula.
5475 **Harnblasenmastdarmfistel**, f. recto-vesical fistula.
5476 **Harnblasenschamfistel**, f. vesico-pudendal fistula.
5477 **Harnblasenscheidenfistel**, f. vesico-vaginal fistula.
5478 **Harnfistel**, f. urinary fistula.
5479 **Harngenitalfistel**, f. urino-genital fistula.
5480 **Harnleiter**, m. 2. ureter, catheter.
5481 **Harnleiterbauchfistel**, f. uretero-abdominal fistula.
5482 **Harnleiterdarmfistel**, f. uretero-intestinal fistula.
5483 **Harnleiterfistel**, f. fistula of the ureter.
5484 **Harnleitergebärmutterfistel**, f. uretero-uterine fistula.
5485 **Harnleiterscheidenfistel**, f. uretero-vaginal fistula.
5486 **Harnröhrenfistel**, f. urethral fistula.
5487 **Harnröhrenscheidenfistel**, f. urethro-vaginal fistula.
5488 **Harnstrangfistel**, f. urachal fistula.
5489 **Hornhautfistel**, f. corneal fistula.
5490 **Kiemenfistel**, f. bronchial fistula.
5491 **Knochenfistel**, f. cloaca (in necrosis).
5492 **Kommunicationsfistel**, f. communication fistula, (as in vesico-vaginal fistula.)
5493 **Larynxfistel**, f. laryngeal fistula.
5494 **Leberfistel**, f. hepatic fistula.
5495 **Luftfistel**, f. aërial fistula.
5496 **Luftröhrenfistel**, f. tracheal fistula.

5497 **Luftspeiseröhrenfistel,** f. laryngo-oesophageal fistula.
5498 **Lungenfistel,** f. pulmonary fistula.
5499 **Lymphfistel,** f. lymphatic fistula.
5500 **Magendünndarmfistel,** f. gastro-enteric fistula.
5501 **Magenfistel,** f. gastric fistula.
5502 **Mastdarmblasenfistel,** f. recto-vesical fistula.
5503 **Mastdarmfistel,** f. rectal fistula.
5504 **Mastdarmharnröhrenfistel,** f. recto-urethral fistula.
5505 **Mastdarmscheidenfistel,** f. recto-vaginal fistula.
5506 **Milchfistel,** f. lacteal or mammary fistula.
5507 **Mutterscheidenfistel,** f. vaginal fistula.
5508 **Nabeldarmfistel,** f. omphalo-intestinal fistula.
5509 **Nackenfistel,** f. cervical fistula.
5510 **Nierenbeckenbauchfistel,** f. reno-pelvic-abdominal fistula.
5511 **Nierenbeckenfistel,** f. fistula of pelvis of kidney.
5512 **Nierenfistel,** f. renal fistula.
5513 **Samenfistel,** f. seminal fistula.
5514 **Scheidenblasenfistel,** f. vesico-vaginal fistula.
5515 **Scheidendammfistel,** f. perineal fistula.
5516 **Scheidendünndarmfistel,** f. enterico-vaginal fistula.
5517 **Scheidenfistel,** f. vaginal fistula.
5518 **Scheidenmastdarmfistel,** f. recto-vaginal fistula.
5519 **Speichelfistel,** f. salivary fistula.
5520 **Speichelgangfistel,** f. salivary duct fistula.
5521 **Steiszfistel,** f. fistula in ano.
5522 **Thoraxfistel,** f. thoracic fistula.
5523 **Thränendrüsenfistel,** f. } lachrymal fistula.
5524 **Thränenfistel,** f. } lachrymal fistula.
5525 **Thränensackfistel,** f. fistula of the lachrymal sac.
5526 **Trachealfistel,** f. tracheal fistula.
5527 **Unterlippenfistel,** f. congenital fissure or sinus of the lower lip.
5528 **Urinfistel,** f. urinary fistula.
5529 **Zahnfistel,** f. dental fistula, etc.
5530 § 21. **Das GEWEBE,** the tissue, in compounds:
5531 **Adergewebe,** n. 1. venous tissue.
5532 **Amnionbindegewebe,** n. 1. amnion connective tissue.
5533 **Balkengewebe,** n. 1. trabecular tissue.
5534 **Beckengewebe,** n. 1. } pelvic connective tissue.
5535 **Beckenzellgewebe,** n. 1. } pelvic connective tissue.
5536 **Bindegewebe,** n. 1. connective tissue.
5537 **Blasengewebe,** n. 1. vesicular tissue.
5538 **Blutgefäszbindegewebe,** n. 1. connective tissue of a blood vessel.
5539 **Brustdrüsengewebe,** n. 1. tissue of breast gland.
5540 **Fasergewebe,** n. 1. fibrous tissue.
5541 **Fettgewebe,** n. 1. adipose tissue.
5542 **Flickgewebe,** n. 1. cicatricial tissue.
5543 **Gallertgewebe,** n. 1. gelatinous tissue.
5544 **Gebärmuttergewebe,** n. 1. uterine tissue.
5545 **Gefäszgewebe,** n. 1. vascular tissue.
5546 **Glashautgewebe,** n. 1. hyaloid tissue.
5547 **Halsbindegewebe,** n. 1. cervical connective tissue.
5548 **Halszellgewebe,** n. 1. cervical cellular tissue.
5549 **Hautzellgewebe,** n. 1. subcutaneous cellular tissue.
5550 **Herzgewebe,** n. 1. tissue of the heart.
5551 **Hirnspinnengewebe,** n. 1. arachnoid membrane.
5552 **Hodengewebe,** n. 1. testicle parenchyma.
5553 **Horngewebe,** n. 1. corneous or horny tissue.
5554 **Hornhautgewebe,** n. 1. cornea tissue.
5555 **Kapselgewebe,** n. 1. capsular tissue.
5556 **Keimgewebe,** n. 1. germinal tissue.

5557 **Klappengewebe**, n. 1. valve tissue.
5558 **Knochengewebe**, n. 1. bony tissue.
5559 **Knorpelgewebe**, n. 1. cartilagenous tissue.
5560 **Körpergewebe**, n. 1. body tissue.
5561 **Krebsgewebe**, n. 1. cancer tissue.
5562 **Lebergewebe**, n. 1. hepatic tissue.
5563 **Lungengewebe**, n. 1. cellular structure of the lung.
5564 **Markgewebe**, n. 1. medullary tissue.
5565 **Maschengewebe**, n. 1. retiform tissue.
5566 **Muskelgewebe**, n. 1. muscular tissue.
5567 **Muttergewebe**, n. 1. uterine tissue.
5568 **Narbenbindegewebe**, n. 1. (from Narbe, f. scar, scar connective tissue.
5569 **Narbengewebe**, n. 1. cicatricial tissue.
5570 **Nervengewebe**, n. 1. nerve tissue.
5571 **Oberhautgewebe**, n. 1. epidermic tissue.
5572 **Ovarialgewebe**, n. 1. ovarian tissue.
5573 **Plattengewebe**, n. 1. lamellar tissue.
5574 **Rindengewebe**, n. 1. cortical tissue.
5575 **Scheidenschwellgewebe**, n. 1. erectile vagina tissue.
5576 **Schilddrüsengewebe**, n. 1. thyroid gland tissue.
5577 **Schleimgewebe**, n. 1. mucous tissue.
5578 **Schwellgewebe**, n. 1. spongy or cavernous tissue.
5579 **Sehnengewebe**, n. 1. tendon tissue.
5580 **Zellgewebe**, n. 1. cellular or alveolar tissue, connective tissue, etc.
5581 § 22. **Das HAAR**, the hair. In compounds:
5582 **Haar**, n. 1. hair. cilium.
5583 **Haarader**, f. capillary vein.
5584 **Haaranlage**, f. hair rudiment.
5585 **Haarausfall**, m. 1. } falling off of the hair.
5586 **Haarausfallen**, n. 2. } falling off of the hair.
5587 **Haarbalg**, m. 1. hair follicle.
5588 **Haarbalgdrüse**, f. sebaceous gland; gland of the hair follicles.
5589 **Haarbalgmilbe**, f. ocarus folliculorum.
5590 **Haarbalgmündung**, f. orifice of a hair follicle.
5591 **Haarbalgmuskeln**, pl. m. 2. muscles of the hair follicles, arrectores pili.
5592 **Haarband**, n. 1. ciliary process.
5593 **Haarbeet**, n. 1. } hair bed (the hair growing from the skin).
5594 **Haarbett**, n. 1. } hair bed (the hair growing from the skin).
5595 **Haarboden**, m. 2. } hair bed (the hair growing from the skin).
5596 **Haarbildung**, f. hair formation.
5597 **Haarbruch**, m. 1. capillary fracture.
5598 **Haarbuschel**, n. 2. hair tuft.
5599 **Haardrüse**, f. gland of hair follicles.
5600 **Haarfaser**, f. filament.
5601 **haarfaserig**, adj. filamentous.
5602 **haarförmig**, adj. capillary, piliform.
5603 **Haargefäsz**, n. 1. capillary vessel.
5604 **Haargefäsznetz**, n. 1. capillary network.
5605 **Haargefäszwand**, f. wall of capillary vessel.
5606 **haarig**, adj. hairy.
5607 **Haarkegel**, m. 2. hair cone.
5608 **Haarkeim**, m. 1. hair papilla.
5609 **Haarknäuel**, m. 2. hairy ball or concretion, mass of hair.
5610 **Haarknopf**, m. 1. } hairbulb.
5611 **Haarkolben**, m. 2. } hairbulb.
5612 **Haarkopf**, m. 1. } tricocephalus dispar.
5613 **Haarkopfwurm**, m. 1. } tricocephalus dispar.
5614 **Haarkrone**, f. hair crown.
5615 **haarlos**, adj. hairless.
5616 **Haarlosigkeit**, f. } baldness.
5617 **Haarmangel**, m. 2. } baldness.
5618 **Haarmark**, n. 1. medulla of hair.
5619 **Haarnerv**, m. 3. ciliary nerve.
5620 **Haaroberhäutchen**, n. 2. hair cuticle.
5621 **Haarpapille**, f. hair papilla.
5622 **Haarrinde**, f. hair cortex.
5623 **Haarröhrchen**, n. 2. / **Haarröhre**, f. } capillary tube.
5624 **Haarsäckchen**, n. 2. / **Haarsack**, m. 1. } hair follicle.

5625 **Haarsackmilbe**, f. acarus folliculorum.
5626 **Haarschaft**, f. hair shaft.
5627 **Haarscheide**, f. hair sheath.
5628 **Haarscheitel**, m. 2. crown of the head, parting of hair.
5629 **Haarschuppen**, f. pl. scurf.
5630 **Haarschwinde**, f. } falling off of the hair, alopecia.
5631 **Haarschwund**, m. 1. }
5632 **Haarspalt**, m. 1. splitting of hair.
5633 **Haarspitze**, f. point of hair.
5634 **Haarstoff**, m. 1. hair forming material.
5635 **Haarstrang**, m. 1. seton.
5636 **Haarstrom**, m. 1. hair whorl.
5637 **Haarwachs**, n. 1. tendinous tissue.
5638 **Haarwachstum**, n. 1. hair growth.
5639 **Haarwarze**, f. hairy mole.
5640 **Haarwirbel**, m. 2. hair whorl.
5641 **Haarwurm**, m. 1. trichina spiralis.
5642 **Haarwürmer**, m. 1. pl. naematodes.
5643 **Haarwurzel**, f. hair root.
5644 **Haarwurzelscheide**, f. sheath of hair root.
5645 **Haarzelle**, f. hair cell; auditory cell.
5646 **Haarzopf**, m. 1. } tuft of hair.
5647 **Haarzotte**, f. }
5648 **Haarzwiebel**, f. hair bulb.
5649 **Barthaar**, n. 1. beard hair.
5650 **Bluthaargefäsz**, n. 1. capillary blood vessel.
5651 **Haupthaar**, n. 1. } hair of the head.
5652 **Kopfhaar**, n. 1. }
5653 **Nasenganghaar**, n. 1. nasal vibrissa.
5654 **Nasenhaare**, pl. n. 1. vibrissae.
5655 **Schamhaar**, n. 1. pubic hair, etc.
5656 § 23. **Die HAUT**. the skin in compounds.
5657 **Haut**, f. skin, integument, cutis membrane, tunic; coat, film, pellicle.
5658 ——, **äuszere**, f. integumentum commune, membra decidua.
5659 ——, **durchsichtige**, f. cornea.
5660 ——, **gefäszhaltige**, f. tunica vasculosa.
5661 ——, **harte**, f. sclerotic.
5662 ——, **hinfällige**, f. membrana decidua.
5663 ——, **weiche**, f. pia mater.
5664 ——, **weisze**, f. tunica albuginea.
5665 **Hautabschilferung**, f. skin exfoliation.
5666 **Hautabschuppung**, f. skin desquamation.
5667 **Hautabschürfung**, f. skin excoriation.
5668 **Hautabsonderung**, f. (from absondern, to secrete), cutaneous secretion or excretion.
5669 **hautähnlich**, adj. } tegumentary, dermoid, membranous.
5670 **hautartig**, adj. }
5671 **Hautanschwellung**, f. skin swelling.
5672 **Hautatmen**, n. 2. } cutaneous respiration.
5673 **Hautatmung**, f. }
5674 **Hautatrophie**, f. skin atrophy.
5675 **Hautausdünstung**, f. skin perspiration.
5676 **Hautausschlag**, m. 1. cutaneous eruption, efflorescence, exanthem. (ata. pl.)
5677 **Hautausschlag**, nässender, m. 1. mit } impetigo.
5678 **Pustelbildung**, f. }
5679 **Hautauswuchs**, m. 1. skin protuberance, skin excrescence.
5680 **Hautbalg**, m. 1. skin follicle.
5681 **Hautbalggeschwulst**, f. cutaneous follicular tumor, molluscum.
5682 **Hautbeschreiber**, m. 2. dermatologist.
5683 **Hautbeschuppung**, f. formation of skin scales.
5684 **Hautbläschen**, n. 2. papule, vesicle.
5685 **Hautblatt**, n. 1. cutaneous or external plate.
5686 **Hautbläuung**, f. cyanosis.
5687 **Hautblutader**, f. cutaneous vein.
5688 **Hautblüte**, f. skin eruption or outbreak, exanthem, cutaneous efflorescence.
5689 **Hautblutgefäsz**, n. 1. cutaneous blood-vessel.
5690 **Hautbrand**, m. 1. burning or tingling of the skin, skin gangrene.

5691 **Hautbrennen**, n. 2. skin burning or tingling.
5692 **Hautbrücke**, f. skin bridge.
5693 **Häutchen**, n. 2. cuticle, membrane, pellicle, film, nebula.
5694 **häutchenartig**, adj. membranous.
5695 **Hautdecke**, f. cutaneous covering, integument.
5696 **Hautdrüse**, f. cutaneous gland.
5697 **Hautdunst**, m. 1. imperceptible perspiration.
5698 **Hautempfindlichkeit**, f. cutaneous sensibility.
5699 **Hautemphysem**, n. 1. subcutaneous emphysema.
5700 **Hautentfärbung**, f. skin decoloration.
5701 **Hautfalte**, f. skin fold.
5702 **Hautfarbe**, f. skin color, complexion.
5703 **Hautfaserblatt**, n. 1. somatic or parietal mesoblast; somatopleure.
5704 **Hautfett**, n. 1. sebaceous skin matter.
5705 **Hautfettgewebe**, n. 1. adipose skin tissue.
5706 **Hautfettdrüse**, f. skin fatt gland (as in mammary.)
5707 **Hautfinne**, f. pimple, acne.
5708 **Hautfläche**, f. skin surface.
5709 **Hautflecken**, m. 2. spot or speck on the skin, macula, pannus.
5710 **Hautgeschwulst**, f. dermoid or cutaneous tumor.
5711 **Hautgeschwür**, n. 1. skin ulcer.
5712 **Hautgries**, m. 1. milium.
5713 **Hauthämorrhagie**, f. cutaneous hemorrhage.
5714 **Hauthärchen**, n. 2. small skin hair.
5715 **Hauthorn**, n. 1. cutaneous horn.
5716 **Hautknorpel**, m. 2. membranous cartilage.
5717 **Hautknötchen**, n. 2. } skin nodule, as in cancer, syphilis, etc.
5718 **Hautknoten**, m. 2. } skin nodule, as in cancer, syphilis, etc.
5719 **Hautlappen**, m. 2. cutaneous flap.
5720 **Hautlehre**, f. dermatology.
5721 **Hautleistchen**, n. 2. cutaneous ridge, normal skin ridge.
5722 **Hautmäuschen**, n. 2. } cutaneous muscle, platysma.
5723 **Hautmuskel**, m. 2. } cutaneous muscle, platysma.
5724 **Hautnabel**, m. 2. integumentary umbilicus part.
5725 **Hautnaht**, f. cutaneous suture.
5726 **Hautnarbe**, f. cutaneous scar, cicatrix.
5727 **Hautnerv**, m. 3. cutaneous nerve.
5728 **Hautoberfläche**, f. cutaneous surface.
5729 **Hautödem**, n. 1. skin œdema.
5730 **Hautpapillen**, pl. f. skin papillae.
5731 **Hautpigment**, n. 1. skin pigment.
5732 **Hautplatte**, f. cutaneous lamella or plate.
5733 **Hautreiz**, m. 1. cutaneous irritation.
5734 **Hautresorption**, f. skin absorption.
5735 **Hautrisz**, m. 1. chap, crack, fissure of the skin.
5736 **Hautrunzel**, f. fold or wrinkle of the skin.
5737 **Hautsalbe**, f. sebaceous matter.
5738 **Hautsalbendrüse**, f. sebaceous gland.
5739 **Hautschicht**, f. from Schicht, layer, cutaneous layer.
5740 **Hautschleimbeutel**, m. 2. cutaneous mucous bursa.
5741 **Hautschrund**, m. 1. fissure, cleft, chap of the skin, rhagades.
5742 **Hautschwiele**, f. skin callosity.
5743 **Hautsekretion**, f. cutaneous secretion.
5744 **Hautsensibilitätsbezirk**, m. 1. region of the cutaneous sensibility.
5745 **Hautsinn**, m. 1. sense of touch.
5746 **Hautstein**, m. 1. calcareous sebaceous cyst.
5747 **Hautstippe**, f. skin stigma, (as in the bite of an insect.)
5748 **Hautstrieme**, f. wheal, bruise, ecchymosis.
5749 **Hauttalg**, m. 1. sebaceous matter.
5750 **Hauttalgdrüse**, f. sebaceous gland.
5751 **Hautthätigkeit**, f. skin activity.

5752 **Hauttransplantation**, f. } skin
5753 **Hautverpflanzung**, f. } grafting.
5754 **Hautvene**, f. cutaneous vein.
5755 **Hautwärzchen**, n. 2. } wart. cutaneous
Hautwarze, f. } papilla.
5756 **Hautwucherung**, f. skin proliferation.
5757 **Hautwulst**, m. 1. skin protuberance, excrescence.
5758 **Hautwurm**, m. 1. farcy, worm invading the skin.
5759 **Hautzellgewebe**, n. 1. subcutaneous cellular tissue.
5760 **Hautzipfel**, m. 2. tag of skin, etc.
5761 *Note* 1. **Die Haut mag sein**, the skin may be:
5762 **aufgeblasen**, (from v. ir,
5763 **aufblasen**, (blasen) to blow open, to dilate by blowing), emphysematous.
5764 **aufgedunsen**, } to be swelled up or puffed
gedunsen, } up.
5765 **aufgeschwollen**, (from v. ir.
5766 **aufschwellen**, (schwellen) to swell up, to become distended), swelled, inflamed.
5767 **bedeckt** (from
5768 **bedecken**, to cover), covered, loaded.
5769 **blasz**, pallid.
5770 **blau**, blue.
5771 **bläulich rot**, violet.
5772 **bleich**, pale.
5773 **braun**, brown.
5774 **bräunlich rot**, brownish red.
5775 **dick**, thick.
5776 **dunkelrot**, dark red.
5777 **dünn**, thin.
5778 **eisigkalt**, icy, as cold as ice.
5779 **empfindlich**, sensitive.
5780 **fahl**, fallow, erdfahl, earth-colored.
5781 **feucht**, moist.
5782 **gelb**, yellow.
5783 **gelbgrün**, yellowish-green.
5784 **geritzt**, (from
5785 **ritzen**, to scratch), scratched.
5786 **gespannt**, tense, tight.
5787 **grindig**, scabby, scabbed, scurfy.
5788 **hart**, hard.
5789 **heisz**, hot.
5790 **sehr heisz und**
5791 **juckend**, (from jucken, to itch), very hot and itching (with itchy feeling).
5792 **hektisch rot**, hectic red.
5793 **hellrot**, light-red.
5794 **kahl**, bald.
5795 **kalt**, cold.
5796 **klebrig**, chammy.
5797 **kühl**, cool.
5798 **locker**, slack, loose.
5799 **ödematisch**, } oedematous,
5800 **ödematös**, } dropsical.
5801 **ölig**, oily.
5802 **rauh**, harsh, rough.
5803 **rot**, red.
5804 **runzlich**, } wrinkled.
runzig, }
5805 **sanft**, soft, tender.
5806 **scharlachrot**, scarlet (red).
5807 **schaudernd**, } shivering,
5808 **schauerig**, } shuddering.
5809 **schlaff**, flabby.
5810 **schmutzig**, dirty, unclean.
5811 **schuppicht**, } scaly,
schuppig, } squamous.
5812 **shweiszig**, sweaty.
5813 **schwielig**, callous.
5814 **schwitzend**, perspiring.
5815 **straff**, tight, rigid.
5816 **strohartig**, straw-colored.
5817 **teigartig**, doughy.
5818 **verletzt**, injured.
5819 **voll**, full.
5820 **wachsähnlich**, } waxy.
5821 **wachsartig**, }
5822 **weich**, soft.
5823 **weisz**, white.
5824 **zart**, delicate, tender, etc.

5825 § 24. **Die HÖHLE**, f. The Cavity. In compounds:

5826 **Absceszhöhle**, f. abscess-cavity.
5827 **Achselhöhle**, f. armpit, axilla.
5828 **Augenhöhle**, f. orbital cavity.
5829 **Bauchfellhöhle**, f. } peritoneal
5830 **Bauchhöhle**, f. } cavity.
5831 **Beckendarmhöhle**, f. pelvic intestinal cavity.
5832 **Beckenhöhle**, f. pelvic cavity.
5833 **Beinhöhle**, f. articular cavity, or bone socket.
5834 **Bindegewebshöhle**, f. connective tissue-cavity.
5835 **Blasenhöhle**, f. bladder cavity.
5836 **Bluthöhle**, f. haematic or blood cavity.

5837 **Brustfellhöhle**, f. } pleura
5838 **Brustfellsack**, f. } cavity.
5839 **Brusthöhle**, f. thoracic cavity.
5840 **Darmhöhle**, f. intestinal cavity.
5841 **Eingeweidehöhle**, f. visceral cavity.
5842 **Eiterhöhle**, f. pus cavity.
5843 **Gebärmutterhöhle**, f. uterine cavity.
5844 **Gesichthöhlen**, f. pl. facial cavities (mouth, pharynx, nose, etc.)
5845 **Gehörhöhle**, f. auditory cavity.
5846 **Gefäszhöhle**, f. lumen of a vessel.
5847 **Gehirnhöhle**, f. cerebral ventricle.
5848 **Gelenkhöhle**, f. articular cavity, acetabulum.
5849 **Halshöhle**, f. throat cavity.
5850 **Herzbeutelhöhle**, f. pericardium cavity.
5851 **Herzhöhle**, f. heart cavity.
5852 **Hirnhöhle**, f. cerebral ventricle.
5853 **Jauchehöhle**, f. suppurating cavity.
5854 **Kehlkopfhöhle**, f. laryngeal cavity.
5855 **Keilbeinhöhle**, f. sphenoidal cavity.
5856 **Keimhöhle**, f. germinal or embryonic cavity.
5857 **Kieferhöhle**, f. } antrum of
5858 **Kinnbacken-höhle**, f. } Highmore.
5859 **Knochenhöhle**, f. bone cavity, cell or lacuna.
5860 **Knochenwundhöhle**, f. wound cavity in a bone.
5861 **Knorpelhöhle**, f. cartilage cavity.
5862 **Kopfhöhle**, f. cranial cavity.
5863 **Leibeshöhle**, f. abdominal cavity of the body.
5864 **Lungenhöhle**, f. pulmonary cavity.
5865 **Magenhöhle**, f. stomach cavity.
5866 **Markhöhle**, f. medullary cavity.
5867 **Mittelfellhöhle**, f. } mediastinum
5868 **Mittelfellraum**, m. 1. } cavity.
5869 **Mundhöhle**, f. oral cavity.
5870 **Mundrachenhöhle**, f. pharyngo-oral cavity.
5871 **Muschelhöhle**, f. hollow of the toncha.
5872 **Nasenhöhle**, f. nasal cavity or fossa.
5873 **Nasenrachenhöhle**, f. nasopharyngeal cavity.
5874 **Nebenhöhle**, f. accessory cavity.
5875 **Oberaugenhöhle**, f. supraorbital cavity.
5876 **Oberkieferhöhle**, f. antrum of Highmore.
5877 **Ohrenhöhle**, f. } aural cavity.
Ohrhöhle, f. }
5878 **Paukenhöhle**, f. tympanic cavity.
5879 **Peritonealhöhle**, f. peritoneal cavity.
5880 **Rumpfhöhle**, f. trunk cavity.
5881 **Schädelhöhle**, f. cranial cavity.
5882 **Scheidenhauthöhle**, f. cavity of the tunica vaginalis.
5883 **Schleimhauthöhle**, f. cavity of mucous membrane.
5884 **Seitenhöhle**, f. lateral ventricle.
5885 **Siebbeinhöhle**, f. ethmoidal cavity.
5886 **Stirnhöhle**, f. frontal sinus.
5887 **Trommelhöhle**, f. tympanic cavity.
5888 **Wespenbeinhöhle**, f. sphenoidal sinus.
5889 **Wirbelhöhle**, f. } vertebral
5890 **Wirbelkanal**, m. 1. } canal.
5891 **Wundhöhle**, f. cavity of a wound, etc.
5892 § 25. **Die NAHT**, The Suture. In compounds:
5893 **Bauchdecken-naht**, f. } suture of abdominal
5894 **Bauchnaht**, f. } wall.
5895 **Balkennaht**, f. raphe of corpus callosum, quilled suture.
5896 **Beinnaht**, f. bone suture.
5897 **Bindehautnaht**, f. conjunctival suture.
5898 **Dammnaht**, f. perineal suture.
5899 **Darmnaht**, f. intestinal suture.
5900 **Gaumennaht**, f. staphylorraphy; palatine suture.
5901 **Gebärmutternaht**, f. uterine suture.
5902 **Harnröhrennaht**, urethra suture.

5903 **Hasenschartennaht**, f. hare-lip suture.
5904 **Hautnaht**, f. cutaneous suture.
5905 **Hinterhauptsnaht**, f. occipital suture; lambdoid suture.
5906 **Hirnschädelnaht**, f. cranial suture.
5907 **Hodensacknaht**, f. raphe of the scrotum.
5908 **Intermaxillarnaht**, f. intermaxillary suture.
5909 **Jochbeinnaht**, f. zygomatic suture.
5910 **Kammnaht**, f. pectinate suture.
5911 **Keilbeinnaht**, f. sphenoidal suture.
5912 **Kinnnaht**, f. symphysis of the lower jaw.
5913 **Kirschnernaht**, f. glover's suture.
5914 **Klammernaht**, f. clamp suture.
5915 **Knochennaht**, f. bone suture.
5916 **Knopfnaht**, f. interrupted suture, button suture.
5917 **Knotennaht**, f. reef-knot suture.
5918 **Kronennaht**, f. coronal suture.
5919 **Lamdanaht**, f. lambdoid suture.
5920 **Leichennaht**, f. postmortem suture (from Leiche, f. corpse).
5921 **Lippenrotnaht**, f. suture of the red portion of the lip (as in hare-lip operation).
5922 **Mastdarmnaht**, f. rectal suture.
5923 **Matratzennaht** f. mattress suture (Hegar).
5924 **Mittelfleischnaht**, f. perineal suture, raphe of perineum.
5925 **Nasennaht**, f. rhinorrhaphy.
5926 **Nervennaht**, f. nerves-suture.
5927 **Perlnaht**, f. shot suture (the wire carried through a bead or perforated shot).
5928 **Pfeilnaht**, f. sagittal suture.
5929 **Plattennaht**, f. leaden plate suture.
5930 **Quernaht**, f. transverse suture.
5931 **Randnaht**, f. uniting suture, surface suture.
5932 **Sagittalnaht**, f. sagittal suture.
5933 **Schädelnaht**, f. cranial suture.
5934 **Schamlefzennaht**, f. labial suture.
5935 **Scheitelnaht**, f. parietal suture.
5936 **Schienennaht**, f. leaden plate suture.
5937 **Sehnennaht**, f. tendon suture.
5938 **Siebbeinnaht**, f. ethmoidal suture.
5939 **Silberdraht-naht**, f. } silver wire suture, silver suture.
5940 **Silbernaht**, f. }
5941 **Stiftnaht**, f. suture by pegs (as of bone).
5942 **Stirnnaht**, f. frontal suture.
5943 **Trockennaht**, f. the adjusting of wounds by plaster.
5944 **Wangennaht**, f. zygomatic suture.
5945 **Zitzennaht**, f. occipito-mastoid suture, etc.
5946 § 26. **Die WAND**, the wall, in compounds:
5947 **Absceszwand**, f. abscess wall.
5948 **Aortenwand**, f. aortic wall.
5949 **Arterienwand**, f. arterial wall.
5950 **Augapfelwand**, f. eyeball surface.
5951 **Augenhöhlenwand**, f. orbital cavity wall.
5952 **Balgwand**, f. cyst wall.
5953 **Bauchwand**, f. } abdominal wall.
Bauchwandung, f. }
5954 **Blasenscheidenwand**, f. vesico-vaginal wall.
5955 **Blasenwand**, f. bladder wall.
5956 **Blutgefäszwand**, f. blood vessel wall.
5957 **Brusthöhlenwand**, f. thoracic wall.
5958 **Brustwand**, f. } thoracic wall.
Brustwandung, f. }
5959 **Darmmuskelwand**, f. iliac muscle wall.
5960 **Darmwand**, f. } intestinal wall.
Darmwandung, f. }
5961 **Gebärmutterwand**, f. uterine wall.
5962 **Gefäszwand**, f. } wall of a vessel.
Gefäszwandung, f. }
5963 **Gehirnscheidewand**, f. septum lucidum.
5964 **Gelenkwand**, f. joint boundary or capsule.
5965 **Haargefäszwand**, f. wall of capillary vessels.

5966 **Harnröhrenscheidewand**, f. urethro-vaginal septum.

5967 **Herzkammerscheidenwand**, f. ventricular septum.

5968 **Herzkammerwand**, f. ventricular wall.

5969 **Herzscheidewand**, f. septum of the heart.

5970 **Herzvorhofscheidewand**, f. auricular septum of the heart.

5971 **Herzwand**, f. } cardiac
Herzwandung, f. } wall.

5972 **Hirnscheidewand**, f. septum lucidum.

5973 **Kammerscheidewand**, f. ventricular septum.

5974 **Kapillarwand** (see 3692), f. capillary wall.

5975 **Kapselwand**, f. capsular wall.

5976 **Knochenwand**, f. } osseous
Knochenwandung, f. } wall.

5977 **Luftröhrenwand**, f. wall of the trachea.

5978 **Magenwand**, f. } coat or wall of the
Magenwandung, f. } stomach.

5979 **Mastdarmscheidenwand**, f. recto-vaginal septum.

5980 **Mittelwand**, f. mediastinum.

5981 **Muskelwand**, f. muscular wall.

5982 **Nasenhöhlenscheidewand**, f. } nasal
5983 **Nasenscheidewand**, f. } septum.

5984 **Paukenhöhlenwand**, f. wall of tympanic cavity.

5985 **Querscheidewand**, f. transverse septum.

5986 **Rachenwand**, f. pharyngeal wall.

5987 **Sackwand**, f. sack wall.

5988 **Schädelwand**, f. } cranial
Schädelwandung, f. } wall.

5989 **Scheidenmastdarmwand**, f. recto-vaginal wall.

5990 **Scheidenwand**, f. vaginal wall.

5991 **Scheidewand**, f. dividing wall, septum, mediastinum, partition, diaphragm.

5992 **Schlundwand**, f. wall of pharynx.

5993 **Schneckenwand**, f. cochlear wall.

5994 **Uteruswand**, f. } uterine
5995 **Uteruswandung**, f. } wall.

5996 **Vorhofsscheidewand**, f. auricular septum of the heart.

5997 **Zellwand**, f. } cell wall,
Zellwandung, f. } etc.

5998 § 27. **Die ZELLE**, the cell. In compounds:

5999 **Zellblutleiter**, m. 2. cavernous sinus.

6000 **Zellchen**, n. 2. cellule.

6001 **Zelle**, f. cell. Zellen in compounds:

6002 **Zellenanhäufung**, f. cell accumulation.

6003 **zellenarm**, adj. poor in cells.

6004 **Zellenausläufer**, m. 2. } process of off-
6005 **Zellenfortsatz**, m. 1. } shoot of cell.

6006 **Zellenauswanderung**, f. emigration of cells.

6007 **Zellenbalken**, m. 2. cellular trabeculum.

6008 **Zellenbalkennetz**, n. 1. a cellular reticulum.

6009 **zellenbildend**, adj. cell forming or making.

6010 **Zellenbildung**, f. cell formation.

6011 **Zellenfaser**, f. cell fibre.

6012 **Zellenflüssigkeit**, f. cell fluid.

6013 **Zellenform**, f. cell form.

6014 **zellenförmig**, adj. cellular, areolar.

6015 **Zellengang**, m. 1. cellular duct.

6016 **Zellengewebe**, n. 1. cellular or areolar tissue.

6017 **Zellenhaufen**, m. 2. accumulation of cells.

6018 **Zellenhaut**, f. cellular membrane.

6019 { **Zellengehalt**, m. 1. } contents
{ **Zelleninhalt**, m. 1. } of cell.

6020 **Zellenkeim**, m. 1. cell germ.

6021 **Zellenkern**, m. 1. cell nucleus, cystoblast.

6022 **Zellenknistern**, n. 2. crepitant râle.

6023 **Zellenknorpel**, m. 2. cellular cartilage.

6024 **Zellenkörper**, m. 2. body of a cell.

6025 **Zellenkrebs**, m. 1. medullary cancer.

6026 **Zellenleib**, m. 1. body of a cell.

6027 **Zellennest**, n. 1. cell nest (of epithelioma).

6028 **Zellensaft**, m. 1. cell fluid.

6029 **Zellenschicht**, f. layer of cells.
6030 **Zellenstrang**, m. 1. column of cells.
6031 **Zellenwucherung**, f. proliferation of cells.
6032 **Zellenzerfall**, m. 1. cell decay.
6033 **Zellfaden**, m. 2. cell fibre.
6034 **Zellfusion**. f. fusion of cells.
6035 **Zellgewebe**, n. 1. cellular or areolar tissue, connective tissue.
6036 **Zellgewebsabscesz**, m. 1. suppuration of cellular tissue.
6037 **Zellgewebsblutung**, f. hemorrhage into cellular tissue.
6038 **Zellgewebsbrand**, m. 1. sloughing of cellular tissue.
6039 **Zellgewebseiterung**, f. suppuration of cellular tissue.
6040 **Zellgewebsentzündung**, f. inflammation of cellular tissue.
6041 **Zellgewebserweichung**. f. softening of cellular tissue.
6042 **Zellgewebsfaser**, f. cellular tissue fibre.
6043 **Zellgewebsfäserchen**, n. 2. cellular tissue fibril.
6044 **Zellgewebsflüssigkeit**, f. fluid of connective tissue.
6045 **Zellgewebshaut**. f. cellular coat or membrane.
6046 **Zellgewebslücke**, f. interstice of cellular tissue.
6047 **Zellgewebspfropfen**, m. 2. slough of cellular tissue (separated in carbuncle).
6048 **Zellgewebsraum**, m. 1. cellular tissue space.
6049 **Zelgewebsscheide**, f. cellular tissue sheath.
6050 **Zellgewebsschicht**, f. cellular tissue layer.
6051 **Zellgewebsschwund**. m. 1. atrophy of cellular tissue.
6052 **Zellgewebsvereiterung**, f. suppuration of cellular tissue.
6053 **Zellgewebsverhärtung**. f. induration of cellular tissue.
6054 **Zellgewebswucherung**, f. proliferation of cellular tissue.
6055 **Zellhaufen**, m. 2. accumulation of cells.
6056 **Zellhaut**, f. cellular membrane, scarolemma.
6057 **Zellhautsscheide**, f. sheath of cellular tissue.
6058 **zellig**, adj. cellular, areolar, alveolar.
6059 **Zellkern**. m. 1. cell nucleus, cystoblast.
6060 **Zellkörper**, m. 2. } body of a
6061 **Zellleib**, m. 1. } cell.
6062 **Zellmembran**, f. cellular membrane.
6063 **Zellnest**. n. 1. cell-nest of epithelium).
6064 **Zellsaft**, m. 1. cell fluid.
6065 **Zellschicht**, f. layer of cells.
6066 **Zellstoff**, m. 1. cellulose, cellular or connective tissue.
6067 **Zellstoffhülle**, f. cellular tissue coat.
6068 **Zellstoffschicht**. f. layer of connective tissue.
6069 **Zellstrang**, m. 1. column of cells.
6070 **Zellteilung**. f. cell division or segmentation.
6071 { **Zellwand**, f. } cell wall,
{ **Zellwandung**. f. } etc.
6072 **Epithelzellenlage**, f. layer of epithelial cells.
6073 **Empfindungszelle**. f. sensory cell, sensitive cell.
6074 **Schwärmzelle**, f. wandering cell.
6075 **Siebbeinzelle**. f. ethmoidal cell
6076 **Sinneszelle**, f. sensory cell.
6077 **Speichelzelle**, f. salivary corpuscle.
6078 { **Zitzenzelle**, f. } mastoid
{ **Zitzenfortsatszelle**, f. } cell, etc.
6079 § 28. **Mehrere unverbundene, einfache und zusammengesetzte medizinische Wörter and Ausdrücke**, several disconnected simple and compound medical terms and expressions.
6080 1. **Anaërobien**, pl. bacteria able to live without air.
6081 **Bacillen**, m. 1. (from bacillus, pl. bacilli), bacilli.
6082 **bacillär**, adj. pertaining to bacilli.
6083 **bacillenhaltig**, adj. containing bacilli.
6084 **Bacillenlehre**, f. bacteriology.
6085 **bacillenreich**, adj. full of bacilli.
6086 **Bakterien**, pl. bakteria (small microscopic organisms producing and developing diseases.)

6087 **Mikroben**, pl. } microbes.
Mikrobien, pl. }

6088 2. a. **Gesund aussehen**, v. ir. to look (appear) hale, healthy, sound, well, from

6089 **gesund**, adj. hale, healthy, sound, well, and

6090 **aussehen**, v. ir. to look, appear, e. g.

6091 **Er sieht sehr gesund aus**, he looks (appears) very well.

6092 **gesund (sich) befinden**, v. ir. & refl. to be hale, healthy, sound, well; *literally*, to find one's self in a good state or condition of health; from gesund, hale, and sich befinden (to find one's self), e. g.

6093 **Ich befinde mich sehr gesund**, I am very well.

6094 **gesund (sich) fühlen**, v. & refl., to feel hale, healthy, sound, well from gesund, hale, and sich fühlen, to feel one's self, e. g.

6095 **Ich fühle, or Ich fühle mich ganz gesund**, I feel very well.

6096 **gesunden**, to recover, to be restored to health.

In compounds:

6097 **Gesund-brunnen**, m. 2. mineral spring containing medicinal water.

6098 **gesundheitlich**, adj. sanitary.

6099 b. **GESUNDHEIT**, f. health.

In compounds.

6100 **Gesundheitsamt**, n. 1. office of the board of health.

6101 **Gesundheitsbeamte**, m. 3. health officer, sanitary inspector.

6102 **Gesundheitskommission**, f. board of health.

6103 **Gesundheitskunde**, f. sanitary science.

6104 **Gesundheitslehre**, f. hygiene.

6105 **Gesundheitspasz**, m. 1. bill or certificate of health.

6106 **Gesundheitspflege**, f. hygiene; sanitation; care of health.

6107 **Gesundheitspflegegesetz**, n. 1. act or law of health.

6108 **Gesundheitspolizey**, f. sanitary police.

6109 **Gesundheitsrat**, m. 1. board of health.

6110 **Gesundheitsregel**, f. regimen of health.

6111 **Gesundheitsvorschrift**, f. sanitary regulation.

6112 **Gesundheitszustand**, m. 1. state or condition of health, etc.

6113 3. **KRANK**, adj. diseased, indisposed, ill, sick, unwell.

6114 **Kranke**, m. 3. } patient, a sick person, (male
6115 **Kranke**, f. } or female.

6116 **Kränkelei**, f. sickliness.

6117 **kränkeln**, to be sickly, to have indifferent health.

6118 4. **KRANKEN**, } to be sick or get indisposed, to
erkranken, } suffer from.

In compounds:

6119 **Krankenanstalt**, f. asylum for the sick, hospital, infirmary.

6120 **Krankenattest**, m. 1. certificate of ill health.

6121 **Krankenbaracke**, f. asylum or hospital on the barack system.

6122 **Krankenbericht**, m. 1. bulletin.

6123 **Krankenbestand**, m. 1. number of patients.

6124 **Krankenbesuch**, m. 1. professional visit.

6125 **Krankenbesucher**, m. 2. medical visitor; attendant.

6126 **Krankenbett**, n. 1. } sick-bed,
6127 **Siechbett**, n. 1. } hospital-bed.

6128 **Krankendiarium**, n. 1. physicians diary or visiting book.

6129 **Krankendiät**, f. sick-diet.

6130 **Krankenexamen**, n. 2. examination of a patient.

6131 **Krankengeschichte**, f. medical history of a patient.

6132 **Krankenhaus**, n. 1. hospital, infirmary.

6133 **Krankenheber**, m. 2. contrivance for raising a patient in bed.

6134 **Krankenkasse**, f. sick-fund, treasury for the sick.

6135 **Krankenkost**, f. sick diet or regimen.

6136 **Krankenlager**, n. 2. sick-couch, bed.

6137 **Krankenleder**, n. 2. waterproof-sheet.

6138 **Krankenliste**, f. sick list.

6139 **Krankenkorb**, m. 1. basket-ambulance.

6140 **Krankenpflege**, f. nursing care of patients.
6141 **Krankenpfleger**, m. 2. sick attendant, male nurse.
6142 **Krankenpflegerin**, f. nurse.
6143 **Krankensaal**, m. 1. ward.
6144 **Krankenschiff**, n. 1. hospital ship.
6145 **Krankenspeise**, f. sick diet.
6146 **Krankenspital**, n. 1. hospital.
6147 **Krankenstube**, f. } sick-
Krankenzimmer, n. 2. } room.
6148 **Krankenstuhl**, m. 1. invalid chair.
6149 **Krankenstuhlwagen**, m. 2. bath chair.
6150 **Krankenthermometer**, m. 2. clinical thermometer.
6151 **Krankentisch**, m. 1. bed table.
6152 **Krankentrage**, f. stretcher, carrying chair for invalids.
6153 **Krankenträger**, m. 2. stretcher-bearer.
6154 **Krankentransport**, m. 1. transport of the sick and wounded.
6155 **Krankenuntersuchung**, f. examination of a patient.
6156 **Krankenwagen**, m. 2. invalid ambulance, carriage, bath-chair.
6157 **Krankenwärter**, m. 2. male-nurse, sick attendant.
6158 **Krankenwärterin**, f. nurse.
6159 **Krankenwartung**, f. attendance upon the sick.
6160 **Krankenwäsche**, f. bed linen and body linen of sick persons.
6161 **Krankenzelt**, n. 1. ambulance or hospital tent.
6162 **Krankenzertrennung**, f. the distribution ot the sick and wounded (during war.)
6163 **Krankenzettel**, m. 2. bulletin.
6164 **Krankenzimmer**, n. 2. } sick-
Krankenstube, f. } room.
6165 **krankhaft**, adj. abnormal, diseased, morbid, unhealthy.
6166 **Krankhaftigkeit**, f. abnormity, diseased state.
6167 5. **KRANKHEIT**, f. disease, illness, malady, sickness, complaint.
6168 ——, englische, rickets. In compounds:
6169 **Krankheitsabnahme**, f. decline of a disease.
6170 **Krankheitsanlage**, f. predisposition to disease.
6171 **Krankheitsausgang**, m. 1. result or termination of a disease.
6172 **Krankheitsbakterien**, pl. bacteria of disease.
6173 **Krankheitsbefund**, m. 1. diagnosis of disease.
6174 **Krankheitsbericht**, m. 1. bulletin, medical report.
6175 **Krankheitsbewusztsein**, n. 1. consciousness of being ill.
6176 **Krankheitsbild**, n. 1. aspect or form of a disease.
6177 **Krankheitsdauer**, f. duration of a disease.
6178 **Krankheitsentscheidung**, f. crisis of a disease.
6179 **Krankheitsentstehung**, f. etiology of disease.
6180 **Krankheitserreger**, m. 2. exciter of disease, (as bacterium parasite).
6181 **Krankheitserscheinung**, f. appearance, symptom, or phenomenon of a disease.
6182 **Krankheitsform**, f. form or variety of a disease.
6183 **Krankheitsforscher**, m. 2. pathologist.
6184 **Krankheitsgeschichte**, f. history of a disease.
6185 **Krankheitsgift**, n. 1. virus of a disease.
6186 **Krankheitsgruppe**, f. group of diseases.
6187 **Krankheitsherd**, m. 1. focus of diseases.
6188 **Krankheitskeim**, m. 1. germ of a disease.
6189 **Krankheitskenner**, m. 2. pathologist.
6190 **Krankheitskunde**, f. } pathol-
6191 **Krankheitslehre**, f. } ogy.
6192 **Krankheitsmarasmus**, m. 1. wasting of disease.
6193 **Krankheitssitz**, m. 1. seat of disease.
6194 **Krankheitsstimmung**, f. phase of disease.
6195 **Krankheitsstoff**, m. 1. morbid matter.
6196 **Krankheitssymptom**, n. 1. symptom.
6197 **Krankheitsträger**, m. 2. vehicle of disease.

6198 **Krankheitsursache**, f. cause of disease.
6199 **Krankheitsverlauf**, m. 1. course of disease.
6200 **Krankheitsvorgang**. m. 1. process of a disease.
6201 **Krankheitswechsel**, m. 2. change or crisis of disease.
6202 **Krankheitszeichen**, n. 2. symptom of disease.
6203 **Krankheitszeichenlehre**, f. symtomatology.
6204 **krankheitszeichnend**, adj. pathognomonic, s y m p t o - matic.
6205 **Krankheitszufall**, m. 1. attack of disease.
6206 **Krankheitszunahme**. f. exacerbation of disease.
6207 **Krankheitszustand**, m. 1. state of disease.
6208 **kränklich**, adj. ailing, infirm, sickly, unhealthy.
6209 **Kränklichkeit**, f. sickliness. infirmity.
6210 **Kranksein**, n. 1. illness, condition of being sick.
6211 **ungesund**, adj. unhealthy, unsound.
6212 **Ungesundheit**, f. ill health, unwholesomeness, etc.
6213 6. **KRANKHEITS-CHARAKTERISTIK**, Characteristic of a disease.

Eine Krankheit mag sein: A disease may be:

6214 **abwechselnd**, intermittent.
6215 **abnorm**, abnormal, irregular.
6216 **abzehrend**, } consumptive.
6217 **auszehrend**, }
6218 **ähnlich**, like, similar.
6219 **akut** (hitzig), acute.
6220 **allgemein**, general, constitutional.
6221 **allmählich**, gradual.
6222 **alternierend**, alternating.
6223 **analog**, } like, similar,
ähnlich. } analog.
6224 **angeboren**, congenital.
6225 **angreifend**, exhaustive.
6226 **anhaltend**, continued.
6227 **ansteckend**, infectious.
6228 **asthmatisch**, asthmatic, short-breathed.
6229 **ausschlagend**, breaking out (into a rash).
6230 **äuszerlich**. external.
6231 **aussetzend**. intermittent.
6232 **bedenklich**, critical. serious.
6233 **bedeutend**, important.
6234 **bösartig**, } malignant, viru-
schlimm, } lent.
6235 **brennend**. burning. stinging.
6236 **central**, central (as in paralysis).
6237 **chronisch**, chronic, slow.
6238 **contagiös**, contagious.
6239 **einfach**. simple.
6240 **eingewurzelt**, inveterate, inbred.
6241 **endemisch**, endemic.
6242 **entkräftigend**, debilitating, enervating.
6243 **entzündlich**, inflammatory
6244 **epidemisch**, epidemic.
6245 **erbfähig**, inheritable.
6246 **erblich**, hereditary.
6247 **erschöpfend**, exhausting.
6248 **fallsüchtig**, epileptic.
6249 **fieberartig**, } feverish, fe-
6250 **fieberisch**, } brile.
6251 **fieberfrei**, free from fever.
6252 **fieberhaft**, feverish, aguish.
6253 **fieberlos**, free from fever, apyretic.
6254 **fluszartig**, } rheumatic.
rheumatisch, }
6255 **funktionell**, functional.
6256 **furibund**, fierce.
6257 **gallenartig**, } bilious.
6258 **gallensüchtig**, } choleric.
6259 **gallertartig**, } gelatinous.
gallertig, }
6260 **gallertig-schleimig**, muco-gelatinous.
6261 **gallicht**, }
gallig, } bilious.
gallsüchtig, }
6262 **gefährlich**, dangerous.
6263 **gewöhnlich**, common.
6264 **gichtisch**, } gouty.
gichtig, }
6265 **gutartig**, benign, non-malignant.
6266 **hartnäckig**, obstinate, stubborn.
6267 **heftig**, violent.
6268 **hektisch**, hectic, consumptive.
6269 **heilbar**, curable.
6270 **hitzig**, acute, inflammatory.
6271 **hysterisch**, hysterical.
6272 **intermittierend**, intermittent.
6273 **kontagiös**, contagious.
6274 **krätzartig**, } itch-like.
6275 **krätzig**, }
6276 **krebsähnlich**, } cancerous.
6277 **krebsartig**, }

6278 **kritisch**, critical.
6279 **langsam**, slow.
6280 **lebensgefährlich**, perilous, mortal.
6281 **leicht**, } light, slight, mild.
mild, }
6282 **lokal**, local.
6283 **momentan**, momentary, (as in unconsciousness.
6284 **nervig**, } nervous.
6285 **nervös**, }
6286 **neuralgisch**, neuralgic.
6287 **nichtansteckend**, non-contagious.
6288 **nicht reducierbar**, irreducible (e. g. hernia).
6289 **örtlich**, local.
6290 **paralytisch**, paralytic.
6291 **peinlich**, agonizing.
6292 **peinvoll**, painful.
6293 **perialgisch**, highly painful.
6294 **periodisch**, periodical.
6295 **pestartig**, pestilential.
6296 **pestähnlich**, } pest-like.
6297 **pestisch**, }
6298 **pockenähnlich**, } varioloid.
6299 **pockenartig**, }
6300 **primär**, primary.
6301 **quälend**, torturing.
6302 **qualvoll**, tormenting.
6303 **secundär**, symptomatic.
6304 **schleichend**, lingering, slow, insidious.
6305 **schnell**, quick, rapid.
6306 **schrecklich**, formidable.
6307 **schwer**, severe, hard.
6308 **selten**, rare.
6309 **serös**, serous.
6310 **seuchenartig**, epidemical.
6311 **simuliert**, feigned.
6312 **still**, quiet (as in delirium).
6313 **sympathetisch**, sympathetic (as headache).
6314 **tötlich**, deadly, fatal.
6315 **traumatisch**, traumatic.
6316 **übertragbar**, transferable.
6317 **unaufhörlich**, incessant.
6318 **unbedeutend**, unimportant.
6319 **ungefährlich**, undangerous.
6320 **ungemein**, uncommon.
6321 **unheilbar**, incurable.
6322 **verzweifelt**, desperate, incurable.
6323 **vorgeblich**, feigned, pretended, etc.
6324 7. a. **Der SCHMERZ, mag sein**: The pain may be:
6325 **andauernd**, continuous, persistent.
6326 **auf und ab schieszend**, (from v. ir. schieszen, to shoot), shooting up and down.
6327 **ausgebreitet**, diffuse.
6328 **äuszerlich**, external.
6329 **ausstrahlend** (nach allen Seiten), radiating on all sides.
6330 **begränzt or beschränkt auf einen Nerven**, *limited* to one nerve.
6331 **blitzgleich**, lightning-like.
6332 **bohrend**, boring.
6333 **brennend**, burning.
6334 **chronisch**, chronic.
6335 **constant**, } continuous.
6336 **dauernd**, }
6337 **dumpf**, dull.
6338 **drückend**, oppressive, pressing.
6339 **erschöpfend**, exhaustive.
6340 **fliegend**, flying, rushing.
6341 **fast unerträglich**, almost intolerable.
6342 **gelinde**, } light.
mild, }
6343 **gering**, slight.
6344 **hämmernd**, hammering.
6345 **hartnäckig**, stubborn, obstinate.
6346 **heftig**, violent.
6347 **innerlich**, internal.
6348 **intensiv**, intensive.
6349 **intermittierend**, intermittent.
6350 **klopfend**, beating, pulsating.
6351 **kneifend**, pinching.
6352 **kneipend**, griping.
6353 **kolikartig**, colic-like.
6354 **krampfähnlich**, } spasmodic, convulsive.
6355 **krampfartig**, }
6356 **krampfhaft**, }
6357 **kribbelnd**, itching.
6358 **kritisch**, critical.
6359 **lancinierend**, lancinating.
6360 **lokal**, local.
6361 **lokalisiert**, localized.
6362 **markiert**, marked.
6363 **marternd**, racking, torturing.
6364 **nagend**, gnawing.
6365 **nervös**, nervous.
6366 **neuralgisch**, neuralgic.
6367 **oberflächlich**, superficial.
6368 **perniciös**, pernicious.
6369 **plötzlich**, sudden.
6370 **quälend**, } torturing.
6371 **qualvoll**, }
6372 **reisend**, tearing.
6373 **reizend**, } irritating.
irritierend, }

6374 **scharf**, sharp.
6375 **schneidend**, cutting.
6376 **spannend**, straining.
6377 **stechend**, pungent.
6378 **symptomatisch**, symptomatic.
6379 **unregelmäszig**, irregular.
6380 **variierend an Intensität**, varying in intensity.
6381 **vermehrt durch**, augmented by.
6382 **vermehrt durch Berührung**, intensified by touch.
6383 **vermehrt durch Druck**, intensified by pressure.
6384 **vermehrt durch Geräusch**, intensified by noise or sound.
6385 **vermehrt durch Paroxysmen**, intensified by paroxysms.
6386 **verstärkt**, exalted.
6387 **ziehend**, pulling or drawing.
6388 **zuckend**, jerking, quivering, twitching.
6389 **zusammenschnierend**, constricting.
6390 **zwickend**, griping, pinching, etc.
6391 b. **WAS der SCHMERZ sein mag:** What the pain may be:
6392 **Augenschmerz**, m. 1. pain in the eyes.
6393 **Backennervenschmerz**, m. 1. neuralgia of the cheek.
6394 **Bauchschmerz**, m. 1. gastralgia, gripes.
6395 **Unterbauchschmerz**, m. 1. hypogastralgia.
6396 **Beckenschmerz**, m. 1. pelvic pain.
6397 **Blasenschmerz**, m. 1. pain in the bladder.
6398 **Brustbeinschmerz**, m. 1. pain in or about the sternum.
6399 **Brustschmerz**, m. 1. pain in the chest.
6400 **Brustschnupfen**, m. 2. cold in the chest.
6401 **Darmschmerz**, m. 1. colic, gripes, pain in the bowels.
6402 **Drüsenschmerz**, m. 1. adenalgia.
6403 **Gebärmutterschmerz**, m. 1. uterine pain, hysteralgia.
6404 **Gebärwehen**, pl. n. 1. } labor pains.
6405 **Geburtsschmerzen**, pl. m. 1. } labor pains.
6406 **Geburtswehen**, pl. n. 1. } labor pains.
6407 **Gelenkbänderschmerz**, m. 1. pain in the ligaments of a joint, desmalgia.
6408 **Gelenkschmerz**, m. 1. arthralgia.
6409 **Genickschmerz**, m. 1. pain in the neck.
6410 **Gichtschmerz**, m. 1. gout pain, arthritic pain.
6411 **Gichtleiden**, n. 2. gout, gouty affection.
6412 **Gliederschmerz**, m. 1. arthralgia, violent joint pain, gout, rheumatism.
6413 **Gliederweh**, n. 1. joint pain, gout, rheumatism.
6414 ——, **hitziges**, acute polyarticular rheumatism.
6415 **Gürtelschmerz**, m. 1. sense of a painful band around the body (as in tabes, etc.)
6416 **Halsschmerz**, m. 1. pain in the neck, sore throat.
6417 **Harnblasenschmerz**, m. 1. pain in the bladder.
6418 **Harnleiterschmerz**, m. 1. pain in the ureter.
6419 **Harnröhrenschmerz**, m. 1. pain in the urethra.
6420 **Hauptschmerz**, m. 1. chief pain, headache.
6421 **Hautschmerz**, m. 1. cutaneous pain.
6422 **Hodenschmerz**, m. 1. testicular pain.
6423 **Höllenschmerz**, m. 1. excruciating pain.
6424 **Hüftgelenkschmerz**, m. 1. } pain in the hip-joint.
6425 **Hüftgelenkweh**, n. 1. } pain in the hip-joint.
6426 **Hüftschmerz**, m. 1. } sciatica, pain in the hip.
6427 **Hüftweh**, n. 1. } sciatica, pain in the hip.
6428 **Intermenstrualschmerz**, m. 1. intermenstrual pain.
6429 **Kinnbackenschmerz**, m. 1. neuralgia of the jaw.
6430 **Knieschmerz**, m. 1. } pain in the knee.
6431 **Knieweh**, n. 1. } pain in the knee.
6432 **Knochenschmerz**, m. 1. bone pain.
6433 **Kolikschmerz**, m. 1. colicky pain.
6434 **Kopfschmerz**, m. 1. headache.
6435 ——, **einseitiger** or **halbseitiger**, hemicrania.

6436 ——, **gastrischer**, headache arising from digestive disturbances.
6437 ——, **nervöser**, nervous headache.
6438 **Krebsschmerz**, m. 1. cancer pain.
6439 **Kreuzschmerzen**, pl. m. 1. } lumbago.
6440 **Kreuzweh**, n. 1. }
6441 **Leberschmerz**, m. 1. hepatalgia.
6442 **Leibschmerz**, m 1. } abdominal pain, colic, griping pain.
6443 **Leibweh**, n. 1. }
6444 **Leibschneiden**, n. 2. }
6445 **Leistenschmerz**. m. 1. groin pain.
6446 **Lendenschmerz**, m. 1. } lumbago, groin pain.
6447 **Lendenweh**, n. 1. }
6448 **Lungenschmerz**, m. 1. pain in the lung.
6449 **Magenschmerz**, m. 1. gastralgia, stomach pain.
6450 **epigastrischer Schmerz**, m. 1. epigastric pain.
6451 **hypogastrischer Schmerz**. m. 1. hypogastric pain.
6452 **Magengrubeschmerz**. m. 1. pain in the pit of the stomach.
6453 **Magen, verdorbener**, m. 2, stomach out of order.
6454 **Magen, überladen**, m. 2. overloaded stomach with food or drink.
6455 **Magenschwäche**, f. dyspepsia.
6456 **Milzschmerz**, m. 1. pain in splenic region.
6457 **Mittelschmerz**, m. 1. intermenstrual pain.
6458 **Mundschmerz**, m. 1. mouth pain.
6459 **Muskelschmerz**, m. 1. muscular pain.
6460 **Mutterschmerz**, m. 1. uterine pain, labor pain.
6461 **Nachgeburtwehen**, n. 1. pl. } after pains.
6462 **Nachwehen**, n. 1. pl. }
6463 **Nackenschmerz**, m. 1. neck pain.
6464 **Nasenschmerz**, m. 1. pain in the nose.
6465 **Nervenkopfschmerz**, m. 1. nervous headache.
6466 **Nervenschmerz**, m. 1. nerve pain, neuralgia.
6467 **Nierenschmerz**, m. 1. renal colic, nephralgia.
6468 **Ohrenschmerz**, m. 1. pain in the ear, otalgia.
6469 **Rippenschmerz**, m. 1. } costalgia, pleuralgia.
6470 **Rippenweh**, n. 1. }
6471 **Rückenmarkschmerz**, m. 1. myelalgia.
6472 **Rückenschmerz**, m. 1. pain in the back, spinal neuralgia.
6473 **Rückenweh**, n. 1. } pain in the spine.
6474 **Rückgratsschmerz**, m. 1. }
6475 **Rückgratweh**, n. 1. }
6476 **Scheidenschmerz**, m. 1. vaginal pain.
6477 **Schenkelschmerz**, m. 1. pain in the thigh.
6478 **Schluckschmerzen**, m. 1. pl. pain in swallowing, dysphagia.
6479 **Schulterschmerz**, m. 1. shoulder - o m a l g i a or shoulder pain.
6480 **Wadenschmerz**. m. 1. pain in the calves of the leg.
6481 **Wasserbrennen**, n. 2. scalding (sensation) in urinating.
6482 **Zahnschmerzen**, pl. m. 1. toothache.
6483 **Zungenschmerz**, m. 1. pain in the tongue, etc.
6484 8. **TOD**, m. 1. death, in compounds:
6485 **todähnlich**, adj. death-like.
6486 **Todesahnung**, f. anticipation of death.
6487 **Todesanzeichen**, n. 2. sign of death.
6488 **Todesanzeige**, f. obituary notice.
6489 **Todesbericht**, m. 1. mortality report.
6490 **Todesfall**, m. 1. case of death.
6491 **Todesgabe**, f. fatal dose (from v. ir. geben, to give.)
6492 **Todesgefahr**, f. danger of death.
6493 **Todeskampf**, m. 1. death struggle.
6494 **Todespein**, f. } death agony or pain.
Todesqual, }
6495 **Todesschlaf**, m. 1. deathsleep.

8

6496 **Todesursache**, f. cause of death.
6497 **Todeswunde**, f. death wound.
6498 **todkrank**, adj. fatally or mortally sick.
6499 **tödlich**, adj. deadly, fatal, mortal.
6500 **Tödlickkeit**, f. deadliness, mortality.
6501 **tot**, adj. dead, inanimate.
6502 **Tote**, m. 3. and f. a dead person.
6503 **totenähnlich**. adj. like the dead.
6504 **Totenbeschau**, f. } official inspection of a dead person.
Totenschau, f.
6505 **Totenbeschauer**, m. 2. medical inspector of the dead (from beschauen, to behold, inspect.)
6506 **Totenbestattung**, f. burial, interment.
6507 **Totenschein**, m. 1. death certificate.
6508 **Totenstarre**, f. rigor mortis.
6509 **Totenverbrennung**, f. cremation.
6510 **totgeboren**, adj. still-born.
6511 **Totschlag**, m. 1. homicide, manslaughter.
6512 **Scheintod**, m. 1. apparent death.
6513 **scheintot**, adj. apparently dead, etc.

§ 29. Various compounds in:

6514 1. **BRAND**, m. 1. (from v. ir.
6515 **brennen**. to burn), gangrene, mortification, necrosis, sphacelus.
6516 **Brand**, feuchter or heiszer, moist, hot or acute gangrene;
6517 **Brand**, kalter or trockener, cold, dry or chronic gangrene.
6518 **Brandader**. f. crural vein.
6519 **Brandbeule**, f. carbuncle.
6520 **Brandbeulenseuche**, f. anthrax.
6521 **Brandblase**, f. blister caused by burn, gangrenous bulba.
6522 **Brandblatter**, f. blister, malignant pustule.
6523 **Brandfieber**, n. 2. inflammatory fever, suppurative fever.
6524 **Brandflecken**, m. 2. gangrenous spot; burn, scald.
6525 **Brandgas**, n. 1. gas produced in gangrene.
6526 **Brandgeschwür**, n. 1. gangrenous ulcer.
6527 **Brandherd**, m. 1. centre of a burn, as by acids.
6528 **Brandhof**, m. 1. areola of a burn.
6529 **brandig**, adj. gangrenous.
Brandigwerden, n. 2. the becoming gangrenous.
6530 **Brandjauche**, f. foul sanies.
6531 **Brandmal**, n. 1. vascular naevus.
6532 **Brandpilze**, m. 1. pl. ustilagineae, blightrust.
6533 **Brandrose**, f. gangrenous erysipelas.
6534 **Brandsalbe**, f. ointment for burns, Carron oil.
6535 **Brandschorf**, m. 1. dry or white gangrene, eschar, scab.
6536 **Brandschwär**, m. 1. carbuncle, anthrax.
6537 **Brandseuche**, f. ergotism.
6538 **Brandstiftungstrieb**, m. 1. impulse to incendiarism.
Brandstiftungswut, f. rage for incendiarism.
6539 **Brandverletzung**, f. injury by burning, etc.
6540 2. **EITER**, m. 2. } pus, ichor (from jauchen, to suppurate) ichor, sanies.
6541 **Jauche**, f. }
6542 **Eiter**, m. 2, bösartiger, (lit. malicious kind) ichor, sanies.
6543 **Eiterabflusz**, m. 1. } pus discharge or pus evacuation.
6544 **Eiterabgang**, m. 1. }
6545 **Eiterablagerung**, f. depositing of pus, deposit of pus.
6546 **eiterabsetzen**, } to suppurate.
6547 **eiteransetzen**, }
6548 **Eiteransammlung**, f. pus collection.
6549 **eiterartig**, adj. } purulent, puriform, ichorous, sanious.
ichorös, adj.
6550 **jauchеartig**, adj.
jauchicht, adj.
jauchig, adj.
6551 **Eiteraufnahme**, f. } absorption of pus (from v. ir.
Jaucheaufnahme, f. }
6552 **aufnehmen**, to receive. absorp.)
6553 **Eiterauge**, n. 1. hypopion or hypopyon.

6554 **Eiterausflusz**, m. 1. evacuation of pus (from v. ir.
6555 **ausflieszen**, to flow out.)
6556 **Eiterauswurf**, m. 1. throwing up of pus, discharge of pus (from v. ir.
6557 **auswerfen**, to throw out.)
6558 **Eiterbakterium**, n. 1. suppuration, bacterium, streptococcus pyogenes.
6559 **Eiterbalg**, m. 1. abscess sac, pyogenic membrane.
6560 **Eiterband**, n. 1. seton.
6561 **Eiterbecken**, n. 2. porringer.
6562 **eiterbefördernd**, adj. suppurative.
6563 **Eiterbeule**, f. abscess, boil, pustule.
6564 **eiterbildend**, adj. forming pus, promoting suppuration.
6565 **Eiterbildung**, f.
6566 **Jauchung**, f. } formation of pus, suppuration, suppuration.
6567 **Eiterbläschen**, n. 2.
Eiterblase, f.
6568 **Eiterblatter**, f. } pustule, impetigo.
6569 **Eiterbrechen**, n. 2. vomiting pus.
6570 **Eiterbrust**, f. empyema.
6571 **Eiterbutzen**, m. 2. core of an abscess or boil.
6572 **Eiterdurchbruch**, m. 1. (from v. ir.
6573 **——durchbrechen**, to break through), bursting through of pus.
6574 **Eiterentleerung**, f. evacuation of pus.
6575 **Eitererbrechen**, n. 2. pus vomiting.
6576 **Eiterergusz**, m. 1. (from v. ir.
6577 **ergieszen**, to effuse), purulent effusion, empyema.
6578 **eitererzeugend**, adj. producing pus, pyogenic, suppurative.
6579 **Eiterfieber**, n. 2 suppurative fever.
6580 **Eiterflechte**, f. impetigo.
6581 **Eiterflusz**, m. 1. discharge of pus, suppuration.
6582 **Eiterflüssigkeit**, f. serum of pus.
6583 **eiterförmig**, adj.
6584 **eiterhaft**, adj.
6585 **eiterig**, adj. } puriform, purulent.
6586 **Eiterfrasz**, m. 1. (from v. ir.
6587 **fressen**, to eat, consume), corrosion caused by an ulcer.
6588 **Eitergang**, m. 1. sinus.
6589 **Eitergelenk**, n. 1. joint abscess.
6590 **Eitergeschwulst**, f. abscess.
6591 **Eitergeschwür**, n. 1. suppurating ulcer.
6592 **Eitergift**, n. 1. the pus virus.
6593 **Eitergrind**, m. 1. impetigo.
6594 **Eiterharnen**, n. 2. pus in the urine.
6595 **Eiterherd**, m. 1. suppurative focus.
6596 **Eiterhöhle**, f. abscess cavity, vomica.
6597 **Eiterhusten**, m. 2. cough with pus discharge.
6598 **Eiterjauche**, f. ichor.
6599 **Eiterkettencoccus**, m. 1. streptococcus pyogenes.
6600 **Eiterklümpchen**, n. 2.
6601 **Eiterklumpen**, m. 2. } concretion of pus.
6602 **Eiterknoten**, m. 2. purulent focus or collection.
6603 **Eiterkokken**, m. 2. pl. pus cocci.
6604 **Eiterkörperchen**, n. 2. pus corpuscle.
6605 **Eiterkügelchen**, n. 2. pus globule.
6606 **eitermachend**, adj. suppurative.
6607 **Eitermenge**, f. amount or quantity of pus.
6608 **eitern**, to fester, to suppurate, to come to a head.
6609 **Eiternabel**, m. 2. sore navel, empyomphalus.
6610 **eiternd**, adj. suppurating.
6611 **Eiterpfropf**, m. 1. core of a boil or abscess.
6612 **Eitersack**, m. 1. abscess cavity, vomica, pyogenic membrane.
6613 **Eiterschale**, f. porringer.
6614 **Eiterschicht**, f. layer of pus.
6615 **Eiterschnur**, f. seton.
6616 **Eitersenkung**, f. furrowing of pus.
6617 **Eiterserum**, n. 1. serum of pus.
6618 **Eiterspeien**, n. 2. expectoration of pus.
6619 **Eiterstauung**, f. purulent infarct.
6620 **Eiterstock**, m. 1. core of a boil or abscess.
6621 **Eiterstoff**, m. 1. pus.

6622 **Eitertraubencoccus**, m. 1. staphylococcus pyogenes.
6623 **Eiterung**, f. } suppuration.
Vereiterung, f. }
6624 **Eiterung**, f. epitheliale or oberflächliche, epithelial or superficial suppuration.
6625 **EITERUNG**, tiefe or parenchymatöse, deep or parenchymatous suppuration.
6626 **Eiterungsfieber**, n. 2. suppurative fever.
6627 **eiterungsgiftig**, adj. virulent.
6628 **Eiterungsmittel**, n. 2. suppurative.
6629 **Eiterverbreitung**, f. spreading of pus, purulent metastasis.
6630 **Eitervergiftung**, f. pyaemia.
6631 **Eiterwasser**, n. 2. watery pus, ichor.
6632 **Eiterzelle**, f. pus corpuscle.
6633 **Eiterzersetzung**, f. pus decomposition, purulent decomposition.
6634 **Eiterziehen**, n. 2. to cause to suppurate.
6635 **eiterziehend**, adj. from v. ir. ziehen, to draw, suppurative, etc.
6636 3. **WUCHERN**, n. 2. (from
6637 **wuchern**, to grow exuberantly, to luxuriate, to proliferate), proliferation.
6638 **wuchernd**, adj. proliferating.
6629 **Wucherung**, f. proliferation.
6640 **Wucherungsgewebe**, n. 1. proliferation tissue.
6641 **Wucherungsherd**, m. 1. proliferation focus.
6642 **Wucherungsvorgang**, m. 1. process of proliferation, etc.
6643 4. **WULST**, f. tuberosity, elevation, eminence.
6644 **Wulstblätterschwamm**, m. 1. agaricus bulbosus (poisonous fungus).
6645 **wulstig**, adj. padded, swelled, tumid.
6646 **Wulstung**, f. puffiness, swelling (like Wulst).
6647 5. **WUNDE**, f. wound, bruise, injury.
6648 **wund**, adj. sore, wounded, raw, chafed, chapped.
6649 **Wundabsonderung**, f. wound secretion.
6650 **Wundarznei**, f. remedy for wounds.
6651 **Wundarzneikunst**, f. art of surgery.
6652 **Wundarzneilehre**, f. } science of surgery.
6653 **Wundarzneiwissenschaft**, f. }
6654 **wundarzneiwissenschaftlich**, adj. according to scientific surgery or the science of surgery.
6655 **wundarzneilich**, adj. } surgical.
6656 **wundärztlich**, adj. }
6657 **Wunddarzt**, m. 1. surgeon.
6658 **Wundbleiben**, n. 2. remaining sore.
6659 **Wundbrand**, m. 1. hospital gangrene.
6660 **Wunddeckverband**, m. 1. bandage to cover a wound.
6661 **Wundiphtherie**, f. hospital gangrene.
6662 **Wunddouche**, f. irrigator.
6663 **Wundeiterung**, f. wound suppuration.
6664 **wundenfrei**, adj. uninjured, unwounded.
6665 **wundenheilend**, adj. wound-healing.
6666 **Wundenmal**, n. 1. scar of a wound.
6667 **Wundfäulnis**, f. hospital gangrene.
6668 **Wundfieber**, n. 2. traumatic fever.
6669 **Wundfläche**, f. wound surface.
6670 **Wundflüssigkeit**, f. discharge from a wound.
6671 **Wundhacken**, m. 2. blunt-hook, wound-hook.
6672 **Wundheilung**, f. healing of a wound.
6673 ——, **mittelbare**, healing by second intention.
6674 ——, **unmittelbare**, healing by first intention.
6675 **Wundheilungsverlauf**, m. 1. process of healing.
6676 **Wundliegen**, n. 2, bed-sore (soreness from lying in bed).
6677 **Wundlippe**, f. wound lip.
6678 **Wundmittel**, n. 2. remedy for wounds.
6679 **Wundnadel**, f. suture needle.
6680 **Wundnarbe**, f. scar by a wound.
6681 **wundennarbig**, adj. cicatrized, cicatricial.

6682 **Wundpflaster**, n. 2. adhesive plaster.
6683 **Wundrand**, m. 1. margin, edge of a wound.
6684 **Wundreinigungsmittel**, n. 2. anticeptic, a wound cleaning remedy.
6685 **Wundrose**, f. traumatic erysipelas.
6686 **Wundschorfverband**, m. 1. dressing of wounds by artificial scab, as applied to Liester's first anticeptic dressing.
6687 **Wundsein**, n. 1. abrasion, excoriation, chafe, intertrigo.
6688 **Wundspalte**, f. cleft of a wound.
6689 **Wundspritze**, f. syringe for washing wounds.
6690 **Wundstar**, m. 1. traumatic cataract.
6691 **Wundstarrkrampf**, m. 1. traumatic tetanus.
6692 **Wundtrichter**, m. 2. the funnel-like track of a deep wound.
6693 **Wundverlauf**, m. 1. course of a wound.
6694 **Wundwatte**, f. wadding for wounds (e. g. in compressions).
6695 **Wund-winkel**, m. 2. angle of a wound, etc.
6696 **Brandwunde**, f. burn, scald.
6697 **Fleischwunde**, f. flesh-wound.
6698 **Herzwunde**, f. wound of the heart.
6699 **Hiebwunde**, f. gash caused by a blow.
6700 **Knochenwunde**, f. wound or injury of bone.
6701 **Meiselwunde**, f. wound produced by a chisel.
6702 **Querwunde**, f. transverse wound, wound dressed with a pledget.
6703 **Quetschwunde**, f. contused wound.
6704 **Riszwunde**, f. lacerated wound (from v. ir.
6705 **reiszen** to tear).
6706 **Schnittverletzung**, f. } incised wound.
6707 **Schnittwunde**, f. }
6708 **Schröpfwunde**, f. (from schröpfen, to scarify), wound made by scarification through
6709 **Schröpfer**, m. 2. **Schröpfschnäpper**, m. 2. or **Schröpfschnepper**, m. 2. } scarificator.
6710 **Schuszwunde**, f. (from v. ir.
6711 **schieszen**, to shoot), gunshot-wound.
6712 **Stichverletzung**, f. } punctured wound.
6713 **Stichwunde**, f. }
6714 **Todeswunde**, f. mortal wound, death wound.
6715 **Verwundung**, f. } (from **Läsion**, f. }
6716 **verwunden**, to wound), wounding, hurting, lesion.
6717 **verletzbar**, adj. vulnerable.
6718 **Verletzbarkeit**, f. } (from **Verletzlichkeit**, f. }
6719 **verletzen**, to hurt, injure, wound), vulnerability.
6720 **verletzlich**, adj. vulnerable.
6721 **Verletzung**, f. } injury, wound, **Läsion**, f. } lesion, etc.
6722 6. **CHARAKTERISTIK DER WUNDEN** characteristic of wounds.
6723 **Eine Wunde mag sein**: A wound may be:
6724 **assimilierend**, assimilating.
6725 **blutend**, bleeding.
6726 **besorgt**, cured for.
6727 **compliciert**, complicated.
6728 **einfach**, simple.
6729 **eiternd**, suppurating.
6730 **entzündet**, inflamed.
6731 **fressend**, ulcerating.
6732 **geätzt**, cauterized.
6733 **gebäht**, fomented.
6734 **gereinigt**, cleaned, purified.
6735 **granulierend**, granulating.
6736 **heilend**, healing.
6737 **klaffend**, gaping (from
6738 **klaffen**, to gape).
6739 **länglich**, longitudinal.
6740 **oberflächlich**, superficial.
6741 **penitrierend**, penetrating.
6742 **purulent**, purulent, suppurative.
6743 **quer**, transverse, diagonal, oblique.
6744 **schief**, oblique.
6745 **schlimm**, bad, very sore.
6746 **schmerzlich**, painful.
6747 **schrunded**, } (from **schrundig**, }
6748 **schrunden**, to split, crack), chapped, e. g., cracked lips.

6749 **schwürig**, ulcerous, suppurating.
6750 **sickernd**, oozing, trickling, (from
6751 **sickern**, to ooze).
6752 **sondiert**, (from
6753 **sondieren**, to probe, sound), probed.
6754 **tief**, deep.
6755 **tödlich or tötlich**, fatal.
6756 **unterbunden**, (from
6757 **unterbinden**, to bandage), bandaged, ligated.
6758 **unterlaufen**, (e. g. mit Blut) (from
6759 **unterlaufen** to run under), suffused (e. g. with blood).
6760 **untersucht**, examined.
6761 **verbunden**, (from
6762 **verbinden**, to dress, unite), dressed, united.
6763 **vergifted** (from
6764 **vergiften**, to poison), poisoned.
6765 **verjaucht**, (from verjauchen, to form putrid or ichorous pus), decomposed, putrified.
6766 **vernarbt**, cicatriced.
6767 **vernäht**, united by suture.
6768 **verklebt**, overspread by adhesive plaster.
6769 **verschwollen** (from v. ir.
6770 **schwellen**, to swell), swollen or closed by swelling.
6771 **verwachsen** (from v. ir.
6772 **verwachsen**, to grow over, heal up), grown over.
6773 **zerteilt**, divided, by resolution effected.
6774 **zusammengezogen**, (from v. ir.
6775 **zusammenziehen**, to contract, to draw together), contracted, etc.
6776 **§30 der ALLGEMEINZUSTAND eines PATIENTEN.**
6777 1. The Patient's general condition.
Der Patient mag, the patient may :
6778 **gehen**, v. ir. walk : go.
6779 **liegen**, v. ir. lie.
6780 **sitzen**, v. ir. sit.
6781 **stehen**, v. ir. stand.
6782 **sterben**, v. ir die, etc., or may be :
6783 **gehend**, walking, going,
6784 **liegend**, lying.
6785 **sitzend**, sitting.
6786 **stehend**, standing.
6787 **sterbend**, dying, etc.
6788 **(a) Sein Gang**, m. 1. (from **gehen, to walk**), gait, walk, may be :
6789 **beschwerlich**, laborious.
6790 **hinkend**, limping, hoppling.
6791 **lahm**, lame, halting.
6792 **mühsam**, painful.
6793 **rüstig**, brisk.
6794 **schnell**, quick.
6795 **schwankend**, staggering.
6796 **sicher**, steady
6797 **steif**, stiff.
6798 **stolpernd**, stumbling.
6799 **taumelig**, **taumelnd**, reeling, tottering.
6800 **ungleich**, uneven.
6801 **unsicher**, unsteady.
6802 **wackelig**, **wackelnd**, shaky.
6803 **zitternd**, trembling, etc.
6804 **(b) Seine Lage**, f. (from v. ir.
6805 **liegen**, to lie) position, posture, attitude may be :
6806 **aufrecht**, e. g.
6807 **sitzend**, (from v. ir.
6808 **sitzen**, to sit), sitting upright, etc.
6809 **ausgestreckt**, e. g.
6810 **liegend**, (from v. ir.
6811 **liegen**, to lie), (from
6812 **ausstrecken**, to stretch out, extend) e. g. mit **ausgestreckten**.
6813 **Gliedern auf dem Sofa, auf** or in **dem Bette**, etc., lying with outstretched limbs on the sofa, on or in bed, etc.
6814 **eingezogen**, (from v. ir.
6815 **einziehen**, to draw in) retracted, drawn in.
6816 **gebeugt**, (from v. ir. & refl. sich
6817 **beugen**, to bend), bent.
6818 **gebückt**, (from v. ir. & refl. sich
6819 **bücken**, to bow, bend, e. g. by rheumatism, etc.,) bowed bent, etc.
6820 (c) The Patient may be :
6821 **beraubt**, (from
6822 **berauben**, to deprive, to rob), deprived, e. g. **der**
6823 **Kraft sich zu bewegen**, deprived of the power to move;
6824 **sich vom**
6825 **Bett or vom**
6826 **Stuhle zu**

(118)

6827 **erheben**, deprived of the power to raise himself from the bed or from the chair, etc., der
6828 **Mittel zur**
6829 **Erhaltung**, deprived of the means for existence, etc.
6830 **ebenbürtig**, of equal birth; enjoying equal rights or privileges, etc.
6831 **erschlafft**, } e. g. durch
6832 **erschöpft**, }
6833 **krankhafte**,
6834 **Zuckungen der**
6835 **Muskeln**, relaxed, enervated, exhausted by convulsive movements of the muscles, etc.
6836 **gebunden**, (from v. ir.
6837 **binden**, to bind), bound, e. g. in **einer** and **derselben Lage liegen zu bleiben),** to be bound to remain lying in one and the same position, etc.
6838 **niedergedrückt**, (from
6839 **nieder drücken**, to press down, prostrate), depressed.
6840 **niedergeschlagen**, (from v. ir.
6841 **niederschlagen**, to beat down) to be depressed.
6842 **schlafsüchtig**, } comatose, lethargic, given to
6843 **lethargisch**, } sleep or stupor.
6844 **schreiend**, (from v. ir.
6845 **schreien**, to cry, shriek, scream), e. g. aus
6846 **Leibeskräften schreien or aufschreien in der Nacht or im Schlaf or vor Angst vor Freude, vor Schrecken vor Schmerzen**, etc., to cry or to scream with all might at night or in sleep for fear, for joy, for terror, for pain, etc.
6847 **sich schneuzen**, to blow one's nose.
6848 **sich unruhig hin and herwerfen**, to throw one's self in restlessness hither and thither, etc.
6849 (d) **Die Beschwerde oder Krankheit mag sein**, the affection or disease may be:
6850 **Abgeschlagenheit**, f. (fr. v. ir.
6851 **abschlagen**, to refuse, defeat, repulse), dejection, depression.
6852 **Abmagerung**, f. emaciation.
6853 **Abnahme**, f. (from v. ir.
6854 **abnehmen**, to decrease), decreasing, e. g. decreasing in weight.
6855 **an Gewicht abnehmen**.
6856 **Abneigung**, f. (from
6857 **abneigen**, to turn aside from), antipathy, disinclination.
6858 **Abspannung**, f. (from
6859 **abspannen**, to relax), languor, e. g. in the face.
6860 **Abzehrung**, f. (from
6861 **abzehren**, to waste), emaciation.
6862 **Alpdrücken**, n. 2. (from
6863 **drücken**, to press), lit. the feeling of pressure like the weight of an Alp., nightmare.
6864 **Altersschwäche**, f. decrepitude, senile tremor.
6865 **Aufgeblasenheit**, f. puffiness (from v. ir.
6866 **aufblasen**, to inflate, swell, blow up).
6867 **Aufgedunsenheit**, f. turgescence (from
6868 **aufdunsen**, to be swelled, puffed up).
6869 **Auszehrung**, f. consumption (from
6870 **auszehren**, to consume, emaciate).
6871 **Besinnungslosigkeit**, f. senselessness.
6872 **Berauschung**, f. drunkenness, intoxication.
6873 **Betäubung**, f. insensibility, stupor (from
6874 **betäuben**, to stun, stupify).
6875 **Betrunkenheit**, f. intoxication, inebriation.
6876 **Bewustlosigkeit**, f. stupor, unconsciousness.
6877 **Blutgeschwür**, n. 1. furuncle.
6878 **Coma**, n. 1. } Coma, pre-
Anlage von - disposition
Schlafsucht, f. } to sleep.
6879 **Delirium**, n. 1. delirium (from
6880 **delirieren**, to rave, to be delirious).
6881 **Dickleibigkeit**, f. corpulency.
6882 **Doppelsehen**, n. 2. double vision.
6883 **Eiterbeule**, f. abscess.
6884 **Eiterbläschen**, n. 2. pustule, blister, pimple.
6885 **Eiterblase**, f. carbuncle.

6886 **Epilepsie**, f. } epilepsy, falling sickness.
6887 **Fallsucht**, f. }

6888 **Ekzem**, n. 1. eczema.

6889 **Elefantenaussatz**, m. 1. Elefantiasis Graecorum, lepra nodosa.

6890 **Elephantenkrankheit**, f. Elephantiasis Arabum.

6891 **Ermattung**, f. exhaustion, lassitude.

6892 **Ermüdung**, f. weariness, lassitude.

6893 **Ermüdungszustand**, m. 1. state of fatigue.

6994 **Erschlaffung**, f. relaxation, debility, laxity.

6895 **Erschöpftheit**, f. } exhaustion, faintness, state of exhaustion.
6896 **Erschöpfung**, f. }
6897 **Erschöpfungszustand**, m. 1. }

6898 **Fettleibigkeit**, f. obesity, corpulence.

6899 **Fleckensehen**, n. 2. fancied seeing of black spots.

6900 **Fliegensehen**, n. 2. seeing of flies, muscae volitantes.

6901 **Flockensehen**, n. 2. seeing of flakes.

6902 **Funkensehen**, n. 2. seeing of sparks.

6903 **Gefühlsbeklemmung**, f. feeling of discomfort.

6904 **Gefühlslähmung**, f. paralysis of sensation.

6905 **Gefühllosigkeit**, f. insensibility.

6906 **Gefühlsnervenstörung**, f. disturbance of sensory nerves.

6907 **Gehörtäuschung**, f. delusion or deception of hearing, e. g.

6908 **Ohrenbrausen**, n. 2. } buzzing in the ear, tinnitus aurium.
6909 **Ohrenklingen**, n. 2. }
Ohrenringen, n. 2. }
6910 **Ohrensausen** n. 2. }
6911 **Ohrensingen**, n. 2. }
6912 **Ohrentönen**, n. 2. }

6913 **Geistesstumpfheit**. f. dulness of intellect.

6914 **Geistesträgheit**, f. torpor, intellectual indolence.

6915 **Gemütsaufregung**, f. } mental excitement.
6916 **Gemütsbewegung**, f. }

6917 **Geruchphantasie**, f. olfactory sensation or impression.

6918 **Geschmackstäuschung**, f. deception of taste.

6919 **Geschwulst**, f. swelling, f. tumor, excrescence.

6920 **Geschwür**, n. 1. abscess, boil, ulcer.

6921 **Halbsehen**, n. 2. seeing only half an object.

6922 **Hallucinationen**, f. pl. hallucinations, illusions.

6923 **Hautröte**, f. erythema, with burning and itching.

6924 **Heiserkeit**, f. hoarseness.

6925 **Hemiopie**, f. seeing only half.

6926 **Kurzsichtigkeit**, f. shortsightedness.

6927 **Lethargie**, f. stupor, lethargy.

6928 **Mückensehen**, n. 2. seeing of gnats.

6929 **Muskelzucken**, n. 2. muscular tremor or jerking.

6930 **Narkosie**, f. narcosis, torpor, illusion, paralysis.

6931 **Notzucht**, f. rape by violence.

6932 **Raserei**, f. frenzy (from rasen, to rave.)

6933 **Säuferwahnsinn**, m. 1. madness of drunkards.

6934 **Schlaflosigkeit**, f. insomnia, sleeplessness.

6935 **Schläfrigkeit**, f. drowsiness, sleepiness.

6936 **Schlafscheu**, f. dread of sleep, hypnophobia.

6937 **Schlafsucht**, f. coma, hypnosis, lethargy.

6938 **Schlaftrunkenheit**. f. sleepiness.

6939 **Schlafwandeln**, n. 2. } somnambulism, (from
Somnambulismus, m. 1. }

6940 **wandeln**, to walk about in sleep.)

6941 **Sinnlichkeit**, f. sensuality.

6942 **Sinnesstörungen**, f. pl. } illusions, deception of the senses.
6943 **Sinnestäuschungen**, f. pl. }

6944 **Sklerose**, f. (from

6945 **sklerosieren**, to harden) sclerosis, hardening of a part or organ, as in tympanic cavity of the ear.

6946 **Spinnensehen**, n. 2. from Spinne, f. spider, seeing of spiders.

6947 **Stimmbeschwerde**, f. voice affection.

Note 1. **Die Stimme**, f. voice, mag

6948 **klingen**, may sound:
6949 **erloschen**, lost (from v. ir.
6950 **erlöschen**, to go out, lit. and fig. to be extinguished.)
6951 **fremdartig**, strangely.
6952 **gebrochen**, broken (from v. ir.
6953 **brechen**, to break.)
6954 **heiszer**, hoarse.
6955 **laut**, loud.
6956 **leise**, soft, whispering.
6957 **näselnd**, nasal, speaking through the nose (from
6958 **näseln**, to snuffle), snuffling.
6959 **rauh**, husky.
6960 **schwach**, weak, faint, etc.
6961 **Stimmung**, f. (from
6962 **stimmen**, to tune), disposition, frame of mind, humor, temper.
6963 **Die Stimmung mag sein**, may be:
6964 **erregt**, irritated in temper, etc.
6965 **gedrückt, niedergedrückt**, depressed in spirits.
6966 **gereizt**, peevish (temper.)
6967 **gute or böse, üble**, good or ill humor, etc.
6968 **Stumpfsinn**, m. 1. } **Stumpfsinnigkeit**, f. } stupidity.
6969 **Taubheit**, f. deafness (from taub, deaf.)
6970 **Taubstummheit**, f. being deaf and dumb.
6971 **Tollheit**, f. }
6972 **Tollsucht**, f. } folly, madness, lunacy, frency, insanity.
6973 **Tollwut**, f. }
6974 **Träumerei**, f. (from
6975 **träumen**, to dream), dreaming, hallucination.
6976 **Triefauge**, n. 1. (from
6977 **triefen**, to drip, to trickle), water flowing from the eyes.
6978 **Tripper**, m. 2. gonorrhoea.
6979 **Tripperkrampf**, m. 1. chordee.
6980 **Trübsinn**, m. 1. dejection, melancholy.
6981 **Übelbefinden**, n. 2. }
6982 **Übelkeit**, f. } indisposition, nausea, being unwell.
6983 **Unwohlsein**, n. 1. }
6984 **Ungeziefer**, n. 2. vermin, see *Würmer* below.
6985 **Verwirrung**, f. }
6986 **Verworrenkeit**, f. } (from v. ir.
6987 **verwirren**, to confuse, to entangle.) confusion, disorder.
6988 **Wahnsinn**, m. 1. madness, insanity.
6989 **Würmer**, m. 1. pl. worms (see Appendix below).
6990 **Zunahme**, f. (from v. ir.
6991 **zunehmen**, to increase, e. g.
6992 ——, **an Gewicht**, to increase in weight.
6993 **Zitterwahnsinn**, m. 1. { madness of drunkards, delirium tremens.
6994 **Appendix**. *Ungeziefer* und *Würmer*, vermin and worms, e. g.
6995 **Askariden**, f. pl. ascarides.
6996 **Bandwurm**, m. 1. tapeworm.
6997 **Binnenwürmer**, m. 1. pl. (from
6998 **binnen**, inner), entocoa.
6999 **Bundwürmer**, m. 1. pl. ascarides.
7000 **Eingeweidenwürmer**, m. 1. pl. {
7001 **Helminthen**, pl. { helminths, small worms living in various parts of the body.
7002 **Fadenwurm**, m. 1. threadworm.
7003 **Finnenwurm**, m. 1. cysticerous cellulosae.
7004 **Floh**, m. 1. flea.
7005 **Hautwurm**, m. 1. skinworm, farcy.
7006 **Helminthen**, pl. intestinal worms.
7007 **Hülsenwurm**, m. 1. echinococcus.
7008 **Laus**, f. louse, pediculus.
7009 **Madenwurm**, m. 1. (from
7010 **Made**, maggot, mite.)
7011 **Mastdarmwurm**, m. 1. }
7012 **Springwurm**, m. 1. } oxyuris vermicularis.
7013 **madig**, adj. magotty, full of mites.
7014 **Parasit**, m. 3. }
7015 **Schmarotzer**, m. 2. } parasite.
7016 **schmarotzerisch**, adj. parasitic.
7017 **Schmarotzertier**, n. 1. animal parasite.
7018 **Peitschenwurm**, m. 1. guinea worm, tricocephalus dispar.
7019 **Plattwürmer**, m. 1. pl. flat worms, platodes.

7020 **Spulwurm**, m. 1. ascaris lumbricoides.
7021 **Trichine**, f. trichina.
7022 **Wanze**, f. bug, etc.

2. **APPETIT**, appetite.

7023 **Appetit**, m. 1.
7024, **Eszlust**, f. (lit. desire to eat.) } appetite.
7025 **Appetit** or **Eszlust haben** or **bekommen** (from v. ir.
7026 **bekommen**, to receive, get), to have or to get an appetite.
7027 **Ekel**, m. 2. disgust, distaste, nausea (from v.
7028 **ekeln**, to feel disgust, to nauseate).
7029 **Ekelgefühl**, n. 1. feeling of nausea, disgust, distaste.
7030 **ekelhaft**, adj. nauseous.
7031 **hungrig**, adj. hungry.
7032 **durstig**, adj. thirsty.
7033 **hungern**, to hunger.
7034 **hungrig** or **durstig sein** or **werden**, to be or to become hungry or thirsty, or to have or to get an appetite for food or for drink.
7035 **Hunger**, m. 2. hunger.
7036 **Durst**, m. 1. thirst.
7037 **Hunger** or **Durst befriedigen** or **stillen**, to stay the appetite, to appease, satisfy or set at rest; to satisfy the hunger and quench the thirst.
7038 **Hunger** or **Durst leiden** (lit. to suffer hunger or thirst), to hunger or to thirst.
7039 **sich berauschen**,
7040 **sich betrinken**, } to get drunk or intoxicated.
7041 **über Gebühr**, or **übermäszig essen** or **trinken**. } to eat or to drink to excess (above measure).
7042 **verschlucken (sich)**, to swallow the wrong way.
7043 **verschmachten**,
7044 **vor Hunger** or **vor Durst**, } to droop, to pine away, for hunger or for thirst, to starve or to die, etc.
7045 **Hungergefühl**, n. 1.
7046 **Durstgefühl**, n. 1. } feeling of hunger or thirst.
7047 **Hungerkur**, f. fasting cure.
7048 **Hungerpest**, f.
7049 **Hungertyphus**, m. 1. } relapsing fever.
7050 **Hungersnot**, f. famine.
7051 **Hungerstod**, m. 1. death from starvation.
7052 **Heiszhunger**, m. 2. morbid desire, craving for food (from
7053 **heisz**, hot).
7054 **hungern**, v. impers. to hunger, to be hungry, e. g. es hungert mich, I am hungry.
7055 **verhungern**, to famish, to starve.
7056 **appetitlich**, adj. exciting the appetite, nice, delicate.
7057 **Appetitabnahme**, f.
7058 **Appetitlosigkeit**, f. } want of appetite, decrease of appetite, anerexia.
7059 **Appetitverlust**, m. 1. loss of appetite (from v. ir.
7060 **verlieren**, to lose.
7061 **Appetitzunahme**, f. (from v. ir.
7062 **zunehmen**, to increase), increase of appetite, etc.
7063 Note: **Der Appetit mag sein:** The appetite may be:
7064 **abgeneigt**,
7065 **abneigend**, } repugnant, having a feeling of disgust for any or for a certain kind of food or drink.
7066 { **begierig**, **gierig**, } craving, ravenous.
7067 **beständig**, constant.
7068 **bitter**, bitter, having a bitter taste in the mouth.
7069 **capriciös**, capricious.
7070 **gereizt**, appetized, excited (from
7071 **reizen**, to irritate, excite).
7072 **gering**, small, feeble.
7073 **geschwächt**, blunted (from
7074 **schwächen**, to weaken).
7075 **gut**, good, hearty.
7076 **sehr gut**, very good.
7077 **ziemlich gut**, tolerably well.
7078 **launisch**, depraved, perverted.
7079 **mangelhaft**, deficient.
7080 **schwach**, weak.
7081 **stark**,
7082 **tüchtig**, } hearty, normal.
7083 **unaufhörlich**, constant, unceasing.
7084 **ungewöhnlich**, uncommon, unusual.

(122)

7085 **unstillbar,**
7086 **nimmersatt,** insatiable, craving for any or for some particular food, e. g. for acids or vegetables, or for drink and beverages; a morbid hunger and thirst.
7087 **vortrefflich,** excellent, etc.
7088 3. **Was die TEMPERATUR sein mag:** What the temperature may be:
7089 **Die Temperatur des Körpers mag:** The temperature of the body may:
7090 **abwechseln,** change, alternate, intermit.
7091 **fallen,**
7092 **herabgehen,** go down, decrease.
7093 **steigen (in die Höhe**
7094 **gehen),** rise.
7095 **allmählich,** gradually.
7096 **nach und nach,** by degrees.
7097 **plötzlich,** suddenly.
7098 **Grad,** m. 1. degree.
7099 **Kälte,** f. cold, coldness, chill.
7100 **Klima,** n. 1. (pl. Klimate) climate.
7101 **Kältegrad,** m. 1. degree of cold.
7102 **Wärme,** f. heat, warmth.
Wärmegrad, m. 1. degree of heat.
7103 **Wärmeabgabe,** f. (from v. ir. abgeben, to give away).
7104 **Wärmeausgabe,** f. (from v. ir.
7105 **ausgeben,** to give out), the quantity of heat lost, (from the body).
7106 **frösteln,** to be chilly, to shiver.
7107 **Frösteln,** n. 2. chill, shiver, shivering.
7108 **Frostschauer,** m. 2. shivering.
7109 **Hitze,** f. heat.
7110 **überlaufen,** v. ir. to run over, spread over, overspread, seize, e. g.:
7111 1. **Frostschauer und Hitze überlaufen den Patienten,** shivering and heat seize the patient.
7112 2. **Frösteln und Hitze wechseln ab,** chill and heat alternate, etc. In compounds:
7113 **Temperaturabnahme,** f. diminution of temperature.
7114 **Temperaturänderung,** f. change of temperature.
7115 **Temperaturempfindung,** f. sense of temperature.
7116 **Temperaturerhöhung,** f. rise of temperature.
7117 **Temperaturerniedrigung,** f. lowering of temperature.
7118 **Temperaturgefühl,** n. 1. sense of temperature.
7119 **Temperaturgrad,** m. 1. degree of temperature.
7120 **Temperaturschwankung,** f. oscillation of temperature.
7121 **Temperatursinn,** m. 1. sense of temperature.
7122 **Temperatursteigerung,** f. rise of temperature.
7123 **Temperaturverhältnis,** n. 1. state of temperature.
7124 § 31. The *names* of the *Diseases* in Compounds:
7125 **ABSCESZ,** m. 1. abscess.
7126 **Bauchfellabscesz,** m. 1. peritoneal abscess.
7127 **Beckenabscesz,** m. 1. pelvic abscess.
7128 **Drüsenabscesz,** m. 1. glandular abscess.
7129 **Gebärmutterabscesz,** m. 1. uterine abscess.
7130 **Gehirnabscesz,** m. 1. cerebral abscess.
7131 **Gelenkabscesz,** m. 1. joint abscess.
7132 **Herzabscesz,** m. 1. cardiac abscess.
7133 **Knochenabscesz,** m. 1. bone abscess.
7134 **Kongestionsabscesz,** m. 1. congestive abscess, burrowing abscess (e. g. psoas abscess).
7135 **Kopfabscesz,** m. 1. abscess of the head, (of the brain or scalp).
7136 **Kotabscesz,** m. 1. faecal abscess.
7137 **Leberabscesz,** m. 1. hepatic abscess.
7138 **Leistenabscesz,** m. 1. inguinal abscess.
7139 **Lendenabscesz,** m. 1. lumbar abscess.
7140 **Lippenabscesz,** m. 1. labial abscess.
7141 **Lungenabscesz,** m. 1. pulmonary abscess, vomica.
7142 **Magenabscesz,** m. 1. gastric abscess.

7143 **Mandelabscesz**, m. 1.
7144 **Mandeleitergeschwulst**, f. } abscess of the tonsil.
7145 **Milarabscesz**, m. 1. miliary abscess.
7146 **Milzabscesz**. m. 1. splenic abscess.
7147 **Nasenwinkelabscesz**, m. 1. lachrymal sac abscess.
7148 **Nierenabscesz**, m. 1. renal abscess.
7149 **Oberkieferhöhlenabscesz**, m. 1. abscess in antrum of Highmore.
7150 **Sackabscesz**, m. 1. encysted abscess.
7151 **Scheidenabscesz**, m. 1. thekal abscess.
7152 **Schlundabscesz**, m. 1. pharyngeal abscess.
7153 **Sehnenabscesz**, m. 1. thekal abscess.
7154 **Urinabscesz**, m. 1. urinary abscess.
7155 **Versenkungsabscesz**. m. 1. abscessus congestivus, burrowing abscess.
7156 **Wurmabscesz**, m. 1. worm abscess.
7157 **Zahnabscesz**, m. 1. dental abscess.
7158 **Zellenabscesz**, m. 1. suppuration of cellular tissue, etc.
7159 2. **ASTHMA**, n. 1. asthma.
7160 **Herzasthma**, n. 1. cardiac asthma.
7161 **Heuasthma**, n. 1.
7162 **Heufieber**, n. 2.
7163 **Heuschnupfen**, m. 2. } hay fever.
7164 **Krampfasthma**, n. 1. asthma.
7165 **Millar'sches Asthma**, n. 1. laryngismus stridulus.
7166 **Schleiferasthma**, n. 1. knife-grinder's asthma (from v. ir.
7167 **schleifen**. to sharpen).
7168 3. **BLUTFLUSZ**, m. 1.
7169 **Blutung**, f. } *hemorrhage*, haematorrhoea, bleeding.
7170 **Afterblutflusz**, m. 1.
7171 **Afterblutung**, f. } hemorrhage of the anus.
7172 **Amenie**, **Amenorrhöe**, f. amenorrhoea.
7173 **Amnionblutflusz**, m. 1.
Amnionblutung, f. } hemorrhage into the amnion.

7174 **Augenblutflusz**, m. 1. intraocular hemorrhage.
7175 **Bauchfellblutung**, f. peritoneal hemorrhage.
7176 **Beckenblutung**, f. pelvic hemorrhage.
7177 **Blasenblutung**, f. vesical hemorrhage.
7178 **Blutgang**, m. 1. flow of blood.
7179 **Darmblutflusz**, m. 1.
7180 **Darmblutung**, f. } intestinal hemorrhage.
7181 **Gebärmutterblutflusz**, m. 1.
7182 **Gebärmutterblutung**, f. } uterine hemorrhage, menorrhagia.
7183 **Gebärmutterblutsturz**, m. 1. uterine flooding (rush of blood.
7184 **Gehirnblutflusz**, m. 1.
7185 **Gehirnblutschlag**, m. 1. } sanguineous apoplexy.
7186 **Gehirnblutung**, f. cerebral hemorrhage, apoplexy.
7187 **Gelenkblutung**, f. hemorrhage into a joint.
7188 **Goldaderflusz**. m. 1. bleeding of the piles.
7189 **Hämorrhoidalblutung**, f. hemorrhage from haemorrhoids.
7190 **Hämorrhoidalflusz**, m. 1. haemorrhoids, piles.
7191 **Harnblasenblutflusz**, m. 1. hemorrhage into the ureter.
7192 **Harnröhrenblutflusz**, m. 1.
7193 **Harnröhrenblutung**, f. } hemorrhage from the urethra.
7194 **Hirnblutergusz**, m. 1.
7195 **Hirnblutflusz**, m. 1.
7196 **Hirnblutung**. f. } cerebral hemorrhage or apoplexy.
7197 **Hirnhautblutung**, f. meningeal hemorrhage.
7198 **Hodenscheidenhautblutung**, f. haematocele of tunica vaginalis.
7199 **Kehlkopfblutung**, f. laryngeal hemorrhage.
7200 **Kindbettblutflusz**, m. 1.
7201 **Kindbettflusz**, m. 1.
7202 **Kindbettreinigung**, f. } lochial discharge.
7203 **Knochenblutung**, f. hemorrhage from bone.

7204 **Leberblutung**, f. hemorrhage from or into the liver.
7205 **Leukorrhöe** (**der weisze Flusz**), f. leucorrhoea, flux albus.
7206 **Lungenblutflusz**, m. 1. } hemorrhage from lungs.
7207 **Lungenblutung**, f. }
7208 **Lungenblutsturz**, m. 1. violent hemoptysis.
7209 **Magenblutung**, f. hemorrhage from the stomach.
7210 **Mastdarmblutflusz**, m. 1. hemorrhoids.
7211 **Mastdarmblutung**, f. hemorrhage from the rectum, hemorrhoids.
7212 **Meningealblutung**, f. meningeal hemorrhage.
7213 **Menstruation**, f. menstruation.
7214 **Milzblutflusz**, m. 1. } splenic hemorrhage.
7215 **Milzblutung**, f. }
7216 **Mundblutflusz**, m. 1. } hemorrhage from the mouth.
7217 **Mundblutung**, f. }
7218 **Mundhöhlenblutung**, f. hemmorrhage from the oral cavity.
7219 **Mutterblutflusz**, m. 1. } flooding metrorrhagia.
7220 **Mutterblutung**, f. }
7221 **Mutterflusz**, m. 1. uterine discharge, lochia, leucorrhoea.
7222 **Mutterscheidenblutflusz**, m. 1. } vaginal hemorrhage.
7223 **Mutterscheidenblutung**, f. }
7224 **Muttertrompetenblutung**, f. hemorrhage into the Fallopian tube.
7225 **Nabelblutflusz**, m. 1. } hemorrhage from umbilicus.
7226 **Nabelblutung**, f. }
7227 **Nachblutung**, f. secondary hemorrhage.
7228 **Nachgeburtsblutung**, f. postpartum hemorrhage.
7229 **Netzhautblutung**, f. retinal hemorrhage.
7230 **Nierenblutflusz**, m. 1. } haematuria.
7231 **Nierenblutung**, f. }
7232 **Ohrblutflusz**, m. 1. } hemorrhage from the ear.
7233 **Ohrenblutflusz**, m. 1. }
7234 **Pankreasblutung**, f. hemorrhage into the pancreas.
7235 **Pharynxblutung**, f. } pharyngeal hemorrhage.
7236 **Rachenblutung**, f. }
7237 **Rutenblutung**, f. hemorrhage from the penis.
7238 **Schamlefzenblutung**, f. hemorrhage into or from the labia pudendi.
7239 **Scheidenblutflusz**, m. 1. } hemorrhage from the vagina, colporrhagia.
7240 **Scheidenblutung**, f. }
7241 **Scheidenhautblutung**, f. haematocele.
7242 **Schlundblutung**, f. hemorrhage from the pharynx.
7243 **Schwangerschaftsblutung**, f. hemorrhage of pregnancy.
7244 **Speiseröhrenblutung**, f. hemorrhage from the oesophagus.
7245 **Tracheablutung**, f. hemorrhage in or from the trachea.
7246 **Tubenblutung**, f. hemorrhage into the Fallopian tube.
7247 **Uterinblutung**, f. uterine hemorrhage (from uterin, adj. uterine, derived from uterus).
7248 **Verblutung**, f. (from verbluten, to bleed to death), bleeding to death, cessation of bleeding.
7249 **Wochenflusz**, m. 1. } lochia.
7250 **Wochenreinigung**, f. }
7251 **Zahnfleischblutung**, f. hemorrhage from the gum.
7252 **Zellgewebsblutung**, f. hemorrhage into cellular tissue.
7253 **Zungenblutung**, f. hemorrhage from the tongue, etc.

7254 4. **ENTZÜNDUNG**, inflammation.

7255 **Aderentzündung**, f. phlebitis.
7256 **Aderhautentzündung**, f. choroiditis.
7257 **Aortenentzündung**, f. aortitis.
7258 **Augapfelentzündung**, f. panophthalmitis.
7259 **Augenbindehautentzündung**, f. conjunctivitis.
7260 **Augendrüsenentzündung**, f. inflammation of the meibomian glands.
7261 **Augenentzündung**, f. inflammation of the eyeball, ophthalmia, ophthalmitis.

7262 **Augenhöhlenentzündung**, f. inflam. of the orbital cavity.
7263 **Augenhornhautentzündung**, f. keratitis, inflam. of the cornea.
7264 **Augenliddrüsenentzündung**, f. inflam. of the glands of the eyelid.
7265 **Augenlidentzündung**, f. } blepharitis.
7266 **Augenlidhautentzündung**, f. }
7267 **Augenlidrandentzündung**, f. } inflammation of tarsal cartilage.
7268 **Augenlidknorpelentzündung**, f. }
7269 **Augenlidzellgewebsentzündung**, f. inflam. of the palpebral cellular tissue.
7270 **Augenmuskelentzündung**, f. inflam. of eye muscle.
7271 **Bauchfellentzündung**, f. peritonitis.
7272 **Bauchfellüberzugsentzündung**, f. (der Gebärmutter), perimetritis, or metroperitonitis.
7273 **Beckenzellgewebsentzündung**, f. parametritis, pelvic cellulitis.
7274 **Beinhautentzündung**, f. periostitis.
7275 **Bindehautentzündung**, f. conjunctivitis, ophthalmia.
7276 **Blasenentzündung**, f. cystitis.
7277 **Blasenhalsentzündung**, f. inflam. of the neck of the bladder.
7278 **Blutleiterentzündung**, f. inflam. of a sinus.
7279 **Brustdrüsenentzündung**, f. mastitis.
7280 **Brustentzündung**, f. inflam. of the chest.
7281 **Brustfellentzündung**, f. pleurisy, pleuritis.
7282 **Brustwarzenentzündung**, f. inflam. of the nipple.
7283 **Darmentzündung**, f. enteritis.
7284 **Darmfellentzündung**, f. peritonitis.
7285 **Darmhautentzündung**, f. inflam. of the wall of intestine.
7286 **Darmnetzentzündung**, f. inflam. of omentum.
7287 **Dünndarmentzündung**, f. enteritis.
7288 **Eierstocksentzündung**, f. oöphoritis, inflam. of ovary.
7289 **Eichelentzündung**, f. } balanitis.
7290 **Eichelkatarrh**, m. 1. }
7291 **Fettgewebsentzündung**, f. inflam. of fatty tissue.
7292 **Fingerentzündung**, f. whitlow, panaritium, paronychia.
7293 **Fingersehnenscheidenentzündung**, f. thecal abscess, panaritium tendinosum.
7294 **Flechsenentzündung**, f. inflam. of a tendon.
7295 **Gallenblasenentzündung**, f. inflam. of gall-bladder.
7296 **Gallenwegeentzündung**, f. inflam. of the biliary passage.
7297 **Gaumenentzündung**, f. inflam. of palate.
7298 **Gastroadenitis**, f. inflam. of the glands of the stomach.
7299 **Gebärmutterbauchentzündung**, f. utero-abdominal inflam.
7300 **Gebärmutterbauchfellüberzugentzündung**, f. perimetritis.
7301 **Gebärmutterentzündung**, f. uterine inflam.
7302 **Gefäszentzündung**, f. inflam. of vessels.
7303 **Gehirnentzündung**, f. encephalitis.
7304 **Gehirnhautentzündung**, f. meningitis.
7305 **Gelenkbänderentzündung**, f. inflam. of the ligaments of a joint.
7306 **Gelenkentzündung**, f. arthritis, inflam. of a joint.
7307 **Gelenkkapselentzündung**, f. inflam. of the capsule of a joint.
7308 **Gliederentzündung**, f. arthritis.
7309 **Gonitis**, f. inflam. of the knee joint.
7310 **Grimmdarmentzündung**, f. colitis.
7311 **Halsbraüne** or **Halsentzündung**, f. quinsy, tonsilitis.
7312 **Halsdrüsenentzündung**, f. inflam. of cervical glands.
7313 **Halsentzündung**, f. inflam. of the throat.
7314 **Halswirbelgelenkentzündung**, f. inflam. of the joints of the (upper) cervical spine.

7315 **Halszellgewebsentzündung**, f. inflammation of the cervical connective tissue.
7316 **Handgelenkentzündung,** f. inflam. of the joints of the hand.
7317 **Harnblasenentzündung,** f. cystitis.
7318 **Harngangentzündung,** f. inflam. of the urinary passage.
7319 **Harnleiterentzündung,** f. inflam. of the ureter.
7320 **Harnröhrenentzündung,** f. urethritis.
7321 **Hauptschlagaderentzündung**, f. aortitis.
7322 **Hautentzündung,** f. dermatitis.
7323 **Herzbeutelentzündung,** f. pericarditis.
7324 **Herzentzündung**, f. carditis.
7325 **Herzfleischentzündung,** f. } myocarditis.
7326 **Herzmuskelentzündung,** f. } myocarditis.
7327 **Herzhautentzündung,** f. endocarditis, pericarditis.
7328 **Herzklappenentzündung**, f. inflam. of the cardiac valves.
7329 **Hirnentzündung**, f. } encephalitis.
7330 **Hirnsubstanzentzündung**, f. } encephalitis.
7331 **Hirnhautentzündung,** f. meningitis.
7332 **Hirnmarkentzündung**, f. encephalitis, involving the medullary brain substance.
7333 **Hirnrindenentzündung,** f. inflam. of the cortex of the brain.
7334 **Hodenentzündung,** f. orchitis.
7335 **Hodensackentzündung,** f. inflam. of the scrotum.
7336 **Hornhautentzündung,** f. corneitis.
7337 **Hüftgelenkentzündung,** f. coxitis, hip disease.
7338 **Kapselentzündung,** f. inflam. of the capsule (e. g. of liver).
7339 **Kehldeckelentzündung,** f. inflam. of the epiglottis.
7340 **Kehlentzündung,** f. } laryngitis.
7341 **Kehlkopfentzündung,** } laryngitis.
7342 **Kinnbackenhöhlenentzündung**, f. inflam. of the antrum of Highmore.
7343 **Kitzlerentzündung,** f. clitoritis.
7344 **Kniegelenkentzündung,** f. inflam. of knee joint.
7345 **Knochenentzündung,** f. osteitis.
7346 **Knochenhautentzündung,** f. periostitis.
7347 **Knochenmarkentzündung,** f. osteo- myelitis.
7448 **Knorpelentzündung,** f. } inflam. of the cartilage.
7349 **Knorpelgewebeentzündung,** f. } inflam. of the cartilage.
7350 **Knorpelhautentzündung**, f. inflam. of perichondrium.
7351 **Leberentzündung**, f. hepatitis.
7352 **Lederhautentzündung,** f. inflam. of the sclerotic.
7353 **Lendenmuskelentzündung,** f. inflam. of the psoas muscle.
7354 **Lidentzündung**, f. blepharitis.
7355 **Linsenentzündung,** f. inflam. of the lens (from Linse, f. lens).
7356 **Linsenkapselentzündung**, f. inflam. of the capsule.
7357 **Lippenentzündung,** f. labial inflammation.
7358 **Luftröhrenentzündung,** f. bronchitis, tracheitis.
7359 **Luftröhrenkopfentzündung,** f. laryngitis.
7360 **Lungenentzündung**, f. pneumonia.
7361 ——, **falsche,** peripneumonia notha.
7362 **Lymphdrüsenentzündung,** f. inflam. of a lymphatic gland.
7363 **Lymphgefäszentzündung**, f. lymphangitis.
7364 **Magendarmentzündung,** f. gastro-enteritis.
7365 **Magendrüsenentzündung,** f. inflam. of the glands of the stomach.
7366 **Magenentzündung**, f. gastritis.
7367 **Magenzwölffingerdarmentzündung,** f. gastro-duodenitis.
7368 **Mandelentzündung,** f. tonsilitis.
7369 **Mastdarmentzündung**, f. proctitis.

7370 **Milchkanalentzündung**, f. inflam. of lactiferous duct.

7371 **Milzentzündung**, f. splenitis. inflam. of the spleen.

7372 **Mittelfellentzündung**, f. inflam. of mediastinum.

7373 **Mittelohrentzündung**, f. | otitis interna.

7374 **Mittelohrkatarrh**, m. 1. | otitis interna.

7375 **Mundentzündung**, f.

7376 **Mundhöhlenentzündung**, f. | stomatitis.

7377 **Mundkatarrh**, m. 1. | stomatitis.

7378 **Mundschleimhautentzündung**, f. | stomatitis.

7379 **Muskelentzündung**, f. myositis.

7380 **Mutterentzündung**, f. metritis.

7381 **Mutterkuchenentzündung**. f. placentitis, inflam. of placenta.

7382 **Mutterscheidenentzündung**. f. inflam. of vagina.

7383 **Muttertrompetenentzündung**, f. salphingitis.

7384 **Nabelvenenentzündung**. f. omphalophlebitis, inflam. of umbilical vein.

7385 **Nagelbettentzündung**. f. onychia.

7386 **Nasenentzündung**, f. rhinitis, inflam. of the nose.

7387 **Nebenhodenentzündung**, f. epididymitis.

7388 **Nervenentzündung**, f. neuritis.

7389 **Netzentzündung**, f. inflam. of omentum, epiploïtis.

7390 **Netzhautentzündung**. f. inflam. of retina, retinitis.

7391 **Nierenbeckenbauchentzündung**, f. inflam. of kidney pelvis, nephropyelitis.

7392 **Nierenkelchentzündung**, f. inflam. of renal calyx.

7393 **Nierenentzündung**, f. kidney inflammation, nephritis.

7394 **Ohrdrüsenbräune**, f. | parotitis, mumps.

7395 **Ohrdrüsenentzündung**, f. | parotitis, mumps.

7396 **Ohrenentzündung**, f. inflam. of the ear, otitis.

7397 **Ohrgefäszentzündung**. f. angiotitis, inflam. of the ear vessels.

7398 **Ohrspeicheldrüsenentzündung**. f. parotitis, inflam. of parotid gland, mumps.

7399 **Ohrtrompetenentzündung**, f. inflam. of Eustachian tube.

7400 **Paukenfellentzündung**, f. inflam. of membrana tympani.

7401 **Paukenhöhlenentzündung**, f. inflam. of tympanic cavity, otitis interna.

7402 **Pfortaderentzündung**, f. inflam. of portal vein

7403 **Phosphorentzündung**, f. inflam. caused by phosphor.

7404 **Rachenentzündung**, f. | pharyngitis.

7405 **Rachenschleimhautentzündung**, f. | pharyngitis.

7406 **Regenbogenhautentzündung**, f. iritis (from Regenbogen, m. 2. rainbow.

7407 **Rippenfellentzündung**, f. pleurisy.

7408 **Rückenmarkentzündung**, f. | spinal meningitis.

7409 **Rückenmarkhautentzündung**, f. | spinal meningitis.

7410 **Saugaderentzündung**, f. inflam. of the lymphatics.

7411 **Schamlefzenentzündung**, f. | inflam. of labia pudendi.

7412 **Schamlippenentzündung**, f. | inflam. of labia pudendi.

7413 **Schamritzenentzündung**, f. inflam. of the vulva.

7414 **Scheidenentzündung**, f. inflam. of the vagina.

7415 **Scheidenhautentzündung**, f. periorchitis.

7416 **Scheidenschleimhautentzündung**, f. vaginitis.

7417 **Scheidenwandentzündung**, f. inflam. of vaginal wall.

7418 **Schilddrüsenentzündung**, f. inflam. of the thyroid gland.

7419 **Schleimbeutelentzündung**, f. bursitis.

7420 **Schleimdrüsenentzündung**. f. inflam. of mucous glands.

7421 **Schleimhautentzündung**, f. inflam. of mucous membrane.

7422 **Schlundentzündung**, f. | pharyngitis.

7423 **Schlundkopfentzündung**, f. | pharyngitis.

7424 **Schultergelenkentzündung,** f. shoulderjoint inflammation.
7425 **Sehnenscheidenentzündung** f. tendon sheath inflammation.
7426 **Selbstentzündung,** f. idiopathic inflammation.
7427 **Speiseröhrenentzündung,** f. inflam. of oesophagus.
7428 **Thränendrüsenentzündung,** f. } inflam. of lachrymal sack.
7429 **Thränensackentzündung,** f. } inflam. of lachrymal sack.
7430 **Tiefenentzündung,** f. (from Tiefe, f. depth) deep-seated inflammation.
7431 **Trommelfellentzündung,** f. myringitis.
7432 **Tubenentzündung,** f. inflam. of Fallopian tube.
7433 **Venenentzündung,** f. phlebitis, inflam. of vein.
7434 **Vorhautentzündung,** f. prepuce inflammation.
7435 **Vorsteherdrüsenentzündung,** f. inflam. of the prostate.
7436 **Wirbelentzündung,** f. } spondylitis.
7437 **Wirbelsäulenentzündung,** f. } spondylitis.
7438 **Wasserhautentzündung,** f. inflam. of hyaloid membrane or of the amnion.
7439 **Zahnwurzelhautentzündung,** f. periodontitis.
7440 **Zellgewebeentzündung,** f. inflam. of cellular tissue, etc.
7441 **Zitzenfortsatzentzündung,** f. inflammation of mastoid process.
7442 5. **FIEBER,** fever.
7443 **Abdominaltyphoid,** n. 1. } enteric fever.
7444 **Abdominaltyphus,** m. 1. } enteric fever.
7445 **Ausschlagsfieber,** n. 2. eruptive or exanthematous fever.
7446 **Binnenfieber,** n. 2. form of malaria in the interior of Holland.
7447 **Blasenfieber,** n. 2. pemphigus.
7448 **Brandfieber,** n. 2. / **Brennfieber,** n. 2. } inflammatory, or suppurative fever.
7449 **Brustfieber,** n. 2. inflammation of the chest (of lung or pleura).
7450 **Darmfieber,** n. 2. enteric fever.
7451 **Eiterfieber,** n. 2. suppurative fever.
7452 **Entzündungsfieber,** n. 2. inflammatory fever.
7453 **Frühjahrsfieber,** n. 2. spring fever.
7454 **Gallenfieber,** n. 2. bilious fever, relapsing fever.
7455 **Gefängnisfieber,** n. 2. jail fever, typhus.
7456 **Gefäszfieber,** n. 2. inflammatory fever.
7457 **Gelbfieber,** n. 2. yellow fever.
7458 **Gieszfieber,** n. 2. brassfounder's ague.
7459 **Guineafieber,** n. 2. guinea fever.
7460 **Harnfieber,** n. 2. catheter fever.
7461 **Herbstfieber,** n. 2. autumnal fever.
7462 **Heufieber,** n. 2. } hay fever.
7463 **Heuschnupfen,** m. 2. } hay fever.
7464 **Heuasthma,** n. 1. } hay fever.
7465 **Hirse or Hirsenfieber,** n. 2. miliary fever.
7466 **Hospitalfieber,** n. 2. / **Spital,** n. 1. } typhus.
7467 **Hustenfieber,** n. 2. catarrhal cough fever.
7468 **Insolationsfieber,** n. 2. dengue fever, (insolation, f. sunbath, sunstroke.)
7469 **Jungfernbleichsucht,** f. } chlorosis.
7470 **Jungfernfieber,** n. 2. } chlorosis.
7471 **Katarrhalfieber,** n. 2. catarrhal fever.
7472 **Katarrh-fieber,** n. 2. epidemisches, influenza.
7473 **Kerkerfieber,** n. 2. jailfever, typhus.
7474 **Kindbetterinfieber,** n. 2. } puerperal fever.
7475 **——enfieber,** n. 2. } puerperal fever.
7476 **Kindbettfieber,** n. 2. } puerperal fever.
7477 **Kopffieber,** n. 2. brain fever.
7478 **Lagerfieber,** n. 2. } camp fever, typhus.
7479 **Lagersucht,** f. } camp fever, typhus.
7480 **Landfieber,** n. 2. endemic fever.

7481 **Leberfieber,** n. 2. hepatic fever.

7482 **Lungenfieber,** n. 2. pulmonary fever.

7483 **Magenfieber,** n. 2. gastric fever.

7484 **Malariafieber,** n. 2. malaria fever.

7485 **Marschfieber,** n. 2. marsh fever.

7486 **Milchfieber,** n. 2. milk fever.

7487 **Milzbrandfieber,** n. 2. anthrax, charbon, malignant pustule, splenic fever, woolsorter's disease.

7488 **Mutterfieber,** n. 2. puerperal fever.

7489 **Nachfieber,** n. 2. secondary fever, protracted fever.

7490 **Nachtfieber,** n. 2. nocturnal fever.

7491 **Nervenfieber,** n. 2. nervous fever, typhus, typhoid.

7492 **Niesfieber,** n. 2. hay fever (from niesen, to sneeze).

7493 **Nieskrampf,** m. 1. spasmodic sneezing.

7494 **Nosokomialfieber,** n. 2. typhus, hospital fever.

7495 **Pestfieber,** n. 2. the plague.

7496 **Petechialfieber,** n. 2.
7497 **Petechial-typhus,** n. 1.
} typhus, petechial fever.

7498 **Pockenfieber,** n. 2.
7499 **Pockenkrankheit,** f.
} small-pox.

7500 **Polkafieber,** n. 2. dengue fever (see above 7468.)

7501 **Porzellanausschlag,** m. 1.
7502 **Porzellanfieber,** n. 2.
7503 **Porzellanfriesel,** m. 2.
} essera urticaria.

7504 **Puerperalfieber,** n. 2. puerperal fever.

7505 **Purpurausschlag,** m. 1.
7506 **Purpurfieber,** n. 2.
7507 **Purpurfriesel,** m. 2.
} purpura.

7508 **Quartanfieber,** n. 2. quartan fever.

7509 **Quintanfieber,** n. 2. quintan fever.

7510 **Quotidienfieber,** n. 2.
tägliches Fieber, n. 2.
} quotidian or daily fever.

7511 **Recurrensfieber,** n. 2. recurrent fever.

7512 **Reizfieber,** n. 2. irritative fever, febris erethica.

7513 **Rosenfleckfieber,** n. 2. roseola.

7514 **Rückfallsfieber,** n.2.
7515 **Rückfallstyphus,** m. 1.
} relapsing fever.

7516 **Savannenfieber,** n. 2. prairie fever.

7517 **Scharlachfieber,** n. 2.
Scharlachfriesel, m. 2.
} scarlet fever, scarlatina.

7518 **Schauerfieber,** n. 2. or (from schauern, to shiver),
Frösteln, n. 2. (from frösteln, to shudder.
} ague, rigor in fever.

7519 **Schüttelfieber,** n. 2. or
Schüttelfrost, m. 1. (from schütteln, to rouse, shake) or
5207 **Frostschauer,** m. 2.
} ague, severe chill.

7521 **Schleichfieber,** n. 2. slow, lingering fever.

7522 **Schleimfieber,** n. 2. febris mucosa, typhoid fever.

7523 **Schnupfenfieber,** n. 2. or
7524 **Grippe,** f.
} influenza, catarrhal fever.

7525 **Schweiszfieber,** n. 2.
} sweating fever.

7526 **Schwitzfieber,** n. 2.
} malarial fever.

7527 **Sumpffieber,** n. 2. marsh fever.

7528 **Typhus,** m. 1. typhus, typhoid fever.

7529 **Unterleibstyphus,** m. 1. typhoid fever.

7530 **Wechselfieber,** n. 2. ague, intermittent fever.

7531 **Wechselfiebermiasma,** n. 1. miasma of ague.

7532 **Wundfieber,** n. 2 traumatic fever.

7533 6. **GESCHWULST, TUMOR.**

7534 **Abdominalgeschwulst,** f. abdominal tumor.

7535 **Adergeschwulst,** f. venous or vascular tumor.

7536 **Augengeschwulst,** f. eye tumor.

7537 **Augenhöhlengeschwulst**, f. orbital tumor.
7538 **Augenlidblutadergeschwulst**, f. naevus of the eyelid.
7539 **Augenliddrüsengeschwulst**, f. meibomian or tarsal cyst.
7540 **Augenlidgeschwulst**, f. oedema of the eyelid.
7541 **Augenwinkelgeschwulst**, f. or
7542 **Nasenwinkelgeschwulst**, f. } swelling of lachrymal sac.
7543 **Balgfasergeschwulst**, f. cystic fibroma.
7544 **Balggeschwulst**, f. encysted tumor, mit wässerigem Inhalt, with watery contents, hygroma.
7545 **Bauchspeicheldrüsengeschwulst**, f. pancreatic tumor.
7546 **Beckengeschwulst**, f. pelvic tumor.
7547 **Beingeschwulst**, f. bony tumor, osteoma.
7548 **Beinhautgeschwulst**, f. periosteal tumor or swelling.
7549 **Beutelgeschwulst**, f. cystic tumor.
7550 **Bindegewebsgeschwulst**, f. connective tissue tumor.
7551 **Blasengeschwulst**, f. vesicular tumor, vesicular tumor cyst.
7552 **Blutadergeschwulst**, f.
7553 **Blutaderknoten**, m. 2. } varix, varicose swelling.
7554 **Blutgefäszgeschwulst**, f. angioma.
7555 **Blutgeschwulst**, f. haematoma, bloodcyst.
7556 **Bruchgeschwulst**, f. hernial tumor.
7557 **Brustdrüsengeschwulst**, f. mammary tumor.
7558 **Brustgeschwulst**, f. thoracic tumor.
7559 **Cystengeschwulst**, f. cystic tumor.
7560 **Darmgeschwulst**, f. intestine tumor.
7561 **Desmoidgeschwulst**, f. soft, fibrous tumor.
7562 **Drüsengeschwulst**, f. gland tumor.
7563 **Eierstocksgeschwulst**, f. ovarian tumor.
7564 **Eitergeschwulst**, f. abscess.
7565 **Fasergeschwulst**, f. fibrous tumor, fibroma.
7566 **Faserkerngeschwulst**, f. fibro-nucleated tumor.
7567 **Faserknorpelgeschwulst**, f. fibro-cartilaginous tumor.
7568 **Fasermuskelgeschwulst**, f. fibro-myoma.
7569 **Faserschleimgeschwulst**, f. fibro-myxoma.
7570 **Fettgeschwulst**, f.
7571 **Fettgewebsgeschwulst**, f.
7572 **Fetthautgeschwulst**, f. } lipoma, fatty tumor, subcutaneous fatty tumor.
7573 **Fleischgeschwulst**, f. sarcoma, myoma.
7574 **Fleischknochengeschwulst**, f. osteo-sarcoma.
7575 **Gallengeschwulst**, f. biliary tumor.
7576 **Gallertgeschwulst**, f. colloid growth.
7577 **Gebärmuttergeschwulst**, f. uterine tumor.
7578 **Gebärmutterwindgeschwulst**, f. distention of uterus by wind.
7579 **Gebärmutterwindsucht**, f. physometra.
7580 **Geburtsgeschwulst**, f. caput succedaneum.
7581 **Gefäszgeschwulst**, f. angioma, vascular tumor.
7582 **Gehirngeschwulst**, f. cerebral tumor.
7583 **Gehirnsandgeschwulst**, f. psammoma.
7584 **Gelenkgeschwulst**, f. joint swelling or tumor.
7585 ——, **weisze**, f. white swelling, tumor albus.
7586 **Gelenkknochengeschwulst**, f. swelling or tumor of articular boneends.
7587 **Gliedergeschwulst**, f. a swelling of the limbs.
7588 **Granulationsgeschwulst**, f. granulation tumor.
7589 **Grützbeutel**, m. 2.
7590 **Grützbeutelgeschwulst**, f.
7591 **Grützbreigeschwulst**, f.
7592 **Grützgeschwulst**, f. } sebaceous or atheromatous cyst, atheroma.

7593 **Hagelgeschwulst**, f. } chalazion, stye, meibomian cyst.
7594 **Hagelkorn**, n. 1. }
7595 **Halsgeschwulst**, f. cervical tumor.
7596 **Harnröhrengeschwulst**, f. urethral tumor or swelling.
7597 **Harnröhrenwulst**, m. 1. urethral prominence (felt through vagina).
7598 **Hauptgeschwulst**, f. primary tumor.
7599 **Hautbalggeschwulst**, f. cutaneous follicular tumor, molluscum.
7600 **Hautgeschwulst**, f. cutaneous or dermoid tumor.
7601 **Hautwulst**, m. 1. skin protuberance, skin excrescence.
7602 **Herzgeschwulst**, f. cardiac tumor.
7603 **Hirngeschwulst**, f. cerebral tumor.
7604 **Hirnsandgeschwulst**, f. psammoma.
7605 **Hodengeschwulst**, f. swelling or tumor of testicles.
7606 **Hodensackgeschwulst**, f. swelling or tumor of the scrotum.
7607 **Hodenspeckgeschwulst**, f. steatoma of the testicle.
7608 **Hohlgeschwulst**, f. tumor with a cavity.
7609 **Honigbalggeschwulst**, f. } meliceris.
7610 **Honiggeschwulst**, f. }
7611 **Horngeschwulst**, f. horny tumor.
7612 **Hornhautgeschwulst**, f. cornea tumor.
7613 **Hydatidengeschwulst**, f. hydatid tumor.
7614 **Infektionsgeschwulst**, f. infection tumor.
7615 **Kehldeckelwulst**, m. 1. cushion of the epiglottis.
7616 **Knochengeschwulst**, f. osteosteatoma.
7617 **Knochenwulst**, m. 1. bony prominence, bony tuberosity.
7618 **Knorpelgeschwulst**, f. enchondroma.
7619 **Kombinationsgeschwulst**, f. mixed tumor.
7620 **Kopfblutgeschwulst**, f. cephalhaematoma.
7621 **Kopfgeschwulst**, f. tumor or swelling of the head.
7622 **Kopfwindgeschwulst**, f. emphysema of the scalp, pneumocele.
7623 **Kotgeschwulst**, f. faecal tumor.
7624 **Krebsgeschwulst**, f. cancerous tumor.
7625 **Kreuzbeingeschwulst**, f. sacrum tumor.
7626 **Kropfgeschwulst**, f. gôitre, bronchocele.
7627 **Krystalwulst**, m. 1. mass of lens fibres.
7628 **Leberblutgeschwulst**, f. liver blood cyst.
7629 **Leistendrüsengeschwulst**, f. bubo.
7630 **Leistengeschwulst**, f. inguinal tumor.
7631 **Leistenring**, m. 1. inguinal ring.
7632 **Lippengeschwulst**, f. labial tumor.
7633 **Luftgeschwulst**, f. emphysema.
7634 **Lufttumor**, m. 2. gaseous tumor.
7635 **Lumbaranschwellung**, f. lumbar enlargement (of spinal cord).
7636 **Lungengeschwulst**, f. lardaceous lung disease.
7637 **Lymphdrüsengeschwulst**, f. swelling of lymphatic gland, lymphoma.
7638 **Lymphgefäszgeschwulst**, f. lymphangioma.
7639 **Lymphgeschwulst**, f. lymphoma.
7640 **Magengeschwulst**, f. stomach tumor, gastric swelling.
7641 **Markgeschwulst**, f. medullary tumor.
7642 **Markwulst**, m. 1. medullary eminence.
7643 **Maulbeergeschwulst**, f. mulberry tumor (naevus).
7644 **Milchgeschwulst**, f. } milk tumor caused by retained milk in the breast.
7645 **Milchknoten**, m. 2. }
7646 **Milzanschwellung**, f. } spleen enlargment.
7647 **Milzschwellung**, f. }
7648 **Milzgeschwulst**, f. spleen tumor.

7649 **Milztumor**, m. 2. splenic tumor.
7650 **Mischgeschwulst**, f. } mixed
7651 **Mischtumor**, m. 2. } tumor.
7652 **Mittelfellgeschwulst**, f. mediastinal tumor.
7653 **Muskelgechwulst**, f. myoma.
7654 **Muskelwulst**, m. 1. muscular elevation.
7655 **Muttergeschwulst**, f. uterine tumor.
7656 **Nabelgeschwulst**, f. umbilical swelling or tumor.
7657 **Nabelwassergeschwulst**, f. umbilical oedema.
7658 **Nagelgeschwulst**, f. nail tumor (on or about.)
7659 **Narbengeschwulst**, f. keloid, cicatrix tumor.
7660 **Nasenwinkelgeschwulst**, f. swelling of lachrymal sac.
7661 **Nervengeschwulst**, f. neuroma.
7662 **Netzgeschwulst**, f. omental tumor.
7663 **Nierenanschwellung**, f. kidney swelling.
7664 **Nierengeschwulst**, f. } renal swelling or tumor.
7665 **Nierentumor**, m. 2. }
7666 **Ohrblutgeschwulst**, f. ear blood tumor, haematoma auris.
7667 **Ohrdrüsengeschwulst**, f. parotid tumor.
7668 **Ohrgeschwulst**, f. ear tumor (of or about).
7669 **Ohrspeicheldrüsengeschwulst**, f. swelling or tumor of parotid gland.
7670 **Pankreasgeschwulst**, f. pancreatic tumor.
7671 **Papillargeschwulst**, f. warty tumor, papilloma.
7672 **Pestgeschwulst**, f. plague bubo or boil.
7673 **Pigmentgeschwulst**, f. melanotic tumor, pigmented growth.
7674 **Pulsadergeschwulst**, f. aneurism.
7675 **Retentionsgeschwulst**, f. retention tumor.
7676 **Retropharyngealgeschwulst**, f. retropharyngeal tumor.
7677 **Rückenwulst**. m. 1. dorsal eminence, medullary ridge (of early embryo.)
7678 **Sackgeschwulst**, f. cyst, encysted tumor.
7679 **Samenadergeschwulst**, f. varicocele.
7680 **Samenstranggeschwulst**, f. spermatic cord tumor.
7681 **Sandgeschwulst**, f. brain-sand tumor, psammoma.
7682 **Schamlefzengeschwulst**, f. swelling or tumor of labia pudendi.
7683 **Scheidengeschwulst**, f. vaginal tumor.
7684 **Scheidenwulst**, m. 1. vaginal fold or ruga
7685 **Scheitelgeschwulst**, f. caput succedanum.
7686 **Schenkelgeschwulst**, f. tumor of the thigh.
7687 **——, weisze**, phlegmasia alba dolens, "white leg."
7688 **Schilddrüsengeschwulst**, f. thyroid gland tumor.
7689 **Schleimbeutelgeschwulst**, f. bursal tumor.
7690 **Schleimgeschwulst**, f. from
7691 **Schleim**, m. 1. mucus, phlegm, mucous tumor, myxoma; ——, bösartige. myxosarcoma.
7692 **Schleimgewebsgeschwulst**, f. mucous or gelatinous tumor.
7693 **Schlüsselbeingeschwulst**, f. clavicle tumor.
7694 **Schwammgeschwulst**, f. fungating tumor.
7695 **Speckgeschwulst**, f. steatoma.
7696 **Speicheldrüsengeschwulst**, f. } salivary tumor.
7697 **Speichelgeschwulst**, f. }
7698 **Steingeschwulst**, f. tumor of stony hardness.
7699 **Stimmritzgeschwulst**, f. glottis oedema (from Stimmritze, f. rima glottidis).
7700 **Talgdrüsengeschwulst**, f. sebaceous cyst or tumor, wen.
7701 **Talgdrüsenwulst**, m. 1. swellings developing sebacious glands.
7702 **Thränendrüsengeschwulst**, f. tumor or swelling of lachrymal gland.
7703 **Thränengeschwulst**, f. } swelling or tumor of lachrymal sac.
7704 **Thränenwinkelgeschwulst**, f. }

7705 **Traubengeschwulst,** f. staphyloma.
7706 **Tubengeschwulst,** f. swelling or tumor of Fallopian tube.
7707 **Tuberkelgeschwulst,** f. tubercular swelling.
7708 **Unterleibsgeschwulst,** f. abdominal tumor.
7709 **Vorsteherdrüsengeschwulst,** f. tumor of the prostate.
7710 **Wassergeschwulst,** f. oedema, oedematous swelling.
7711 **Windgeschwulst,** f. traumatic-emphysema.
7712 **Wirbelgeschwulst,** f. vertebra tumor.
7713 **Zellgewebsgeschwulst,** f. connective tissue tumor or new growth, etc.
7714 7. **GESCHWÜR,** *Ulcer.*
7715 **Augengeschwür,** n. 1. cornea ulcer.
7716 **Augenwinkelgeschwür,** n. 1. aegilops, an eyelid abscess opening at the inner anthus.
7717 **Beingeschwür,** n. 1. bone ulceration, caries.
7718 **Bindehautverschwärung,** f. conjunctiva ulceration.
7719 **Blutgeschwür,** n. 1. furuncle, phlegmon.
7720 **Brandgeschwür,** n. 1. gangrenous ulcer.
7721 **Brustdrüsengeschwür,** n. 1. mammary ulcer.
7722 **Brustgeschwür,** n. 1. emphysema.
7723 **Darmgeschwür,** n. 1. intestinal ulcer.
7724 **Eitergeschwür,** n. 1. suppurating ulcer.
7725 **Fingergeschwür,** n. 1. paronychia, whitlow.
7726 **Gallenblasengeschwür,** n. 1. gallbladder ulcer.
7727 **Gefäszgeschwür,** n. 1. blood-vessel ulcer.
7728 **Gelenkgeschwür,** n. 1. joint ulceration.
7729 **Gichtgeschwür,** n. 1. sore caused by the breaking of the skin over a chalk stone.
7730 **Gürtelgeschwür,** n. 1. circular ulcer.
7731 **Halsgeschwür,** n. 1. neck or throat ulcer.
7732 **Harnröhrgeschwür,** n. 1. urethral ulcer.
7733 **Hautgeschwür,** n. 1. skin ulcer.
7734 **Herzgeschwür,** n. 1. heart ulcer.
7735 **Hirngeschwür,** n. 1. fungus cerebri.
7736 **Hohlgeschwür,** n. 1. excavated ulcer fistula.
7737 **Hornhautgeschwür,** n. 1. corneal ulcer.
7738 **Infektionsgeschwür,** n. 1. infection ulcer.
7739 **Kehlkopfgeschwür,** n. 1. laryngeal ulcer.
7740 **Knorpelgeschwür,** n. 1. erosion or ulcer of cartilage.
7741 **Kopfgeschwür,** n. 1. head ulcer.
7742 **Krebsgeschwür,** n. 1. cancerous ulcer.
7743 **Längengeschwür,** n. 1. longitudinal ulcer.
7744 **Lippengeschwür,** n. 1. labial ulcer.
7745 **Lungengeschwür,** n. 1. abscess of the lung, vomica.
7746 **Magengeschwür,** n. 1. stomach ulcer.
7747 **Mastdarmgeschwür,** n. 1. rectum ulcer.
7748 **Mundgeschwür,** n. 1. mouth ulcer.
7749 **Mundhöhlengeschwür,** n. 1. ulcer of the oral cavity.
7750 **Muttergeschwür,** n. 1. uterine ulcer or abrasion.
7751 **Muttermundgeschwür,** n. 1. ulcer of os uteri.
7752 **Nabelgeschwür,** n. 1. umbilical ulcer.
7753 **Nagelgeschwür,** n. 1. onychia, whitlow.
7754 **Nasengeschwür,** n. 1. ulcer in nose.
7755 **Nasenwinkelgeschwür,** n. 1. lachrymal sack abscess or sinus.
7756 **Nierengeschwür,** n. 1. kidney ulceration.
7757 **Ohrgeschwür,** n. 1. ear ulceration.
7758 **Puerperalgeschwür,** n. 1. puerperal ulcer (at vaginal orifice.)
7759 **Pustelgeschwür,** n. 1. pustular ulcer (such as Aleppo boil.)
7760 **Reizgeschwür,** n. 1. irritable ulcer.

7761 **Riszgeschwür**, n. 1. linear ulcer, fissure ulcer.
7762 **Röhrengeschwür**, n. 1. } fis-
7763 **Röhrgeschwür**, n. 1. } tula.
7764 **Runzelgeschwür**. n. 1. (from Runzel. f. fold. ruga, wrinkle) fissured ulcer, rhagades.
7765 **Saharageschwür**, n. 1. Aleppo boil.
7766 **Schamlippengeschwür**. n. 1. lymphae or labia ulcer.
7767 **Scheidengeschwür**, n. 1. vagina ulcer.
7768 **Schleimhautgeschwür**, n. 1. ulcer of mucous membrane.
7769 **Speiseröhrengeschwür** n. 1. oesophagus ulcer.
7770 **Thränensack-geschwür**, n. 1. } ulceration of lachrymal sac.
7771 **Thränenwinkel-geschwür**, n. 1. }
7772 **Tuberkelgeschwür**, n. 1. tubercular ulcer.
7773 **Unterschenkelgeschwür**, n. 1. ulcer of the leg, etc.
7774 **Vorsteherdrüsengeschwür**. n. 1. ulcer of the prostate.
7775 8. **GICHT**, *Gout.*
7776 **Augengicht**, f. eye gout.
7777 **Ballengicht**, f. palm or sole gout.
7778 **Darmgicht**, f. colic, ileus.
7779 **Ellbogengicht**, f. gout in the ellbow joint.
7780 **Gliedergicht**, f. articular gout.
7781 **Halsgicht**, f. neck or throat gout.
7782 **Handgicht**, f. Hand gout, chiragra.
7783 **Hüftgicht**, f. hip gout.
7784 **Kindergichte**, f. pl. } eclampsia infantum, infantile convulsions
7785 **Kinderkrämpfe**, m. 1. pl. }
7786 **Kinnbackengicht**, f. gout in maxilla.
7787 **Kniegicht**, f. gonagra, gout in knee.
7788 **Knotengicht**, f. chronic rheumatic arthritis, malum senile articulorum.
7789 **Kopfgicht**, f. rheumatic headache.
7790 **Lendengicht**, f. lumbago.
7791 **Magengicht**, f. gout of the stomach.
7792 **Muttergicht**, f. uterine gout.
7793 **Nackengicht**, f. gout in neck, trachelagra.
7794 **Rückgratsgicht**, f. gout of the spine.
7795 **Schultergicht**, f. shoulder gout.
7796 **Trippergicht**, f. gonorrhoeal rheumatism.
7797 **Gicht, laufende**, f. flying gout.
7798 **——, reiszende**, f. gout, articular disease.
7799 **——, bruch**, m. 1. palsy.
7800 **gichtbrüchig**, adj. palsied. paralytic.
7801 **Gichtbrüchige**, m. 3. (f. declined like adjectives) palsied person, paralytic.
7802 **Gichtbrüchigkeit**, f. palsy.
7803 **Gichtfieber**, n. 2. arthritical fever.
7804 **gichtheilend**, adj. } anthar-
7805 **gichtlindernd**, adj. } tritic.
7806 **Gichtknoten**, m. 2. tophus, gouty deposit.
7807 **Gichtkolik**, f. arthritical gripes, stomach gout.
7808 **Gichtkörner**, n. 1. pl. grains of peony.
7809 **gichtkrank**, adj. gouty, ill, sick with the gout.
7810 **Gichtleiden**, n. 1. gouty affection.
7811 **Gichtschmerzen**, m. 1. pl. gout pains.
7812 **Gichtstoff**, m. 1. gouty matter, communicating gout matter, etc.
7813 9. **KATARRH**, catarrh.
7814 **Abdominalkatarrh**, m. 1. abdominal catarrh.
7815 **Bindehautkatarrh**, m. 1. conjunctivitis, ophthalmia.
7816 **Blasenkatarrh**, m. 1. cystitis, catarrh of the bladder.
7817 **Bronchialkatarrh**, m. 1. bronchitis.
7818 **Gaumenkatarrh**, m. 1. sore throat.
7819 **Gebärmutterkatarrh**, m. 1. catarrh of the uterus, leucorrhoea.
7820 **Harnblasenkatarrh**, m. 1. cystitis.
7821 **Harnröhrenkatarrh**, m. 1. } gonorrhoea.
7822 **Harnröhrenschleimflusz**. m. 1. }
7823 **Harnröhrentripper**, m. 2. }

7824 **Kehlkopfkatarrrh**, m. 1. larynx catarrh.
7825 **Kopfflusz**, m. 1. catarrh of the head.
7826 **Luftröhrenkatarrh**, m. 1. bronchial catarrh.
7827 **Lungenkatarrh**, m. 1. pulmonary catarrh.
7828 **Magendarmkatarrh**, m. 1. gastro-intestinal catarrh,
7829 **Magenkatarrh**, m. 1. gastric catarrh.
7830 **Magenschleimflusz**, m. 1. stomach catarrh.
7831 **Mastdarmkatarrh**, m. 1. } catarrh of the rectum.
7832 **Mastdarmschleimflusz**, m. 1. }
7833 **Mundkatarrh**, m. 1. stomatitis.
7834 **Mutterkatarrh**, m. 1. uterine catarrh.
7835 **Nasenkatarrh**, m. 1. nasopharyngeal catarrh.
7836 **Ohrenkatarrh**, m. 1. otorrhoea.
7837 **Rachenkatarrh**, m. 1. pharyngitis.
7838 **Rachenkroup**, m. 1. pharyngeal croup.
7839 **Roggenkatarrh**, m. 1. summer catarrh.
7840 **Schwellungskatarrh**, m. 1. congestive catarrh.
7841 **Speiseröhrenkatarrh**, m. 1. catarrh of the oesophagus.
7842 **Steckflusz**. m. 1. suffocating catarrh.
7843 **Stickflusz**, m. 1. suffocative catarrh, etc.
7844 10. **KRAMPF**, *cramp, spasm.*
7845 **Atemkrampf**, m. 1. respiratory spasm.
7846 **Augapfelstarrkrampf**. m. 1. ophthalmospasmus, tetanus oculi.
7847 **Augenkrampf**, spasm of accommodation.
7848 **Augenlidkrampf**, m. 1. blepharospasm, blepharophimosis.
7849 **Augenmuskelkrampf**. m. 1. spasm of an eye muscle.
7850 **Blasenkrampf**. m. 1. bladder spasm.
7851 **Bronchialkrampf**, m. 1. } asthma.
7852 **Brustkrampf**, m. 1. }
7853 **Darmkrampf**, m. 1. intestinal spasm.
7854 **Fingerkrampf**, m. 1. writer's or scrivener's palsy.
7855 **Gefäszkrampf**, m. 1. vascular spasm.
7856 **Genickkrampf**, m. 1. epidermic cerebro-spinal meningitis.
7857 **Gesichtskrampf**, m. 1. facial spasm.
7858 —, mimischer, convulsive tic.
7859 **Gewohnheitskrampf**, m. 1. habitual spasm, as in asthma, epilepsy, etc.
7860 **Gliederkrampf**, m. 1. cramp or spasm in the limbs.
7861 **Glottiskrampf**, m. 1. glottis spasm.
7862 **Halsstarrkrampf**, m. 1. rigid neck spasm.
7863 **Harnröhrenkrampf**, m. 1. urethral spasm.
7864 **Hautkrampf**, m. 1. cutis anserina.
7865 **Herzkrampf**, m. 1. angina pectoris.
7866 **Hustenkrampf**, m. 1. spasmodic cough.
7867 **Inspirationskrampf**, m. 1. inspiratory spasm (as in hydrophobia).
7868 **Kaumuskelkrampf**, m. 1. masticatory spasm. trismus.
7869 **Kehlkopfkrampf**, m. 1. } glottis spasm.
7870 **Kehlkopfmuskelkrampf**, m. 1. }
7871 **Kehlkrampf**, m. 1. }
7872 **Kinderkrämpfe**. pl. m. 1. infantile convulsions.
7873 **Kinnbackenkrampf**, m. 1. lockjaw, trismus.
7874 **Klavierspielerkrampf**, m. 1. pianoforte player's cramp.
7875 **Kopfgenickkrampf**, m. 1. cerebro-spinal meningitis.
7876 **Krampf**, m. 1. cramp, convulsion, spasm.
7877 **Laufkrampf**, m. 1. runner's cramp.
7878 **Lidkrampf**, m. 1. blepharospasm.
7879 **Luftröhrenkrampf**, m. 1. bronchial asthma.
7880 **Lungenkrampf**, m. 1. asthma.
7881 **Magenkrampf**. m. 1. gastralgia, stomach spasm.

7882 **Mastdarmkrampf**, m. 1. spasm of rectum.

7883 **Melkerkrampf**, m. 1. milkmaid's cramp.

7884 **Mundkrampf**, m. 1. spasmodic distortion of the mouth.

7885 **Muskelkrampf**, m. 1. muscular spasm.

7886 **Mutterkornkrampf**, m. 1. convulsive spasm from ergotism.

7887 **Mutterkrampf**, m. 1. uterine spasm.

7888 **Nackenmuskulaturkrampf**, m. 1. spasm of the cervical muscles, trachelismus.

7889 **Nähekrampf**, m. 1. sewer's cramp.

7890 **Nickkrampf**, m. 1. (from nicken, to nick), wry-neck, torticollis, spasmus nutans.

7891 **Nieskrampf**, m. 1. spasmodic sneezing.

7892 **Puerperalkrampf**, m. 1. puerpereal convulsion.

7893 **Respirationskrampf**, m. 1. respiratory muscle spasm.

7894 **Rutenkrampf**, m. 1. priapism.

7895 **Salaamconvulsionen**, f. pl. } salaam convulsions.

7896 **Salaamkrampf**, m. 1. } salaam convulsions.

7897 **Scheideneingangskrampf**, m. 1. } vaginismus.

7898 **Scheidenkrampf**, m. 1. } vaginismus.

7899 **Speiseröhrenkrampf**, m. 1. oesophagus spasm.

7900 **Starrkrampf**, m. 1. tetanus, trismus, lock-jaw.

7901 **Stimmkrampf**, m. 1. vocal spasm.

7902 **Stimmritzenkrampf**, m. 1. glottis spasm (from Stimmritze. f. rima glottidis).

7903 **Stotterkrampf**, m. 1. stutter-spasm.

7904 **stotternd**, adj. stuttering

7905 **Streckkrampf**, m. 1. (from strecken, to stretch), tetanic spasm (as in strychnia poisoning).

7906 **Trigeminuskrampf**. m. 1. spasm of the fifth cranial nerve.

7907 **Weinkrampf**, m. 1. hysterical crying (from weinen, to weep, to cry).

7908 **Wundstarrkrampf**, m. 1 traumatic tetanus.

7909 **Wurmkrampf**, m. 1. convulsions produced by worms.

7910 **Zahnkrampf**, m. 1. convulsions caused by teething.

7911 **Zungenkrampf**, m. 1. tongue spasm, etc.

7912 11. **KRANKHEITEN DISEASES**, including:

7913 **Affektion**, f. affection.

7914 **Anschwellung**, f. enlargement.

7915 **Atrophie**, f. atrophy.

7916 **Beschwerde**, f. affection.

7917 **Bräune**, f. quinsy.

7918 **Erkältung**, f. cold, chill.

7919 **Erkrankung**, f. sickness, disease.

7920 **Kolic**, f. colic.

7921 **Leiden**, n. 1. suffering.

7922 **Pest**, f. pestilence.

7923 **Rheumatismus**, m. 1. rheumatism.

7924 **Röte**, f. redness, rash.

7925 **Rotlauf**, m. 1. } erysipelas.

7926 **Rose**, f. } erysipelas.

7927 **Ruhr**, f. flux, diarrhoea.

7928 **Seuche**, f. plague, pestilence.

7929 **Skrofel**, f. scrofula.

7930 **Schwund**, m. 1. atrophy, withering.

7931 **Sucht**, f. sickness, chronic disease.

7932 **Tuberkulose**, f. tuberculosis.

7933 **Typhus**, m. 1. typhus.

7934 **Übel**, n. 1. malady, ailment, complaint.

7935 **Verhärtung**, f. induration, hardening.

7936 **Weh**, n. 1. woe, pain, etc.

7937 **Abmagerung**, f. emaciation, atrophy.

7938 **Abweichen**, n. 2. diarrhoea; anomaly.

7939 **Abzehrung**. f. } consumption, wasting disease.
Abzehrungskrankheit. f. } consumption, wasting disease.

7940 **Adenosis**, f. gland affection.

7941 **Adenosklerose**, f. induration of a gland.

7942 **Aerosklerose**, f. gland induration.

7943 **Agrypnie**, f. sleeplessness.

7944 **Allgemeinerkrankung**, f. general or constitutional disorder.

7945 **Allgemeinleiden**, n. 2. general affection.

7946 **Altermarasmus**, m. 1. senile wasting.
7947 **Anämie** (Blutarmut), f. anaemia.
7948 **Apepsie**, f. disturbed digestion.
7949 **apeptisch**, adj. indigestible.
7950 **Apoplexie**, f. appolexy.
7951 **Armeekrankheit**, f. disease of armies.
7952 **Atembeschwerde**, f. } dyspnoea.
Atemnot, f.
7953 **Atmungsbeschwerde**, f.
7954 **Atrophie**, f. atrophy.
7955 **Aufgeblasenheit**, f. } inflation, turgescence, puffiness, emphysema.
7956 **Aufgedunsenheit**, f.
7957 **Augenblennorrhöe**, f. catarrhal ophthalmia.
7958 **Augenkrankheit**, f. eye disease.
7959 **Augenlidrose**, f. erysipelas of the eyelids.
7960 **Augenschleimflusz**, m. 1. } catarrhal ophthalmia.
7961 **Augenschnupfen**, m. 2.
7962 **Augenweh**, n. 1. pain in the eye.
7963 **Auszehrung**, f. } phthsisis, consumption, wasting disease.
7964 **Auszehrungskrankheit**, f.
7965 **Ballismus**, m. 1. St. Vitus' dance.
7966 **Bauchbeschwerde**, f. abdominal complaint.
7967 **Bauchgrimmen**, n. 2. } colic.
7968 **Bauchkneipen**, n. 2.
7969 **Bauchkrankheit**, f. abdominal disease.
7970 **Bauchnervenkrankheit**, f. hypochondriasis.
7971 **Bauchschwindsucht**, f. abdominal phthisis, gastrophthisis.
7972 **Bauchskrofeln**, pl. scrofulous disease of the mesenteric glands.
7973 **Bauchweh**, n. 1. belly-ache, colic.
7974 **Bauchwindsucht**, f. tympanitis.
7975 **Barbadoesbein**, n. 1. } Barbadoes-leg, Elephantiasis Arabum.
7976 **Barbadoeskrankheit**, f.
7977 **Barbadoesschenkel**, m. 2.
7978 **Beinweh**, n. 1. bone pain, ostealgia.
7979 **Bergkrankheit**, f. mountain climbers and aëronauts' disease (above from 2-4000 miles.)
7980 **Bergsucht**, f. miners' phthisis.
7981 **Blähsucht**, f. flatulence.
7982 **Blähungsbeschwerde**, f. flatulency.
7983 **Blasenbeschwerde**, f. bladder troubles.
7984 **Blasenerkrankung**, f. } bladder disease, pemphigus.
7985 **Blasenkrankheit**, f.
7986 **Blasenrose**, f. } erysipelas.
7887 **Blasenrotlauf**, m. 1.
7988 **Blattern**, pl. } variolae, small-pox.
7989 **Blatterkrankheit**, f.
7990 **Pockenkrankheit**, f.
7991 **Pocken**, f.
7992 **Bleichsucht**, f. chlorosis.
7993 **Bleikrankheit**, f. lead poisoning.
7994 **Blennosis**, f. catarrh of membrane.
7995 **Blutgefäszkrankheit**, f. disease of blood vessels.
7996 **Brustkrankheit**, f. } pulmonary or thoracic disease, chest disease, pain in the chest.
7997 **Brustleiden**, n. 2.
7998 **Brustweh**, n. 1.
7999 **Darmkrankheit**, f. } intestinal disease.
8000 **Darmleiden**, n. 2.
8001 **Darmschwindsucht**, intestinal tuberculosis, tabes mesenterica.
8002 **Darmtyphus**, m. 1. enteric fever.
8003 **Darrsucht**, f. tabes mesenterica, marasmus, consumption.
8004 ——, f. der Berg-und Hüttenleute, miners' phthisis.
8005 **Eierstockschwindsucht**, f. ovarian phthisis.
8006 **Eingeweideleiden**, n. 2. visceral or intestinal disease.
8007 **Fallsucht**, f. epilepsy or falling sickness.
8008 **Faserstofferkrankung**, f. fibrin degeneration.
8009 **Flechsenweh**, n. 1. tendon pain.

8010 **Gallenkolik**, f. } bilious
8011 **Gallenkrampf**, m. 1. } colic, cholera.
8012 **Gallenkrankheit**, f. gallbladder disease, bilious disease.
8013 **Gallenlosigkeit**, f. } acholia.
8014 **Gallenmangel**. m. 2. }
8015 **Gallensteinkrankheit**, f. gallstone disease.
8016 **Gallensucht**, f. bile-apparatus disease.
8017 **Gastralgia**, f. gastralgia.
8018 **Gastrodynie**. f. stomach pain.
8019 **Gebärmutterkolik**, f. uterine colic, hysteralgia.
8020 **Gebärmutterschwindsucht**, f. uterine phthisis.
8021 **Gefäszerkrankung**, f. disease of vessels.
8022 **Gehirnerkrankung**, f. } cerebral disease.
8023 **Gehirnkrankheit**, f. }
8024 **Gehörkrankheit**, f. } ear disease, ear affection.
8025 **Gehörleiden**, n. 2. }
8026 **Geilheit**, f. lasciviousness.
8027 **Geilsucht**, f. nymphomania, satyriosis.
8028 **Gekrösschwindsucht**, f. tabes mesenterica.
8029 **Gelbsucht**, f. jaundice, icterus.
8030 **Gelenkkrankheit**, f. } joint disease.
8031 **Gelenkleiden**, n. 2. }
8032 **Geschlechtskrankheit**, f. disease of the sexual organs.
8033 **Gewohnheitskrankheit**, f. disease acquired by custom or habit.
8034 **Gichtbrüchigkeit**, f. palsy.
8035 **Gichtkolik**. f. stomach gout.
8036 **Gliederbeschwerde**. f. pain in the limbs or joints.
8037 **Gliederflusz**, m. 1. rheumatism.
8038 **Gliederkrankheit**, f. articular disease, arthritis.
8039 **Gliedersucht**, f. arthritis.
8040 **Gotthardkrankheit**, f. disease effected by the parasite dochmius duodenalis.
8041 **Grind**, m. 1. scab, scurf, crust.
8042 **Gröszenwahn**, m. 1. mania for greatness, etc.
8043 **Grübelkrankheit**, f. "the spleen," a mental disease.
8044 **Grübelsucht**, f. metaphysical mania, caused by inquisitiveness into metaphysical subjects; by the French called "folie du doute," doubting insanity.
8045 **Grundkrankheit**, f. } primary disease.
8046 **Grundleiden**, n. 2. }
8047 **Grünsucht**, f. clorosis.
8048 **Gürtelkrankheit**, f. } herpes, zoster, shingles.
8049 **Gürtelrose**, f. }
8050 **Haargefäszkrankheit**, f. disease of capillaries.
8051 **Haarkrankheit**, f. hair disease.
8052 **Halsbräune**, f. croup, quinsy.
8053 **Halskrankheit**, f. } neck or throat disease.
8054 **Halsleiden**, n. 2. }
8055 **Halsschwindsucht**, f. laryngeal or tracheal phthisis.
8056 **Halsweh**, n. 1. sore throat or pain in the neck.
8057 **Hämorrhoidalbeschwerde**, f. } haemorrhoidal affection.
8058 **Hämorrhoidalleiden**, n. 2. }
8059 **Hämorrhoidalflusz**, m. 1. haemorrhoids, piles.
8060 **Handgelenkkrankheit**, f. wrist joint disease.
8061 **Harnkrankheit**, f. urinary disease.
8062 **Harnröhrentripper**, m. 2. gonorrhoea.
8063 **Harnruhr**, f. diabetes.
8064 **Harnsteinkrankheit**, f. stone in the bladder.
8065 **Hasenhaarschneiderkrankheit**, f. furrier's, disease.
8066 **Hauptkrankheit**, f. primary on chief disease.
8067 **Hauterkrankung**, f. skin disease.
8068 **Hautjucken**, n. 2. itch, itching.
8069 **Hautkrebs**, m. 1. carcinoma cutis, epithelioma.
8070 **Hautleiden**, n. 2. cutaneous affection.
8071 **Hautrose**, f. erysipelas.
8072 **Hautröte**, f. erythema.
8073 **Hautschwindsucht**, f. subcutaneous emphysema.
8074 **Heftigheit**, f. acuteness, violence of disease.
8075 **heimsiech**, adj. homesick.
8076 **Heimweh**, n. 1. home-sickness.

8077 **Herdkrankheit**, f. }
8078 **Herderkrankung**, f. } metastatic disease.
8079 **Herzklopfen**, n. 2. heart palpitation.
8080 **Herzkrankheit**, f. }
8081 **Herzleiden**, n. 2. } cardiac disease.
8082 **Herzmuskelerkrankung**, f. disease of the cardiac muscle.
8083 **Herzneuralgie**, f. angina pectoris.
8084 **Herzostienerkrankung**, f. disease of the heart orifices.
8085 **Herzweh**, n. 1. cardialgia.
8086 **Hirnkrankheit**, f. }
8087 **Hirnleiden**, n. 2. } cerebral disease or affection.
8088 **Hodenkrankheit**, f. testicles disease.
8089 **Hüftkrankheit**, f. }
8090 **Hüftleiden**, n. 2. } hip disease.
8091 **Hühnerpest**, f. chicken cholera.
8092 **Hühnerpocke**, f. chicken-pox.
8093 **Hüsteln**, n. 2. a little cough, (from hüsteln, to cough a little).
8094 **Husten**, m. 2. cough, coughing (from husten, to cough).
8095 **Hustenanfall**, m. 1. attack or paroxism of cough.
8096 **Hustenkitzel**, m. 2. tickling sensation causing coughing.
8097 **Hustenkrampf**, m. 1. spasmodic coughing.
8098 **Hydromanie**, f. craze for water.
8099 **Hydropathie**, f. hydropathy.
8100 **hydropathisch**, adj. hydropathic.
8101 **Hydropisie**, f. dropsy.
8102 **Hysteropathie**, f. womb disease.
8103 **Ichorrhämie**, f. bloodpoisoning.
8104 **Ichthysmus**, m. 1. poisoning by fish.
8105 **Idiopathie**, f. independent or primary disease.
8106 **Idiotie**, f. idiocy.
8107 **Infektionskrankheit**, f. infections disease.
8108 **Invasionskrankheit**, f. infectious disease, due to parasite, as in itch, etc.
8109 **Involutionskrankheit**, f. disease from involuntary actions of old age.
8110 **Irresein**, n. 1. insanity.
8111 **Jungfernkrankheit**, f. chlorosis.
8112 **kachektisch**, adj. cachectic.
8113 **Kachektik**, f, }
Kachexie, f. } cachexia; bad nutrition condition of the body
8114 **Karbunkelkrankheit**, f. anthrax.
8115 **Katatomie**, f. insanity with muscle rigidity.
8116 **Kehlkopfschwindsucht**, f. }
Kehlkopftuberkulose, f. } laryngeal phthisis.
8117 **Keuchhusten**, m. 2. (from keuchen, to gasp, wheeze) whooping cough.
8118 **Kieferleiden**, n. 2. jaw disease.
8119 **Kinderkrankheit**, f. disease of children.
8120 **Klappenerkrankung**, f. }
8121 **Klappenkrankheit**, f. }
8122 **Klappenleiden**, n. 2. } valvular disease.
8123 **Klaustrophobie**, f. morbid dread of having doors and windows closed.
8124 **Knochenhautübel**, n. 2. }
8125 **Knochenkrankheit**, f. }
8126 **Knochenleiden**, n. 2. } bone disease.
8127 **Knochenweh**, n. 1. bone pain.
8128 **Knollenkrankheit**, f. elephantiasis Arabum.
8129 ——, (from Knollen, m. 2. lump, nodule, tubercle).
8130 **Knotenkrankheit**, f. carbuncle.
8131 ——, (from Knoten, tubercle, node, knot, knob, condyle).
8132 **Kohlensucht**, f. coal-miner's phthisis, anthrakosis.
8133 **Kolik**, f. colic.
8134 **Königskrankheit**, f. }
8135 **Königsübel**, n. 2. } king's evil.
8136 **Konsumtion**, f. consumption, phthisis.
8137 **Kopfkrankheit**, f. headache.
8138 **Kopfrheumatismus**, m. 1. rheumatic headache.
8139 **Kopfschnupfen**, m. 2. cold in the head.
8140 **Krampfkrankheit**, f. convulsive disease.
8141 **Krampfsucht**, f. epilepsy, ergotism.

8142 **Krampfübel**, n. 2. convulsive affection.
8143 **Krampfwehen**, n. 1. pl. spasmodic labor pains.
8144 **Krebserkrankung**, f. } cancerous disease.
8145 **Krebskrankheit**, f. } cancerous disease.
8146 **Kriebelkrankheit**, f. } ergotism.
8147 **Kriebelsucht**, f. } ergotism.
8148 **Kriebeln**, n. 2. fretting, tingling, irritation, itching.
8149 **Kriegspest**, f. } typhus.
8150 **Kriegstyphus**, m. 1. } typhus.
8151 **Kriegsseuche**, f. epidemic due to war.
8152 **Landkrankheit**, f. } epidemic disease prevalent everywhere in a country.
8153 **Landseuche**, f. } epidemic disease prevalent everywhere in a country.
8154 **Leberanschwellung**, f. liver enlargement.
8155 **Leberatrophie**, f. liver atrophy.
8156 **Leberbeschwerde**, f. liver complaint, liver disease.
8157 **Leberkolik**, f. hepatic colic.
8158 **Leberkrankheit**, f. } liver disease.
8159 **Leberleiden**, n. 2. } liver disease.
8160 **Lebersucht**, f. } liver disease.
8161 **Leberschwund**, m. 1. liver atrophy.
8162 **Libersteinkrankheit**, f. gallstone disease.
8163 **Lebervergröszerung**, f. liver enlargement.
8164 **Leberverhärtung**, f. liver induration.
8165 **Leberverkleinerung**, f. liver shrinking.
8166 **Leberverletzung**, f. injury to the liver.
8167 **Leberverstopfung**, f. hepatic obstruction.
8168 **Lendenkrankheit**, f. lumbago.
8169 **Leukorrhöe**, f. leucorrhœa, flux albus.
8170 **Löwenkrankheit**, f. } leontiasis.
Löwenaussatz, m. 1. } leontiasis.
8171 **Luftröhrenschwindsucht**, f. laryngeal or tracheal phthisis.
8172 **Lumpensammlerkrankheit**, f. } rag-sorter's disease.
8173 **Lumpensorterkrankheit**, f. } rag-sorter's disease.
8174 **Lungenaffektion**, f. pulmonary affection.
8175 **Lungenbeschwerde**, f. pulmonary disorder.
8176 **Lungenkrankheit**, f. pulmonary disease.
8177 **Lungenleiden**, n. 2. pulmonary affection.
8178 **Lungenschwindsucht**, f. pulmonary phthisis.
8179 **Lungensucht**, f. consumption.
8180 **Lungentuberkulose**, f. lung tuberculosis.
8181 **Lustseuche**, f. venereal disease.
8182 **Magenbeschwerde**, f. stomach disorder, indigestion.
8183 **Magenkrankheit**, f. stomach disease.
8184 **Magenleiden**, n. 2. stomach affection.
8185 **Magenschwindsucht**, f. gastric phthisis.
8186 **Magentuberkulose**, f. stomach tuberculosis.
8187 **Magenweh**, n. 1. stomach pain.
8188 **Malariaerkrankung**, f. disease caused by malaria.
8189 **Malerkolik**, f. } painter's colic.
8190 **Malerkrankheit**, f. } painter's colic.
8191 **Mandelbräune**, f. tonsilitis, cynanche, angina.
8192 **Marschkrankheit**, f. malarial disease.
8193 **Masern**, pl. } rubeola, morbilli, measles.
8194 **Masernkrankheit**, f. } rubeola, morbilli, measles.
8195 **Massenerkrankung**, f. disease attacking large numbers of people.
8196 **Mastdarmkrankheit**, f. rectum disease,
8197 **Merkurialkrankheit**, f. mercurial poisoning.
8198 **Metalkolik**, f. metallic colic.
8199 **Miasma**, n. 1. (pl. en.) miasma.
8200 **Mikrobiohaemie**, f. disease caused by absorption of micro-organisms into the blood.
8201 **Milzbeschwerde**, f. } spleen affection.
Milzleiden, n. 2. } spleen affection.
8202 **Milzkrankheit**, f. disease of the spleen.
8203 **Milzschwindsucht**, f. splenic phthisis.

8204 **Milzsucht**, f. hypochondriasis.
8205 **Milzweh**, n. 1. spleen pain, splenalgia.
8206 **Minenkrankheit**, f. miners' disease.
8207 **Misopaedie**, f. dislike of one's own children (symptom of melancholia).
8208 **Misopsychie**, f. being tired of life.
8209 **Modekrankheit**, f. fashionable or prevalent disease.
8210 **Monatliche Reinigung**, f. } menstruation, menses.
8211 **Monatsflusz**, m. 1. }
8212 **Mundfäule**, f. } cancer of the mouth (cancrum oris).
8213 **Mundfäulnis**, f. }
8214 **Mundkrankheit**, f. mouth disease.
8215 **Muskelerkrankung**, f. muscle disease.
8216 **Muskelkrankheit**, f. affection or disease of muscles.
8217 **Muskelleiden**, n. 2. disease of muscles.
8218 **Mutterbeschwerde**, f. hysterics.
8219 **Muttergrimmen**, n. 2. uterine colic.
8220 **Mutterkrankheit**, f. uterine disease.
8221 **Muttersucht**, f. hysteria.
8222 **Mutterweh**, n. 1. uterine pain, labor pain.
8223 **Nabelkrankheit**, f. umbilicus disease.
8224 **Nachkrankheit**, f. secondary or consequent disease.
8225 **Nackenweh**, n. 1. neck pain.
8226 **Nagelkrankheit**, f. disease of nails.
8227 **Nebenkrankheit**, f. secondary or accessory disease.
8228 **Nebennierenerkrankung**, f. suprarenal disease, Addison's disease.
8229 **Nervenbeschwerde**, f. nerve complaint, neurosis.
8230 **Nervenerkrankung**, f. disease of nerves.
8231 **Nervenkrankheit**, f. disease of the nerves, neuropathy, neurosis.
8232 **Nervenleiden**, n. 2. } disease of the nerves, neuropathy, neurosis.
8233 **Nervenübel**, n. 2. }
8234 **Nesselbrand**, m. 1. } urticaria, nettle-rash.
8235 **Nesselfieber**, n. 2. }
8236 **Nesselfriesel**, m. 2. }
8237 **Nesselkrankheit**, f. **Nesselsucht**, f. }
8238 **Neuralgie**, f. neuralgia.
8239 **Nierenbeschwerde**, f. } kidney trouble, kidney disease, renal disease.
8240 **Nierenerkrankung**, f. }
8241 **Nierenkrankheit**, f. }
8242 **Nierenweh**, n. 1. } renal colic, nephralgia, renal affection.
8243 **Nierenkolik**, f. }
8244 **Nierenleiden**, n. 2. }
8245 **Nosophobie**, f. morbid dread of disease.
8246 **Nostalgie**, f. home-sickness.
8247 **Ödem**, n. 1. oedema.
8248 **Ohrenkrankheit**, f. } aural disease.
8249 **Ohrenleiden**, n. 2. }
8250 **Ohrenweh**, n. 1. ear pain, otalgia.
8251 **Perlfriesel**, m. 2. miliary fever.
8252 **Pestkrankheit**, f. the plague.
8253 **Pilzerkrankung**, f. } disease caused by fungus.
8254 **Pilzkrankheit**, f. }
8255 **Pneumonie**, f. } pneumonia.
8256 **Pneumonitis**, f. }
8257 **Primärerkrankung**, f. primary disease.
8258 **Puerperal Krankheit**, f. puerperal disease.
8259 **Quecksilberkrankheit**, f. disease caused by mercury.
8260 { **Rachenkrankheit**, f. pharyngeal disease. **Rachenkroup**, f. pharyngeal croup.
8261 **Respirationsbeschwerde**, f. respiratory trouble.
8262 **Respirationskrankheit**, f. respiratory disease.
8263 **Rostkrankheit**, f. disease of plants produced by uredineae.
8264 **Röteln**, pl. German measles.
8265 **Rotlauf**, m. 1. } erysipelas.
8266 **Rotlauffieber**, n. 2. }
8267 **Rückenschmerz**, m. 1. } back pain, spinal neuralgia.
8268 **Rückenweh**, n. 1. }
8269 **Rückenmarkserkrankung**, f. spinal cord disease.

8270 **Rückenmarksnervenschwäche**, f. spinal neurasthenia.

8271 **Rückenmarksschwäche**, f. spinal debility.

8272 **Rückenmarksschwindsucht**, f. tabes dorsalis.

8273 **Rückgratskrankheit**, f. disease of the spinal column.

8274 **Rülpen**, n. 2. (from

8275 **rülpen**, to belch, eructate), belching, eructation.

8276 **Sartenkrankheit**, f. an affection like or identical with Aleppo boil.

8277 **Säuferkrankheit**, f. chronic alcoholism (from

8278 **saufen**, to drink excessively.)

8279 **Scharlachbräune**, f. angina, scarlatinosa, sore throat in scarlet fever patients.

8280 **Scheinkrankheit**, f. illusive, fictitious illness, malingering.

8281 **Schlafkrankheit**, f.
8282 **Schlafsucht**, f.
} coma, lethargy.

8283 **Schleimhautkrankheit**, f.
8284 **Schleimhautleiden**, n. 2.
8285 **Schleimkrankheit**, f.
} disease of mucous membrane. catarrhal disease.

8286 **Schultergelenkkrankheit**, f. shoulderjoint disease.

8287 **Schweiszseuche**, f.
8288 **Schweiszsucht**, f.
} sweating sickness, sudor anglicus.

8289 **Schwindelsucht**, f. vertigo.

8290 **Seekrankheit**, f. sea-sickness.

8291 **seekrank**, adj. sea-sick.

8292 **seelenkrank**, adj. mentally diseased.

8293 **Seelenkrankheit**, f.
8294 **Seelenkummer**, m. 2.
8295 **Seelenleiden**, n. 2.
} mental disease, mental grief, anguish, sorrow, disorder of mind.

8296 **Sklerose**, f. hardening of a part or organ.

8297 **Skrofelkrankheit**, f.
Skrofulose, f.
} scrofula.

8298 **Sommerflecken**, m. 2. pl.
Sommersprossen, f. pl.
} freckles.

8299 **sommerfleckig**,
sommersprossig,
} frekled.

8300 **Somnambulismus**, m. 1. somnambulism, walking in sleep.

8301 **Somnolenz**, f. stupor.

8302 **Speckkrankheit**, f. lardeous disease.

8303 **Speiseröhrenkrankheit**, f. oesophageal disease.

8304 **Starrsucht**, f. catalepsy.

8305 **Staubkrankheit**, f. disease due to inhaling of dust.

8306 **Steckhusten**, m. 2. whooping cough.

8307 **Steckschnupfen**, m. 2. suffocative coryza.

8308 **Steinkolik**, f. nephritic colic.

8309 **Steinkranke**, m. 3. & f. patients suffering from stone.

8310 **Steinkrankheit**, f.
8311 **Steinleiden**, n. 2
} calculous disease, lithiasis.

8312 **Stickhusten**, m. 2. whooping cough.

8313 **Tachykardie**, f. heart palpitation.

8314 **Tanzkrankheit**, f. (**St. Veitstanz**, m. 1.)
8315 **Tanzsucht**, f.
8316 **Tanzwut**, f.
} chorea, St. Vitus dance. an epidemic of the Middle Ages incessant dancing caused by religious exhalation

8317 **Tastkrankheit**, f. (from

8318 **tasten**, to feel), disease of the sense of touch.

8319 **Tierseuche**, f. epizootic.

8320 **Tobsucht**, f. mania, frenzy, (from toben, to rage).

8321 **Trommelsucht**, f.
8322 **Windsucht**, f.
8323 **Tympanie**, f.
} tympanitis.

8324 **Trunkfälligkeit**, f.
8325 **Trunksucht**, f.
} dipsomania, chronic alcoholism.

8326 **Tuberkelkrankheit**, f.
8327 **Tuberkelsucht**, f.
} tuberculosis.

8328 **Tympanie**, f. tympanitis.

8329 **Unterleibsschwindsucht**, f. abdominal phthisis.

8330 **Urinbeschwerde**, f. urinary affection or troubles.

8331 **Venusseuche**, f. syphilis.

8332 **Verpestung**, f. infection.

8333 **Wachstumskrankheit**, f. disease of development or growth.

8334 **Wahnsinn**, m. 1. insanity.
8335 **Wassersucht**, f. dropsy.
8336 **Wirbelkrankheit**, f. } vertebrae disease.
8337 **Wirbelleiden**, n. 2. } Pott's spine disease.
8338 **Pott'sche**, }
8339 **Wirbeltuberkulose**, f. vertebrae tubercular disease.
8340 **Wochenbettkrankheit**, f. puerperal disease.
9341 **Wöchnerinnenfriesel**, m. 2. miliary rash, during puerperal period.
8342 **Wunddiphtherie**, f. } hospital gangrene
8343 **Wundfäulnis**, f. }
8344 **Wundkrankheit**, f. (any) wound disease.
8345 **Wundrose**, f. traumatic erysipelas.
8346 **Wurmkrankheit**, f. (any) worm disease.
8347 **Wüstenwahnsinn**, m. 1. } insanity from isolation caused by brain exhaustion (in deserts) in travelers.
8348 **Wüstenhallucination**, }
8349 **Wutkrankheit**, f. hydrophobia, from
8350 (**wüten**, to rage, rave).
8351 **Xerosis**, f. trachoma or a change in the cornea and conjunctiva.
8352 **Zahnerkrankung**, f. } disease of teeth.
8353 **Zahnkrankheit**, f. }
8354 **Zahnleiden**, n. 2. }
8355 **Zahnschmerzen**, pl. m. 1. toothache.
8356 **Zehrkrankheit**, f. wasting disease, etc.
8357 12. **KREBS**, *Cancer*.
8358 **Augenkrebs**, m. 1. eye cancer.
8359 **Augenlidkrebs**, m. 1. eyelid cancer.
8360 **Bauchfellkrebs**, m. 1. peritoneal cancer.
8361 **Beinkrebs**, m. 1. bone cancer.
8362 **Blutkrebs**, m. 1. fungus haematodes.
8363 **Brustkrebs**, m. 1. mammary gland cancer.
8364 **Darmkrebs**, m. 1. intestinal cancer.
8365 **Drüsenkrebs**, m. 1. carcinoma of glands.
8366 **Drüsenzellenkrebs**, m. 1. primary cancer of glandular organ.
8367 **Dünndarmkrebs**, m. 1. cancer of the small intestines.
8368 **Faserkrebs**, m. 1. scirrhus.
8369 **Gallenblasenkrebs**, m. 1. cancer of the gall bladder.
8370 **Gallengangkrebs**, m. 1. } bileduct cancer.
8371 **Gallenwegekrebs**, m. 1. }
8372 **Gallertkrebs**, m. 1. colloid, alveolar or reticular carcinoma.
8373 **Gebärmutterkrebs**, m. 1. uterine cancer.
8374 **Gehirnkrebs**, m. 1. cancer of the brain.
8375 **Gesichtskrebs**, m. 1. cancer of the face.
8376 **Harnröhrenkrebs**, m. 1. urethra cancer.
8377 **Hautkrebs**, m. 1. epithelioma.
8378 **Hodenkrebs**, m. 1. testicle cancer.
8379 **Hodensackkrebs**, m. 1. scrotum cancer.
8380 **Kehlkopfkrebs**, m. 1. larynx cancer.
8381 **Knochenkrebs**, m. 1. bone cancer.
8382 **Knollenkrebs**, m. 1. keloid.
8383 **Kopfhautkrebs**, m. 1. scalp cancer.
8384 **Leberkrebs**, m. 1. liver cancer.
8385 **Lippenkrebs**, m. 1. labial cancer.
8386 **Lumbarkrebs**, m. 1. lumbar cancer.
8387 **Lungenkrebs**, m. 1. lung cancer.
8388 **Magenkrebs**, m. 1. stomach cancer.
8389 **Markkrebs**, m. 1. medullary cancer.
8390 **Mastdarmkrebs**, m. 1. rectum cancer.
8391 **Medullarkarcinom**, n. 1. } medullary cancer.
8392 **Medullarkrebs**, m. 1. }
8393 **Milzkrebs**, m. 1. spleen cancer.
8394 **Mundkrebs**, m. 1. mouth cancer.
8395 **Mutterhalskrebs**, m. 1. cancer of cervix uteri.
8396 **Mutterkrebs**, m. 1. uterine cancer.

8397 **Narbenkrebs**, m. 1. from Narbe, f. cicatrix, scar, cicatrix cancer (narbig, adj. cicatrised).
8398 **Nasenkrebs**, m. 1. nose cancer.
8399 **Nervenkrebs**, m. 1. nerve cancer.
8400 **Ohrspeicheldrüsenkrebs**, m. 1. cancer of parotid gland.
8401 **Osteoidkrebs**, m. 1. bone cancer.
8402 **Pankreaskrebs**, m. 1. pancreas cancer.
8403 **Pflasterepithelkrebs**, m. 1. squamous epithelioma.
8404 **Pfortaderkrebs**, m. 1. cancer of the portal vein.
8405 **Pigmentkrebs**, m. 1. melanotic cancer.
8406 **Plattenepithelkrebs**, m. 1. squamouscelled epithelioma.
8407 **Pleurakrebs**, m. 1. pleura cancer.
8408 **Ruszkrebs**, m. 1. chimney-sweeper's cancer.
9409 **Scheidenkrebs**, m. 1. vagina cancer.
8410 **Schleimhautkrebs**, m. 1. cancer of mucous membrane.
8411 **Speicheldrüsenkrebs**, m. 1. salivary gland cancer.
8412 **Speiseröhrenkrebs**, m. 1. oesophagus cancer.
8413 **Strahlenkrebs**, m. 1. radiated sarcoma (as in liver).
8414 **Vorsteherdrüsenkrebs**, m. 1. prostate cancer.
8415 **Wirbelkrebs**, m. 1. vertebra cancer.
8416 **Zellenkrebs**, m. 1. medullary cancer.
8417 **Zottenkrebs**, m. 1. villous cancer.
8418 **Zungenkrebs**, m. 1. cancer of the tongue.
8419 13. **STEIN**, *Stone.*
8420 **Augenstein**, m. 1. lapis divinus.
8421 **Blasenstein**, m. 1. vesical calculus.
8422 **Bronchialstein**, m. 1. pulmonary concretion.
8423 **Gallenblasenstein**, m. 1. gallstone.
8424 **Gallenstein**, m. 1. gallstone, biliary calculus.
8425 **Gallitzenstein**, m. 1. sulphate of zinc.
8426 **Gebärmutterstein**, m. 1. uterus concretion.
8427 **Gehörsteinchen**, n. 2. otoconia, otolith.
8428 **Griesstein**, m. 1. gravel.
8429 **Harnblasenstein**, m. 1. vesical calculus.
8430 **Harnleiterstein**, m. 1. stone in ureter.
8431 **Harnröhrenstein**, m. 1. urethral calculus.
8432 **Harnstein**, m. 1. urinary calculus.
8433 **Hautstein**, m. 1. calcareous sebaceous cyst.
8434 **Hirnstein**, m. 1. brain concretion.
8435 **Höllenstein**, m. 1. nitrate of
8436 silver, —, mitigated (equal parts of nitrate of silver and nitrate of potassium.)
8437 **Kotstein**, m. 1. enterolith, faecal concretion.
8438 **Leberstein**, m. 1. gallstone.
8439 **Lendenstein**, m. 1. renal calculus.
8440 **Luftröhrenstein**, m. 1. tracheal or bronchial concretion.
8441 **Lungenstein**, m. 1. pulmonary concretion.
8442 **Magenstein**, m. 1. gastric concretion.
8443 **Mandelstein**, m. 1. tonsilar calculus.
8444 **Maulbeerstein**, m. 1. mulberry calculus.
8445 **Mutterstein**, m. 1. uterine concretion.
8446 **Nasenstein**, m. 1. rhinolith.
8447 **Nierenbeckenstein**, m. 1. calculus of kidney pelvis.
8448 **Nierenstein**, m. 1. renal calculus.
8449 **Ohrenstein**, m. 1. } otolith.
8450 **Ohrstein**, m. 1. }
8451 **Ohrsteinchen**, n. 2. }
8452 **Pankreasstein**, m. 1. pancreatic concretion.
8453 **Pigmentstein**, m. 1. pigmented stone (in gall bladder.)
8454 **Prostatasand**, m. 1. } prostatic concretion, or gravel.
8455 **Prostatastein**, m. 1. }
8456 **Prostatasteinchen**, n. 2. }
8457 **Silberätzstein**, m. 1. lunar caustic.

8458 **Thränenstein**, m. 1. } lachrymal calculus.
8459 **Thränensackstein**, m. 1. } lachrymal calculus.
8460 **Tonsillarstein**, m. 1. tonsillar calculus.
8461 **Urinstein**, m. 1. urinary calculus.
8462 **Uterusstein**, m. 1. uterine concretion.
8463 **Venenstein**, m. 1. phlebolith
8464 **Vorhautstein**, m. 1. preputial calculus.
8465 **Zahnstein**, m. 1. } tartar on teeth, etc.
8466 **Zahnweinstein**, m. 1. } tartar on teeth, etc.
8467 14. **WASSERSUCHT**, *Dropsy.*
8468 **Augapfelwassersucht**, f. dropsy of the globe.
8469 **Augenwassersucht**, f. hydrophthalmia.
8470 **Bauchfellwassersucht**, f. } ascites.
8471 **Bauchhöhlenwassersucht**, f. } ascites.
8472 **Bauchwassersucht**, f. } ascites.
8473 **Blutwassersucht**, f. anaemia.
8474 **Brustfellwassersucht**, f. } hydrothorax.
8475 **Brustwassersucht**, f. } hydrothorax.
8476 **Eierstockwassersucht**, f. ovarian dropsy.
8477 **Gallenblasenwassersucht**, f. ovarian cyst, dropsy of gallbladder.
8478 **Gebärmuttersackwassersucht**, f. hydrometra.
8479 **Gebärmutterwassersucht**, f. dropsy of uterus, hydrometra.
8480 **Gehirnhöhlenwassersucht**, f. dropsy of cerebral ventricles.
8481 **Gehirnwassersucht**, f. hydrocephalus.
8482 **Gelenkwassersucht**, f. hydrops articuli.
8483 **Gliederwassersucht**, f. hydrops articuli.
8484 **Harnleiterwassersucht**, f. ureter distention.
8485 **Hautwassersucht**, f. anasarca, oedema.
8486 **hautwassersüchtig**, adj. anasarcous, oedematous.
8487 **Herzbeutelwassersucht**, f. hydrops pericardii.
8488 **Hirnhöhlenwassersucht**, f. congenital internal hydrocephalus.
8489 **Hirnwassersucht**, f. hydrocephalus.
8490 **Hodenscheidenhautwassersucht**, f. hydrocele of tunica vaginalis.
8491 **Hodenwasserbruch**, m. 1. } hydrocele.
8492 **Hodenwassersucht**, f. } hydrocele.
8493 **Hodenwassergeschwulst**, f. } hydrocele.
8494 **Kopfwassersucht**, f. hydrocephalus.
8495 **Leibwassersucht**, f. ascites.
8496 **Lungenwassersucht**, f. lung oedema.
8497 **Mutterkuchenwassersucht**, f. chronic oedema of placenta.
8498 **Muttertrompetenwassersucht**, f. hydrosalpinx, dropsy of Fallopian tube.
8499 **Mutterwassersucht**, f. hydrometra, dropsy of uterus.
8500 **Nierenbeckenwassersucht**, f. } hydronephrosis.
8501 **Nierenwassersucht**, f. } hydronephrosis.
8502 **Ohrwassersucht**, f. ear oedema.
8503 **Rückenmarkswassersucht**, f. hydro-rachis.
8504 **Rutenwassersucht**, f. penis oedema.
8505 **Sackwassersucht**, f. encysted dropsy.
8506 **Scharlachwassersucht**, f. scarlatinal dropsy.
8507 **Scheidenhautwassersucht**, f. (des Hodens), hydrocele.
8508 **Schleimbeutelwassersucht**, f. enlarged bursa, housemaid's knee.
8509 **Thränensackwassersucht**, f. dropsy of lachrymal sac.
8510 **Tubenwassersucht**, f. dropsy of Fallopian tube.
8511 **Wurmfortsatzwassersucht**, f. dropsy of vermiform process.
8512 **Zellengewebswassersucht**, f. oedema of cellular tissue, etc.

PART SECOND.

8513 **MASZREGELN und MITTEL**, measures and means, e. g.:
8514 **gesundheitliche**, hygienic,
8515 **medizinische**, medical,
8516 **chirurgische**, surgical,
häusliche, domestic, etc. etc.
§ 32. Hygienic, medical and surgical means.
8517 1. **APOTHEKE**, f. apothecary's store, or officin, office. In compounds:
8518 **Apothekerwesen**, n. 2. all pertaining to a drugstore, etc.
8519 **Apotheker**, m. 2. apothecary, druggist, chemist.
8520 **Apothekerbuch**, n. 1, dispensatory, pharmacopoeia.
8521 **Apothekergehülf**, m. 3. druggist's assistant.
8522 **Apothekergewicht**. n. 1. apothecary's weight, troy-weight.
8523 **Apothekerkunst**, f. pharmacy.
8524 **Apothekerladen**, m. 2. druggist's store.
8525 **Apothekerlaboratorium**, n. 1. apothecary's laboratory.
8526 **Apothekerlehrling**, m. 1. apothecary's apprentice.
8527 **Apothekerrechnung**, f. apothecary's bill.
8528 **Apothekertaxe**, f. price of drugs by law.
8529 **Apothekerwage**, f. apothecary's scales.
8530 **Apothekerware**, f. a drug.
8531 **Apothekerwissenschaft**, f. pharmacology.
8532 **Feldapotheke**, f. field dispensary.
8533 **Hausapotheke**. f. domestic medicine chest.
8534 **Reiseapotheke**, f. medicine chest, used in travels.
8535 **Schiffsapotheke**, f. ship's medicine chest.
8536 **Analyse**, f. analysis (from analysieren, to analyze).
8537 **Zergliederung**, f. } analysis.
8538 **Zerzetzung**, f. }
8539 **Analytiker**, m. 2. analytic.

8540 **Chemie**, f. } chemistry.
8541 **Scheidekunst**, f. }
8542 **Chemist**, m. 3. } chemist.
8543 **Scheidekünstler**, m. 2. }
8544 **specifisch**, adj. specific. (Gewicht, weight.)
8545 **Unze**, f. ounce, etc.
8546 { **verdünnen**, **attenuieren**, { to attenuate, dilute, reduce, make thin. **Verdünnung**, f. attenuation, dilution, reduction.
8547 3. **ARZNEI**, f. **Medizin**, f. } medicine, physic. In compounds:
8548 **Arzneianwendung**, f. method of administering drugs.
8549 **Arzneibiscuit**, n. 1. medicated biscuit.
8550 **Arzneidose**, f. } dose of medicine.
8551 **Arzneidosis**, pl. dosen, }
8552 **Arzneidöschen**, n. 2. }
8553 **Arzneiessige**, pl. m. 1. medicated vinegars, etc.
8554 **Arzneiform**, f. formula.
8555 **Arzneiformel**, f. recipe, medical prescription.
8556 **Arzneigabe**, f. dose.
8557 **Arzneigebrauch**, m. 1. use of medicine.
8558 **Arzneigelehrsamkeit**, f. } science, knowledge, or art of medicine, therapeutics.
8559 { **Arzneikunde**, f. **Arzneikunst**, f. }
8560 { **Heilkunde** f. **Heilkunst**, f. }
8561 **arzneilich**, adj. } medicinal.
8562 **medikamentös**, adj. }
8563 **medizinisch**, adj. }
8564 **Arzneigewicht**, n. 1. officinal weight.
8565 **Arzneimasz**, n. 1. officinal measure.
8566 3. **ARZNEIMITTEL**, n. 2. remedy, medicine, physic.
8567 —**kunde**, f. } pharmacology.
8568 —**lehre**, f. }
8569 **Arzneimittel**, **abführendes**, cathartic.
8570 —, **ableitendes**, derivative, epispastic.

8571 —, **anastaltisches**, blood staunching remedy, stytic, astringent.
8572 —, **appetitmachendes**, stomachic.
8573 —, **ätzendes**, caustic, escharotic.
8574 —, **auflösendes**, resolvent.
8575 —, **ausleerendes**, evacuant.
8576 —, **austrocknendes**, desiccant.
8577 —, **auswurfbeförderndes**, expectorant.
8578 —, **bähendes**, a remedy by fermentation.
8579 —, **belebendes**, restorative stimulant.
8580 —, **beräucherndes**, fumigating remedy.
8581 —, **berauschendes**, intoxicant.
8582 —, **beruhigendes**, sedative.
8583 —, **betäubendes**, narcotic, sedative, stupefactive.
8584 —, **blähungstreibendes**, carminative.
8585 —, **blasenbewirkendes**, vesicant, epispastic.
8586 —, **blutgefäszlähmendes**, general vasomotor depressant.
8587 —, **blutstillendes**, haemostatic, styptic.
8588 —, **brechenerregendes**, emetic.
8589 —, **einblasendes**, remedy by insufflation.
8590 —, **einhüllendes**, enveloping or disguising remedy.
8591 —, **einschläferndes**, hypnotic, soporific.
8592 —, **einspritzendes**, a remedy by syringing, e. g. subcutaneous injection.
8593 —, **einträufelndes**, remedy by instillation.
8594 —, **eisenhaltiges**, ferruginous remedy.
8595 —, **eiterungbeförderndes**. remedy promoting suppuration.
8596 —, **ekelbewirkendes**, nauseant.
8597 —, **enthaarendes**, depilatory.
8598 —. **entzündungswidriges**, antiphlogistic remedy.
8599 —, **erfrischendes**, refreshing, cooling, refrigerating remedy.
8600 —, **erhitzendes**, stimulant, effecting animal heat.
8601 —, **erregendes**, excitant.
8602 —, **erschlaffendes**, relaxant.
8603 —, **erweichendes**, emollient by baths, poultices, etc.
8604 —, **fäulniswidriges**, antiseptic, antizymotic, disinfectant.
8605 —, **fruchtabtreibendes**, abortive.
8606 —, **gährungswidriges**, antizymotic.
8607 —, **harntreibendes**, —, **diuretisches**, diuretic.
8608 —, **hautrötendes**, rubefacient.
8609 —, **herzstärkendes**, cardiac stimulant.
8610 —, **incidierendes**, drastic remedy.
8611 —, **klebendes**, agglutinant.
8612 —, **konsolidierendes**, fixing loose, or hardening soft parts by surgical means.
8613 —, **konstipierendes**, producing constipation.
8614 —, **kopfstärkendes**, strengthening brain or head.
8615 —, **kräftigendes**, tonic.
8616 —, **krampflindernd**, or stillendes, antispasmodic.
8617 —, **kropfverkleinerndes**, reducing gôitre (by iodine).
8618 —, **kühlendes**, refrigerant,
8619 —, **labendes**, refreshing, recreating.
8620 —, **lähmendes**, producing paralysis (by chloroform).
8621 —, **laxierendes**, purgative.
8622 —, **linderndes**, palliative.
8623 —, **magermachendes**, a remedy producing emaciation.
8624 —, **menstruationbeförderndes**, emmenagogue.
8625 —, **milchbewirkendes**, milk producing remedy.
8626 —, **milchtreibendes**, galactagogue.
8627 —, **milderndes**, mitigant, alleviating, demulcent.
8628 —, **muskelbewegendes**, muscular exercise, gymnastics.

8629 —, **muskelerregendes,** muscle stimulant.

8630 —, **nährendes,** nutrient.

8631 —, **narkotisches,** narcotic.

8632 —, **niederschlagendes,** sedative.

8633 —, **niesenerregendes,** errhine or sternutatory.

8634 —, **präservatives,** preservative.

8635 —, **purgierendes,** purgative.

8636 —, **radikalisches,** specific. radical.

8637 —, **reinigendes,** cleansing remedy.

8638 —, **reizendes,** irritant.

8639 —, **reizmilderndes,** emollient.

8640 —, **resorbierendes,** resorbant removing of morbid fluids or deposits.

8641 —, **roborierendes,** roborant.

8642 —, **säuretilgendes,** antacid.

8643 —, **schlafbewirkendes,** hypnotic.

8644 —, **schleimlösendes,** loosening mucus (alkalies).

8645 —, **schmerzstillendes,** anodyne.

8646 —, **schützendes,** prophylactical remedy.

8647 —, **schweiszaufhebendes,** antihydrotic.

8648 —, **schweisztreibendes,** sudorific. diaphoretic.

8649 —, **speichelabsonderndes,** sialagogue, ptyalagogue.

8650 —, **stärkendes,** roborant, restorative.

8651 —, **steinlösendes,** lithontriptic.

8652 —, **traumatisches,** traumatic, woundhealing remedy.

8653 —, **verdauungbefördernndes,** digestive.

8654 —, **verhütendes,** preventative, preservative.

8655 —, **verklebendes,** emplastic remedy.

8656 —, **vernarbungbeförderndes,** remedy promoting cicatrisation.

8657 —, **verschönerndes,** cosmetic.

8658 —, **versuchendes,** testing, trying.

8659 —, **verstopfendes,** obstruent remedy.

8660 —, **verwahrendes,** preservative.

8661 —, **wehenerregendes,** } ecbolic.
—, **wehentreibendes,** } ecbolic.

8662 —, **vertreibendes,** } ecbolic.

8663 —, **wurmtreibendes,** or } anthelmintic, vermifuge.

8664 —, **wurmtötendes,** } anthelmintic, vermifuge.

8665 —, **zusammenziehendes,** astringent.

8666 **Arzneipapiere,** n. 1. pl. medicated papers, chartae.

8667 **Arzneipflanze,** f. medicinal or officinal plant.

8668 **Arzneipflaster,** n. 2. plaster.

8669 **Arzneirecept,** n. 1. recipe.

8670 **Arzneisyruppe,** pl. m. 1. medicated syrups.

8671 **Arzneistift,** m. 1. medicated point, e. g. caustic point.

8672 **Arzneisucht,** f. physic mania.

8673 **Arzneitrank,** m. 1. draught, potion.

8674 **Arzneiverordnung,** f. } prescription, receipt.

8675 **Arzneiverschreibung,** f. } prescription, receipt.

8676 **Arzneiwarenkunde,** f. pharmacognosis.

8677 **Arzneiwein,** m. 1. medicated wine.

8678 **Arzneiwesen,** n. 2. things pertaining to pharmacy.

8679 **Arzneiwirkung,** f. effect or result of medicine.

8680 **Arzneiwissenschaft,** f. medicine, medical science.

8681 **arzneiwissenschaftlich,** adj. medical.

8682 **Hausarznei,** f. domestic remedy, etc.

8683 **Quacksalbereiarznei,** f. quack medicine, etc.

8684 4. **ARZT,** m. 1. } physician, doctor. In compounds:

8685 **DOKTOR,** m. 2. } physician, doctor. In compounds:

8686 **Mediziner,** m. 2. } physician, doctor. In compounds:

8687 —, **ausübender,** } practicing physician, practitioner.

8688 —, **praktizierender,** } practicing physician, practitioner.

8689 —, **ordinierender,** assistant physician, surgeon to a hospital.

8690 **Arztgebühr,** f. physician's fee.

(149)

8691 **ärztlich**, adj. medical.
8692 **ärztliche Behandlung**, f. medical treatment.
8693 **ärztlicher Rat**, m. 1. medical advice, etc.
8694 **Allopath**, m. 3. allopathic doctor.
8695 **allopathisch**, adj. allopathic.
8696 **Amtsarzt**, m. 1. district medical officer.
8697 **Armenarzt**, m. 1. poor-law med. officer.
8698 **Augenarzt**, m. 1. } oculist.
8699 **Okulist**, m. 3. }
8700 **Feldarzt**, m. 1. army surgeon.
8701 **Geburtsarzt**, m. 1. } accoucheur, obstetrician.
8702 **Geburtshelfer**, m. 2. }
8703 **Geburtshelferin**, f. }
8704 **Accoucheur**, m. 1. }
8705 **Hausarzt**, m. 1. family doctor.
8706 **Homoeopath**, m. 3. homöopathist, homöopathic doctor.
8707 **homoeopathisch**, adj. homöopathic.
8708 { **Hühneraugenarzt**, m. 1. / **Hühneraugendoktor**, m. 2. } corn doctor, chiropodist.
8709 **Impfarzt**, m. 1. vaccinator.
8710 **Kurarzt**, m. 1. doctor attending a watering place.
8711 **Landarzt**, m. 1. country doctor.
8712 **Leibarzt**, m. 1. physician in ordinary (in royalty).
8713 **Massage-doctor**, m. 2. massage-treatment practitioner.
8714 **Militärarzt**, m. 1. military surgeon.
8715 **Militäroberarzt**, m. 1. } chief surgeon or surgeon general.
8716 **Oberwundarzt**, m. 1. }
8717 **Ohrenarzt**, m. 1. aurist.
8718 **Quacksalber**, m. 2. quackery practitioner.
8719 **Quacksalberei**, f. quackery.
8720 **quacksalbern**, v. to practice quackery.
8721 **Regimentarzt**, m. 1. regimental surgeon.
8722 **Specialarzt**, m. 1. specialist.
8723 **Tierarzt**, m. 1. } horse doctor, veterinary surgeon.
Veterinarian, m. 1. }
8724 **Wundarzt**, m. 1. } surgeon.
Chirurg, m. 3. }
8725 **Zahnarzt**, m. 1. } dentist, etc.
8726 **Dentist**, m. 3. }
8727 5. **BAD**, n. 1. *bath*, in compounds:
8728 **Aschenbad**, n. 1. the enclosing of the diseased part in fresh, dry wood-ashes.
8729 **Augenbad**, n. 1. ophthalmic bath, eye-douche.
8730 **Dampfbad**, n. 1. vapor bath.
8731 **Douchebad**, n. 1. douche bath by sprinkling or pouring.
8732 **Dunstbad**, n. 1. vapor bath.
8733 **Eisenbad**, n. 1. bath containing iron, either natural or artificial iron-water.
8734 **Essigsäurebad**, n. 1. acetic acid bath.
8735 **Fichtennadelbad**, n. 1. pine-tree bath.
8736 **Fuszbad**, n. 1. footbath.
8737 **Gieszbad**, n. 1. douche bath (from v. ir. gieszen, to pour.)
8738 **Gliedbad**, n. 1. bath for a limb.
8739 **Handbad**, n. 1. hand bath.
8740 **Heilbad**, n. 1. medical or mineral water bath (from
8741 **heilen**, to heal.)
8742 **Heiszwasserbad**, n. 1. hot water bath.
8743 **Jodkalibad**, n. 1. iodide of potassium bath.
8744 **Kopfbad**, n. 1. head bath.
8745 **Kräuterbad**, n. 1. warm bath, prepared through medicinal or aromatic herbs.
8746 **Laubad**, n. 1. tepid bath.
8747 **Laubbad**, n. 1. leaf bath, dry leaves of birch or pine-trees covering diseased parts of the body.
8748 **Luftbad**, n. 1. air bath.
8749 **Malzbad**, n. 1. malt bath.
8750 **Medizinalbad**, n. 1. medicated bath.
8751 **Qualmbad**, n. 1. vapor bath.
8752 **Rachenbad**, n. 1. pharyngeal douche.
8753 **Rauchbad**, n. 1. vapor bath.
8754 **Salzbad**, n. 1. saltwater bath.
8755 **Sandbad**, n. 1. sand bath.
8756 **Schauerbad**, n. 1. shower bath.
8757 **Schneebad**, n. 1. snow bath.

8758 **Schwefelbad**, n. 1. sulphur bath.

8759 **Schweiszbad**, n. 1.
8760 **Schwitzbad**, n. 1. (from schwitzen, to sweat). } hot-air bath, steam. sweating bath.

8761 **Seebad**, n. 1. sea bath.

8762 **Seifenbad**, n. 1. soap bath.

8763 **Sitzbad**, n. 1. hip bath, sitting bath.

8764 **Sonnenbad**, n. 1. sun bath.

8765 **Sprudelbad**, n. 1. shower bath.

8766 **Staubbad**, n. 1. shower bath (by sprinkling like dust.)

8767 **Sturzbad**, n. 1. shower bath (by jumping into the water.)

8768 **Traufbad**, n. 1. shower bath, (from
8769 **träufeln**, to drop.)

8770 **Tropfbad**. n. 1. shower bath (by drops falling slowly.)

8771 **Überraschungsbad**, n. 1. bath (by surprise.)

8772 **Warmbad**, n. 1. warm bath.

8773 **Wasserbad**, n. 1.
8774 **Wasserdampfbad**, n. 1. } vapor bath, etc.

8775 6. **BAND**,
8776 **Binde**, } *Bandage*. Band.

8777 **Band**, n. 1. (from v. ir.
8778 **binden**, to bind), band, bandage, ligature, ligament, fraenum, filament, commissure. In compounds :

8779 **Bandagenlehre**, f. science of bandaging.

8780 **bandagieren**, to bandage.

8781 **Bandagierung**, f. bandaging.

8782 **Bandagist**, m. 3, truss bandage maker.

8783 **bandförmig**, adj. band-shaped, ribbon-formed.

8784 **Bauchbruchband**, n. 1. truss for abdominal hernia.

8785 **Bruchband**, n. 1. suspender, truss.

8786 **Compressionsband**, n. 1. bolster, compress.

8787 **Kopfband**, n. 1. head band or bandage.

8788 **Laszband**, n. 1. bandage after bleeding.

8789 **Nabelbruchband**, n. 1. umbilical truss.

8790 **Schnürverband**, m. 1. elastic ligature.

8791 **Hirnband**, n. 1. frontal bandage.

8792 **Tragband**, n. 1. brace, sling, suspensor, strap.

8793 **Verband**, m. 1. binding up, bandage, dressing.

8794 **Verbandklemme**, f. clamp for elastic bandage.

8795 **Verbandpappe**, f. starch prepared for bandaging.

8796 **Verbandstoff**, m. 1. bandage or dressing material.

8797 **Verbandtechnic**, f. bandaging technic.

8798 **Verbandtorf**, m. 1. peat for dressing, etc.

8799 7. **BINDE**, f. *band, bandage*, belt, ligature, roller, sling, fascia.

8800 **BINDE**, grosze, handkerchief bandage. In compounds :

8801 **Aderbinde**, f. bandage, ligature.

8802 **Aderlaszbäuschchen**, n. 2. compress used in bloodletting.

8803 **Aderlaszbinde**, f. bandage used after bloodletting.

8804 **Armbinde**, f. sling or bandage for the arm, fascia of the arm.

8805 **Augenbinde**, f. eye bandage.

8806 **Aufhebebinde**, f. suspensor, truss.

8807 **Bauchbinde**, f. abdominal bandage, fascia abdominalis.

8808 **Bauchbruchbinde**, f. bandage or truss for abdominal hernia.

8809 **Bruchbinde**, f. bandage for hernia, or fracture, sling.

8810 **Brustbinde**, f. chest bandage.

8811 **Fuszbinde**, f. foot bandage.

8812 **Hauptbinde**, f. head bandage.

8813 ——, **vierköpfig**, four-headed or four-tailed head bandage.

8814 **Hobelbinde**, f.
8815 **Hobelspanbinde**, f. } dolabra bandage, reversed spiral roller.

8816 **Kinnbinde**, f. chin bandage, jaw bandage.

8817 **Kniebinde**, f. knee-cap bandage.

8818 **Knotenbinde**, f. star bandage, packer's bandage.

8819 **Kopfbinde**, f. head band or bandage.

8820 **Laszbinde**, f. bandage after bleeding.
8821 **Leibbinde**, f. body bandage, belt.
8822 **Nabelbinde**, f. umbilical binder.
8823 **Nasenbinde**, f. nose bandage.
8824 **Querbinde**, f. transverse band or bandage.
8825 **Querfalte**, f. transverse fold.
8826 **Rollbinde**, f. roller bandage.
8827 **Schlinge**, f. hanging bandage or sling.
8828 **sechsköpfig**, adj. six-headed (bandage).
8829 **Stirnbinde**, f. frontal bandage.
8830 **Tragbinde**, f. sling, suspensory sling or bandage.
8831 **Tragbeutel**, m. 2. suspender for scrotum.
8832 **Umschlingung**, f. twisting into loops, (volvulus).
8833 **Umschnürung**, f. ligation, tie lying round.
8834 **Unterbindung**, f. ligation, binding up.
8835 **Venenunterbindung**, f. ligation of a vein.
8836 **Verbindung**, f. (from v. ir.
8837 **verbinden**, to dress, bandage, apply a bandage or dressing, to take up, e. g. an artery, etc.
8838 8. **BEHANDLUNGSART**, f. method of treatment, cure;
8839 ——, **allgemeine**, general or constitutional treatment.
8840 ——, **allopathische**, allopathic treatment.
8841 ——, **homoeopathische**, homöopathic treatment.
8842 ——, **hydropathische**, hydropathic treatment.
8843 ——, **klimatische**, climatic treatment.
8844 ——**magnetische**, magnetic treatment.
8845 ——, **durch Massage**, treatment by massage.
8846 ——, **sympathetische**, sympathetic treatment.
8847 **Genesung**, f. (from
8848 **genesen**, to recover) convalescence, recovery.
8849 **Genesungsfall**, m. 1. case of convalescence.
8850 **Genesungsperiode**, f. period of convalescence.
8851 **Heilmethode**, f. (from
8852 **heilen**, to heal), method of healing, cure.
8853 **Heilmittel**, n. 1. remedy.
8854 **Heilung**, f. cure, healing, remedy.
8855 **Heilverfahren**, n. 2. treatment.
8856 **Heilversuch**, m. 1. attempted treatment.
8857 **Heilzweck**, m. 1. therapeutic purpose.
8858 **Labe** or **Labungsmittel**, n. 2. refreshment.
8859 **Radikalheilung**, f. } radical
8860 **Radikalkur**, f. } cure.
8861 **Kur**, f. (from
8862 **kurieren**, to cure, treat), cure, treatment, idiomatic : in der Kur sein, to be under treatment ; or
8863 **eine Kur gebrauchen**, to use a treatment ;
8864 **Rückfall**, m. 1. (from v. ir.
8865 **zurückfallen**, to fall back, i. e. relapse,) to relapse.
8866 **Schutzmittel**, n. 2. (from schützen, to protect), preventative.
8867 **Stärkungsmittel**, n. 2. } (from stärken and kräftigen, to strengthen,) tonic, restorative.
8868 **Kräftigungsmittel**, n. 2. }
8869 **Wiederherstellung**, f. (from
8870 **wiederherstellen**, to restore). restoration.

Compounds with *Kur* closing the words :

8871 **Abmagerungskur**, f. cure by emaciation.
8872 **Arsenkur**, f. treatment by arsenic.
8873 **Atmungskur**, f. respiratory cure.
8874 **Badekur**, f. hydropathic cure.
8875 **Brunnenkur**, f. treatment at watering places, etc.
8876 **Eisenkur**, f. cure by iron.
8877 **Hungerkur**, f. treatment by fasting.
8878 **Kaltwasserkur**, f. cold water treatment.
8879 **Klimakur**, f. climatic cure.
8880 **Kräuterkur**, f. treatment by herbs (extracts.)
8881 **Luftheilkunde**, f. treatment by air or vapors, atmiatrics.
8882 **Luftkurort**, m. 1. climatic health resort.
8883 **Massagekur**, f. treatment by
8884 (**Massieren**, n. 2.), massage.

8885 **Merkurialkur**, f. } cure by mercury, quicksilver.
8886 **Quecksilberkur**, f. }
8887 **Milchkur**, f. milk cure.
8888 **Molkenkur**, f. whey-cure.
8889 **Nachkur**, f. after-cure.
8890 **Obstkur**, f. fruit cure.
8891 **Palliativkur**, palliative treatment.
8892 **Quecksilberkur**, f. treatment by mercury.
8893 **Speichelkur**, f. treatment by salivation.
8894 **Stahlkur**, f. cure by iron.
8895 **Traubenkur**, f. grape cure.
8896 **Trinkkur**, f. treatment by waters at a spring or spa.
8897 **Vorkur**, f. preparatory treatment.
8898 **Wunderkur**, f. miraculous cure.
8899 **Zauberkur**, f. magic cure.
8900 9. **SURGICAL INSTRUMENTS AND MEANS, etc.**
8901 **Aderlasz**, m. 1. phlebotomy, venesection.
8902 **Aderlaszanhänger**, m. 2. } advocate, friend of bleeding, phlebotomist.
8903 **Aderlaszfreund**, m. 1. }
8904 **Aderlaszbäuschchen**, n. 2. compress used after bloodletting.
8905 **Aderlaszbecken**, n. 2. basin for bloodletting.
8906 **Aderlaszbinde**, f, bandage used in bloodletting.
8907 **Aderlaszgerät**, n. 1. bleeding instrument.
8908 **Aderlaszkunst**, f. art of bloodletting.
8909 **Aderlaszlanzette**, f. bleeding lancet.
8910 **Aderlaszlehre**, f. science of bloodletting.
8911 **Aderlasznarbe**, f. scar left after bloodletting.
8912 **Aderlaszschnäpper** or **schnepper**, m. 2. phlebotome, springlancet.
8913 **Aderlaszverband**, m. 1. dressing after bloodletting.
8914 **Aderlaszzeug**, n. 1. instruments for bloodletting.
8915 **Schröpfkopf**, m. 1. **Schröpfglas**, n. 1. } the lancet or the glass, cucurbita.
8916 **Ambulanz**, f. field hospital.
8917 **Amt**, n. 1. } office, study.
8918 **Amtsstube**, f. }
8919 **Amtszubehör**, n. 1. **Amtszubehörzeug**, n. 1. } appurtenances, all that belongs to the office.
8920 **Amputationsmesser**, n. 2. amputation knife, (from
8921 **amputieren**, to amputate.)
8922 **Ätzstifthalter**, m. 2. the case with the caustic stick.
8923 **Charpie**, f. charpie;
8924 ——, **gezupfte**, picked or unraveled lint, (from
8925 **zupfen**, to pluck, or unravel.)
8926 **Charpie-watte**, f. patent lint.
8927 **Englisches Pflaster**, n. 2. court plaster.
8928 **Feile**, f. file.
8929 **Einspritzer**, m. 2. syringe.
8930 **Gummiröhrchen**, n. 2. bougie.
8931 **Heftnadel**, f. suture needle.
8932 **Heftpflaster**, n. 2. } adhesive, sticking plaster.
8933 **adhäsiv Pflaster**, n. 2. }
8934 **adhäsiv Streif**, m. 1. strip of adhesive plaster.
8935 **adhäsiv Pflasterverband**, m. 1. dressing with adh. plaster.
8936 **Heilpflaster**, n. 2. healing plaster.
8937 **Höllensteinhalter**, m. 2. case with the caustic stick.
8938 **Impfen**, n. 2. (from
8939 **impfen**, to inoculate, vaccinate), inoculation, vaccination.
8940 **Impfer**, m. 2. vaccinator.
8941 **Impfgegner**, m. 2. opponent to vaccination.
8942 **Impfgesetz**, n. 1. law for vaccination.
8943 **Impfinstitut**, n. 1. vaccination institute.
8944 **Impfinstrument**, n. 1. inoculation, vaccination instrument.
8945 **Impfling**, m. 1. the person to be vaccinated.
8946 **Impflymphe**, f. } vaccine.
8947 **Impfstoff**, m. 1. }
8948 **Impfmesser**, n. 2. inoculation knife.
8949 **Impfnadel**, f. vaccination needle.

8950 **Impfnotwendigkeit**, f. } necessity for inoculation.
Notimpfung, f. }
8951 **impfpflichtig**, adj. obliged by law to be vaccinated.
8952 **Impfpocken**, pl. f. cow-pox, variolae.
8953 **Impfpustel**, f. inoculation pustule.
8954 **Impfröhrchen**, n. 2. vaccine tube.
8955 **Impfrotlauf**, m. 1. erysipelas after vaccination.
8956 **Impfschein**, m. 1. vaccination certificate.
8957 **Impfschutz**, m. 1. protection through vaccination.
8958 **Impfstelle**, f. the part or place vaccinated.
8959 **Impftrephine**, f. vaccination instrument.
8960 **Impfversuch**, m. 1. inocculation experiment.
8961 **Impfwesen**, n. 2. all pertaining to vaccination.
8962 **Impfwunde**, f. vaccination wound.
8963 **Impfzwang**, m. 1. compulsary vaccination.
8964 **Incissionslanzette**, f. abscess lancet.
8965 ——, **messer**, n. 2. scalpel.
8966 ——, **schere**, f. surgeon's scissors.
8967 **Injektion**, f. injection ; ——, spritze, f. syringe.
8968 **Katheter**, m. 2. catheter.
8969 **Kehlkopfspiegel**, m. 2. laryngo-scope.
8970 **Kettensäge**, f. chain saw.
8971 **Klystierpumpe**, f. clyster pump, enema apparatus.
8972 **Klystierspritze**, f. squirt, syringe (Spritze from spritzen, to gush, inject, syringe.)
8973 **Klystierröhre**, f. } clyster pipe, tube, hose.
8974 **Klystierschlauch**, m. 1. }
8975 **Knochenfeile**, f. bone file.
8976 **Knochensäge**, f. bone saw.
8977 **Knochenschneidewerkzeug**, n. 1. osteotome.
8978 **Knochenzange**, f. bone forceps.
8979 **Kopfsäge**, f. skull saw.
8980 **Kreissäge**, f. circular saw.
8981 **Krückenzange**, f. crutch-shaped forceps, scraping forceps.
8982 **Kugelbohrer**, m. 2. ball gimlet.
8983 **Kugelzange**, f. bullet forceps, ball extractor.
8984 **Lancette**, f. } lancet.
Lanzette, f. }
8985 **Leitsonde**, f. } director.
8986 **Leitungssonde**, f. }
8987 **Magenpumpe**, f. } stomach pump.
8988 **Magenspritze**, f. }
8889 **Milchpumpe**, f. breast or nipple glass.
8990 **Mundspiegel**, m. 2. speculum or dilator oris, stomatoscope.
8991 **Mutterspiegel**, m. 2. vaginal speculum.
8992 **Mutterspritze**, f. uterine syringe.
8993 **Nadel**, f. needle.
8994 **Nadelsonde**, f. exploring needle.
8995 **Nasenspiegel**, m. 2. rhinoscope.
8996 **Nasenspritze**, f. nasal syringe.
8997 **Ohrenspiegel**, m. 2. } speculum auris.
Ohrspiegel, m. 2. }
8998 **Ohrenspritze**, f. } ear syringe.
Ohrspritze, f. }
8999 **Pincette**, f. pincette, surgeon's forceps.
Pincettenschere, f. forceps scissors.
9000 **Punktiernadel**, f. acupuncture needle.
9001 **Rachenschnürer**, m. 2. pharynx constrictor.
9002 **Rachenspiegel**, m. 2. pharyngeal mirror or speculum.
9003 **Ringmesser**, n. 2. ring or annular knife.
9004 **Ritzmesser**, n. 2. lancet. scarificator.
9005 **Rupfzange**, f. (from rupfen, to pluck, to pull), tweezers.
9006 **Säge**, f. saw.
9007 **Schabeeisen**, n. 2. } raspatory.
9008 **Schabemesser**, n. 2. }
9009 **Schädelbohrer**, m. 2. trephine, perforator.
9010 **Schere**, f. scissors.
9011 **Schielnadel**, f. strabismus needle.
9012 **Schlitzmesser**, n. 2. } bistoury, lancet.
9013 **Schnittmesser**, n. 2. }

9014 {**Schnäpper**, m. 2. / **Schnepper**, m. 2.} spring-lancet, scarificator.
9015 **Schlundkopföffner**, m. 2. pharyngeotome.
9016 **Schlundkopfstoszer**, m. 2. probang.
9017 **Schlundsonde**, f. pharyngeal catheter.
9018 **Schwammhalter**, m. 2. spongeholder.
9019 **Seciersaal**, m. 1. (from
9020 **secieren**, to dissect) dissecting room.
9021 **Sichelnadel**, f. sickle needle.
9022 **Skalpel**, n. 2. scalpel.
9023 **Spekulum**, n. 1. speculum.
9024 **Sperrpincette**, f. (from **sperren**, to close, obstruct, shut), forceps with a catch.
9025 **Splitterzange**, f. splinter forceps, (fr. v. ir.
9026 **spleiszen**, to split),
9027 **Spritzröhrchen**, n. 2. injection-pipe.
9028 **Stichlanzette**, f. thumb-lancet.
9029 **Streckbett**, n. 1. stretcher.
9030 **Streckstuhl**, m. 1. extension chair.
9031 **Trepan**. m. 1. / 9032 **Trepanbogen**, m. 2. } trepan, hohle, f. grooved, probe.
9033 **Trepanschlüssel**, m. 2. trepan-key.
9034 **Vaccination**, f. vaccination, (for compounds see **Impfen**.)
9035 **vaccinieren**, to vaccinate.
9036 **Wachssonde**, f. / 9037 **Wachsröhrchen**, n. 2. } catheter.
9038 **Wundeisen**, n. 2. probe.
9039 **Wundfäden**, m. 2. pl. charpie, lint.
9040 **Wundnadel**, f. suture needle.
9041 **Wundpflaster**, n. 2. adhesive plaster.
9042 **Wundpulver**, n. 2. wound powder.
9043 **Wundspritze**, f. syringe to wash out wounds.
9044 **Wundwatte**, f. wadding for wounds.
9045 **Zahnarznei**, f. dental remedy.
9046 **Zahnarzneikunde**, f. / 9047 **Zahnarzneikunst**, f. } dentistry.
9048 **Zahnausbruch**, m. 1. dentition.
9049 **Zahnausnehmen**, n. 2. / 9050 **Zahnausziehen**, n. 2. } extraction of teeth.
9051 **Zahnausnehmer**, m. 2. / 9052 **Zahnauszieher**, m. 2. } tooth drawer, tooth puller.
9053 **Zahnbürste**, f. tooth brush.
9054 **Zahneisen**, n. 2. forceps.
9055 **Zahninstrument**, n. 1. dental instrument.
9056 **Zahnoperation**, f. dental operation.
9057 **Zahnputzer**, m. 2. dental rugine.
9058 **Zahnstocher**, m. 2. toothpick.
9059 **Zahntherapie**, f. dental therapeutics.
9060 **Zahnverband**, m. 1. tooth dressing.
9061 **Zahnwurzelschraube**, f. screw for removing stumps of teeth.
9062 **Zahnzange**, f. tooth forceps.
9063 **Zahnzangenlöffel**, m. 2. blade of tooth forceps, etc.
9064 10. **MATERIA MEDICA or MEDICAL MEANS,** etc. In compounds:
9065 **Alaun**, m. 1. alum ;——, gebrannter, burned alum.
9066 **Alaunerde**, f. alumina, oxide of aluminium.
9067 **Alaunmolken**, f. pl. serum lactis aluminatum, (Germ. Pharm.).
9068 **Alaunstift**, m. 1. alum point (applied locally).
9069 **Alkohol**, m. 1. alcohol.
9070 **Alkoholgährung**, f. alcoholic fermentation.
9071 **alkoholisch**, adj. alcoholic.
9072 **Alkoholvergiftung**, f. alcoholic poisoning.
9073 **Aloë**. f. aloes.
9074 **aloëhaltig**, adj. aloetic.
9075 **Aloëtinktur, zusammengesetzte**, f. tinctura aloës composita (Germ. Pharm.).
9076 **Altheeblätter**, n. 1. pl. marsh-mallow leaves (folia Althaeae).
9077 **Altheesaft**, m. 1. syrupus Althaeae.
9078 **Altheesalbe**, f. unguentum flavum. (Germ. Pharm.).
9079 **Altheewurzel**, f. marsh-mallow root.

9080 **Ammoniak**, m. 1. smelling salt.

9081 **Anästhesie**, f. anaesthesia in operations (in Operationen, f. from operieren, to operate.)

9082 **anästhesieren**, to anaesthetise.

9083 **Anisöl**, n. 1. anis-seed oil.

9084 **Anissäure**, f. anisic acid.

9085 **Arnikablüten**, f. pl. flores arnicae.

9086 **Arnikaöl**, n. 1. oil or essence of arnica.

9087 **Arnikawurzel**, f. radix arnicae.

9088 **Arsenik, weiszer**, m. 1. arsenious acid.

9089 **arsenikalisch**, adj. arsenical.

9090 **Arsenikräucherung**, f. arsenical fumigation.

9091 **Arseniksalbe**, f. arsenic ointment.

9092 **Arsensäure**, f. arsenious acid.

9093 **Ätherbesprühung**, f. (from

9094 **Äther**, m. 2, ether, and

9095 **sprühen**, to spray), spraying with ether.

9096 **Ätherdampf**, m. 1. ether vapor.

9097 **Ätherdouche**, f. ether spray apparatus.

9098 **Athereinatmung**, f. ether inhalation.

9099 **ätherisieren**, to etherise.

9100 **Ätherisierung**, f. ether administration.

9101 **Augenpulver**, n. 2. eye powder.

9102 **Augensalbe**, f. eye-salve ;

9103 **——, zusammengesetzte rote**, unguentum ophthalmicum compositum (Germ. Pharm.).

9104 **Augenwasch-wasser**, n. 2. eye-wash, collyrium.

9105 **Baldrianöl**, n. 1. valerian oil (oleum valeriani).

9106 **Baldriansäure**, f. valerian acid.

9107 **Baldriantinktur**, f. tincture of valerian.

9108 **Baldrianwasser**, n. 2. valerian water.

9109 **Baumöl**, n. 1. olive oil.

9110 **Baumwolle**, f. } cotton wool.
9111 **Watte**, f. }

9112 **Bergamottöl**, n. 1. bergamot oil.

9113 **Bergner-Leberthran**, m. 1. cod-liver oil.

9114 **Bernsteinöl**, n. 1. oil of amber (oleum succini).

9115 **Bernsteinsäure**, f. succinic acid.

9116 **Bertramwurzel**, f. radix pyrethri.

9117 **Bilsenkraut**, n. 1. hyoscyamus leaves, henbane leaves.

9118 **Bilsenkrautöl**, n. 1. fettes, oleum hyoscyami infusum.

9119 **Bilsenpflaster**, n. 2. } emplastrum hyoscyami, unguentum hyoscyami (Germ. Pharm.).
9120 **Bilsensalbe**, f. }

9121 **Bilsensamen**, m. 2. hyoscyamus seed.

9122 **Blasensalbe**, f. blistering ointment.

9123 **Bleioxyd**, n. 1. essigsaures, plumbum aceticum.

9124 **Bleipflaster**, n. 2. emplastrum lethargyri simplex.

9125 **Bleisalbe**, f. unguentum plumbi ;

9126 **Bleisalbe**, gerbsaure, unguentum plumbi tannici (Germ. Pharm.).

9127 **Branntwein**, m. 1. brandy, spirit.

9128 **Branntweinhefe**, f. saccharomyces, cerevisiae of alcohol.

9129 **Brausepulver**, n. 1. } effervescing powder.
9130 **Seidlitzpulver**, n. 1. }

9131 **——, abführendes**, Seidlitz-powder ;

9132 **——, englisches**, pulvis aërophorus Anglicus (Germ. Pharm.).

9133 **Brecharznei**, f. (from v. ir. & refl, sich brechen, sich würgen, to vomit), emetic.

9134 **brechenerregend**, adj. emetic.

9135 **brechenstillend**, adj. antiemetic.

9136 **Brechmittel**, n. 2. an emetic.

9137 **Brechneigung**, f. inclination to vomit.

9138 **Brechnusz**, f. nux vomica.

9139 **Brechpille**, f. emetic pill.

9140 **Brechpulver**, n. 2. emetic powder.

9141 **Brechtrank**, m. 1. emetic.

9142 **Brechwein**, m. I. antimonial wine.

9143 **Brechweinstein**, m. 1. tartar emetic.
9144 **Brechwurzel**, f. ipecacuanha.
9145 **Brechwurzelwein**, m. 1. vinum ipecacuanhae.
9146 **Brom**. n. 1. bromine.
9147 **Bromkalium**, n. 1. bromide of potash.
9148 **Bromkampfer**, m. 2. bromated camphor.
9149 **Bromsalze**, n. 1. pl. bromides.
9150 **Bromsäure**, f. bromic acid.
9151 **Bromwasserstoffsäure**, f. bromal hydrate.
9152 **Brustpulver**, n. 2. compound liquorice powder (Germ. Pharm.).
9153 **Brustsaft**, m. 1. linctus, } pectoral syrup,
9154 **Brustsyrup**, m. 1. } pectoral
9155 **Brustthee**, m. 1. } tea.
9156 **Brusttropfen**, m. 2. pectoral drops.
9157 **Carbolsäure**, f. carbolic acid.
9158 **Chilisalpeter**, m. 2. nitrate of soda.
9159 **Chinarinde**, f. cinchona bark.
9160 **Chinatinktur**, f. tincture of cinchona.
9161 **Chinawein**, m. 1. quinine wine, cinchona wine.
9162 **Chinawurzel**, f. rhizoma chinae.
9163 **Chinin**, n. 1. quinia;
9164 ——, **baldriansaures**, valerianate of quinine;
9165 ——, **gerbsaures**, tannate of quinine;
9166 ——, **salzsaures**, muriate of quinine;
9167 ——, **schwefelsaures**, sulphate of quinine.
9168 **Chinineisen**, n. 2. citronensaures, citrate of iron and quinine.
9169 **Chloräther**, m. 2. chlorine.
9170 **Chloralhydrat**, n. 1. chloral hydrate.
9171 **Chloreisentinktur**, f. tincture of perchloride of iron.
9172 **Chlorgoldpulver**, n. 2. chloride of gold powder.
9173 **Chlorkalk**, m. 1. chlorinated lime.
9174 **Chlorkohlenstoff**, m. 1 tetrachloride of carbon.
9175 **Chlornatron**, n. 1. chlorinated soda.
9176 **Chloroformanäthesierung**, f. anaesthesia from chloroform.
9177 **Chlorräucherung**, f. fumigation by chlorine.
9178 **Chlorsilber**, n. 2. chloride of silver.
9179 **chlorür**, adj. sub-chloride.
9180 **Chlorwasser**, n. 2. liquor chlori.
9181 **Chlorwasserstoffsäure**, f. hydro-chloric acid.
9182 **Chlorzink**, n. 1. choride of zinc.
9183 **Chlorzinkstift**, m. 1. chloride of zink point (caustic).
9184 **Chromsäure**, f. chromic acid.
9185 **Chryophansäure**, f. chryophanic acid.
9186 **Citronenöl**, n. 1. oleum citri.
9187 **Citronensaftsyrup**, m. 1. syrupus succi citri.
9188 **Citronensäure**, f. citric acid.
9189 **Cocablätter**, n. 1 pl. coca leaves.
9190 **Cocainanästhesie**, f. anaesthesia by cocaine.
9191 **Condurangorinde**, f. condurango bark.
9192 **Copaivabalsam**, m. 1. balsam of copaiba.
9193 **Crotonöl**, n. 1. croton oil.
9194 **Cyankalium**, n. 1. cyanide of potassium.
9195 **Cyanquecksilber**, n. 2. cyanide of mercury.
9196 **Cyanwasserstoffsäure**, f. prussic acid.
9197 **Cyanzink**, n. 1. cyanide of zinc.
9198 **Egel**, m. 2. leech.
9199 **Eibischkraut**, n. 1. folia althaeae, mash-mallow leaves.
9200 **Eibischsaft**, m. 1. syrupus althaeae.
9201 **Eibischwurzel**, f. radix althaeae.
9292 **Eichenrinde**, f. oakbark.
9203 **Eichenrindeabkochung**, f. (from abkochen, to decoct,) decoction of oak bark.
9204 **Eisen**, n. 2. iron.
9205 **Eisen, citronensaures**, n. 2. citrate of iron.
9206 **Eisen, reduciertes**, n. 2. reduced iron.
9207 **Eisen, zuckerhaltiges, kohlensaures**, n. 2. saccharated carbonate of iron.

9208 **Eisenalaun**, m. 1. ammoniakalischer, sulphate of iron and ammonium.

9209 **Eisenarznei**, f. ferruginous remedy.

9210 **Eisenbromid**, n. 1. bromide of iron.

9211 **Eisenchinin**, n. 1. citronensaures, citrate of iron and quinine.

9212 **Eisenchlorid**, n. 1. flüssiges, liquor ferri chloridi (Germ. Pharm.) solution of perchloride of iron.

9213 ——, **krystallisches** or **krystallisiertes**, chloride of iron.

9214 **Eisencyanide**, n. 1. ferro-cyanogen.

9215 **Eisenextract**, m. & n. 1. apfelsaures, extractum ferri pomatum.

9216 **Eisenfeilspäne**, m. 1. pl. steel filings.

9217 **Eisenflüssigkeit**, f. essigsaure, liquor ferri acetici.

9218 **Eisenhut**, m. 1 aconite.

9219 **Eisenhutextract**, m. & n. 1. extract of aconite.

9220 **Eisenhutknollen**, m. 2. aconite root.

9221 **Eisenhuttinktur**, f. tincture of aconite.

9222 **Eisenjodidlösung**, f. solution of iodide of iron.

9223 **Eisenoxyd-Ammonium**, n. 1. citronensaures, citrate of iron and ammonia.

9224 **Eisenoxid-Am., schwefelsaures**, n. 1. sulphate of iron and ammonia.

9225 **Eisenoxyd**. n. 1. citronensaures, citrate of iron.

9226 ——, **flüssiges schwefelsaures**, solution of sulphate of iron.

9227 **Eisenoxydul**, n. 1. entwässertes schwefelsaures, ferri sulphas exsiccata.

9228 ——, **milchsaures**, lactate of iron.

9229 ——, **phosphorsaures**, phosphate of iron.

9230 ——, **schwefelsaures**, sulphate of iron.

9231 **Eisenpillen, italienische**, f. pl. pills of aloes and iron.

9232 **Eisenpulver**, n. 2. ferrum pulveratum.

9233 **Eisensalmiak**, m. 1. ammonium chloratum ferratum.

9234 **Eisensäuerlingquelle**, f. chalybeate spring, where the water is rich in iron and carbonic acid, as in Pyrmont.

9235 **Eisenschokolade**, f. chocolate mixed with iron.

9236 **Eisentinktur**, f. ätherische, essigsaure, tinctura ferri acetici aetherea.

9237 **Eisenvitriol**, m. 1. crude sulphate of iron;

9238 **reiner**, pure sulphate of iron.

9239 **Eisenwasser**, n. 2. chalybeate water.

9240 **Eisenwein**, m. 1. iron wine.

9241 **Eisenweinstein**, m. 1. tartarated iron.

9242 **Eisenzucker**, m. 2. ferrum oxydatum saccharatum solubile.

9243 **Essigsäure**, f. acetic acid:

9244 ——, f. gewürzliche, aromatic acetic acid;

9245 ——, verdünnte (from verdünnen, to dilute, attenuate, see 8546), dilute acetic acid.

9246 **Fenchelholz**, n. 1. sassafras wood.

9247 **Fenchelöl**, n. 1. oleum foeniculi.

9248 **Fichtenharz**, n. 1. pine resin.

9249 **Fichtennadelöl**, n. 1. pine oil.

9250 **Fichtensäure**, f. pinic acid.

9251 **Fieberkleeblätter**, n. 1. pl. folia trifolii fibrini.

9252 **Fieberkleeextract**, m. & n. 1. extractum trifolii fibrini.

9253 **Fieberpulver**, n. 2. ague powder.

9254 **Fieberrinde**, f. Peruvian bark.

9255 **Fingerhut**, m. 1. digitalis.

9256 **Fingerhutessig**, m. 1. acetum digitalis.

9257 **Fingerhutkraut**, n. 1. folia digitalis.

9258 **Fingerhutsalbe**, f. unguentum digitalis.

9259 **Fingerhuttinktur**, f. tincture of digitalis.

9260 **Flachssamenthee**, m. 1. flaxseed tea.

9261 **Fliederblumen**, f. pl. flores sambuci.

9262 **Fliedermus**, n. 1. succus sambuci (Germ. Pharm.).

9263 **Fliederthee**, m. 1. elder-flower tea.
9264 **Fliege**, f. fly;
9265 —, **spanische**, cantharides.
9266 **Fliegenpflaster**, n. 2. blistering plaster from cantharides.
9267 **Fluorwasserstoffsäure**, f. hydro-fluoric acid.
9268 **Galläpfel**, m. 1. pl. gall apples.
9269 **Galläpfelgerbsäure**, f. tannic acid.
9270 **Galläpfeltinktur**, f. tincture of galls.
9271 { **Gallerte**, f. gelatin, jelly.
gallertig, adj. gelatinous.
gallertig-schleimig, adj. muco-gelatinous. }
9272 **Gaskalk**, m. 1. hydro-sulphate of lime.
9273 **Gelatine**, f. gelatin.
9274 **gelatinös**, adj. } gelatinous.
gallertig, }
9275 **Gerstenkrütze**, f. } pearl
9276 **Graupen**, f. } barley.
9277 **Gerstenschleim**, m. 1. } barley water, ptisane.
9278 **Gerstentrank**, m. 1. }
9279 **Gipsbrei**, m. 1. plaster of Paris mixed with water for use prepared.
9280 **Glaubersalz**, n. 1. Glauber's salt.
9281 **Glaubersalzwässer**, n. 2. pl. mineral waters containing Glauber's salt, as in
9282 **Carlsbad, Baden.**
9283 **Glycerin**, n. 1. glycerine.
9284 **Glycerinsalbe**, f. unguentum glycerini (G. Ph.).
9285 **Granatblüten**, f. pl. pomegranate blossoms.
9286 **Granatrinde**, f. pomegranate bark.
9287 **Granatwurzelrinde**, f. cortex radicis granati.
9288 **Gummi, arabisches**, n. 1. gum arabic.
9289 **Gummiharz**, n. 1. gum resin.
9290 **Gummiknoten**, m. 2. gumma.
9291 **Gummipflaster**, n. 2. diachylon plaster.
9292 **Gummipulver**, n. 2. compound powder of tragacanth.
9293 **Haferbrei**, m. 1. oatmeal porridge.
9294 **Haferschleim**, m. 1. oatmeal water.
9295 **Hanfextract**, m. & n. 1. indischer, extract of Indian hemp
9296 **Hanfkörner**, n. 1. pl. } hemp-
9297 **Hanfsamen**, m. 2. } seed.
9298 **Hanföl**, n. 1. hemp-seed oil.
9299 **Hefe**, f. dregs.
9300 **Hirschhornsalz**, n. 1. hartshorn.
9301 **Hoffmann'scher Lebensbalsam**, m. 1. mixtura oleosa-balsamica (Germ. Pharm.).
9302 **Hoffmannstropfen**, m. 2. Hoffmann's anodyne.
9303 **Höllenstein**, m. 1. nitrate of silver.
9304 **salpeterhaltiger**, mitigated nitrate of silver (equal parts of silver and nitrate of potassium).
9305 **Holzsäure**, f. acetic acid.
9306 **Honig**, m. 1. } honey.
Honig, gereinigter, m. 1. } purified honey.
9307 **Hopfenöl**, n. 1. essential oil of hops.
9308 **Impflymphe**, f. } vaccine.
9309 **Impfstoff**, m. 1. }
9310 **Isländisch Moosgallerte**, f. Iceland moss jelly.
9311 **Jalapenharz**, n. 1. jalapin.
9312 **Jalapenknollen**, m. 2. tubera jalapae.
9313 **Jalapenpille**, f. jalap pill.
9314 **Jodblei**, n. 1. iodide of lead.
9315 **Jodeisen**, n. 2. iodide of iron.
9316 **zuckerhaltiges**, saccharated iodide of iron.
9317 **Jodkali**, n. 1. iodide of potassium.
9318 **Kaffeesäure**, f. caffeic acid.
9319 **Kali**, n. 1. potash.
9320 —, **chlorsaures**, chlorate of potash.
9321 —, **doppelt kohlensaures**, bicarbonate of potash.
9322 —, **essigsaures**, acetate of potash.
9323 —, **gereinigtes kohlensaures**, purified carbonate of potash.
9324 —, **neutrales weinsaures**, tartrate of potash.
9325 —, **reines kohlensaures**, carbonate of potash.
9326 —, **rohes kohlensaures**, crude carbonate of potash (from woodashes).

9327 ——, **saures**, bicarbonate of potash.
9328 ——, **schwefelsaures**, sulphate of potash, etc.
9329 **Kalilauge**, f. liquor potassae.
9330 **Kalisayrinde**, f. cortex chinae calisayae (Germ. Pharm.).
9331 **Kalium**, n. 1. potassium.
9332 **Kalk**, m. 1. lime.
9333 ——, **gebrannter**, quicklime,
9334 ——, **reiner kohlensaurer**, precipitated carbonate of lime.
9335 ——, **phosphorsaurer**, phosphate of lime.
9336 **Kalkerde**, f. phosphorsaure, phosphate of calcium.
9337 **Kalkstein**, m. 1. carbonate of lime stone.
9338 **Kalmusöl**, n. 1. oil of sweet flag.
9339 **Kamillenöl**, n. 1. ätherisches, etherial oil of chamomile.
9340 **Kamillenthee**, m. 1. chamomile tea.
9341 **Kampferliniment**, n. 1. flüchtiges, compound camphor liniment.
9342 **Kampferöl**, n. 1. camphorated (sweet) olive oil.
9343 **Kampferspiritus**, m. 1. spirit of camphor.
9344 **Kampferwein**, m. 1. camphorated wine.
9345 **Karbolsäure**, f. carbolic acid.
9346 **Kinderpulver**, n. 2. magnesia and rhubarb.
9347 **Klauenfett**, n. 1. } neat's foot
9348 **Knochenöl**, n. 1. } oil.
9349 **Klebpflaster**, n. 2 adhesive plaster, courtplaster.
9350 **Kleesäure**, f. oxalic acid.
9351 **Kohlenölsäure**, f. carbolic acid.
9352 **Kohlensäure**. f. carbonic acid.
9353 **Koriandersamen**, m. 2. coriander seed.
9354 **Krähenaugenextract**, m & n. 1. extract of nux vomica.
9355 **Krausenminzöl**, n. 1. curled mint oil.
9356 **Kräuterarznei**, f. herb medicine.
9357 **Kräuterauszug**, m. 1. tincture of herbs or extract of herbs.
9358 **Kräuterthee**, m. 1. herb tea.
9359 **Kreide**, f. chalk.
9360 ——, **bereitet**, prepared chalk.
9361 **Leberthran**, m. 1. cod-liver oil.
9362 **Leinöl**, n. 1. linseed oil.
9363 **Leinsamenthee**, m. 1. linseed tea.
9364 **Lindenblüten**, f. pl. linden flowers, lime-tree flowers.
9365 **Lobeliatinktur**, f. tincture of lobelia.
9366 **Lobelienkraut**, n. 1. lobelia.
9367 **Majoran**, m. 1. sweet majoram.
9368 **Majoranöl**, n. 1. oil of majoram.
9369 **Mandelöl**, n. 1. almond oil.
9370 **Malz**, n. 1. malt.
9371 **Melisenblätter**, n. 1. pl. balm mint.
9372 **Merkur**, m. 1. quicksilver, mercury.
9373 **Milchsäure**, f. lactic acid.
9374 **Milchzucker**, m. 2. sugar of milk.
9375 **Mohnköpfe**, m. 1. pl. poppy heads.
9376 **Mohnsaft**, m. 1. opium.
9377 **Mohnsamen**, m. 2. poppy seed.
9378 **Morphin, salzsaures**, n. 1. hydro-chlorate of morphia.
9379 ——, **schwefelsaures**, sulphate of morphia.
9380 **Moschus**, m. 1. musk.
9381 ——, **tinktur**, f. tincture of musk.
9382 **Muskatblütenöl**, n. 1. oil of mace.
9383 **Muskatbutter**, f. oleum myristicae.
9384 **Muskatnusz**, f. nutmeg.
9385 **Muskatnuszöl**, n. 1. oleum myristicae.
9386 **Mutterkorn**, n. 1. ergot of rye.
9387 ——, **extract**, n. & m. 1. extractum ergotae liquidum.
9388 **Myrrhentinktur**, f. tincture of myrrh.
9389 **Nelkenöl**, n. 1. oil of cloves.
9390 **Oliveöl**, n. 1. } olive oil.
9391 **Baumöl**, n. 1. }
9392 **Opiat**, n. 1. opiate.
9393 **Opiumextract**, n. & m. 1. extract of opium.
9394 **Opium pflaster**, n. 2. opium plaster.
9395 **Opium salbe**, f. opium ointment.

9396 **Opium syrup**, m. 1. syrupus opiatus (Germ. Pharm.)
9397 **Oxalsäure**, f. oxalic acid.
9398 **Pastillen**, f. pl. pastilles, lozenges.
9399 **Pfefferminze**, f. peppermint.
9400 **Pfefferminzöl**, n. 1. oil of peppermint.
9401 **Pfefferminzthee**, m. 1. peppermint tea.
9402 **Pflaster**, n. 2. plaster.
9403 **Pechpflaster**, n. 2. pitch plaster.
9404 **Pille**, f. pill.
9405 —, **italienische**, pl. pills of aloes and iron.
9406 **Peruvischer balsam**, m. 1. balsam of Peru.
9407 **Petersiliensamen**, m. 2. parsley seed.
9408 **Pomeranzenblätter**, n. 1. pl. orange leaves.
9409 **Pulver**, n. 2. powder.
9410 **Quacksalbereiarznei**, f. medicin of quackery.
9411 **Quasiaholz**, n. 1. } Quassia.
9412 **Bitterholz**, n. 1. }
9413 **Quecksilber**, n. 2. mercury;
9414 —, **pflaster**, mercurial plaster;
9415 —, **chlorid**, n. 1. ätzendes, corrosive sublimate.
9416 **Rettig**, m. 1. radish.
9417 **Meerrettig**, m. 1. horse-radish.
9418 **Rhabarbersaft**, m. 1. syrupus rhei.
9419 **Rhabarbertinktur**, f. wässerige, tinctura rhei;
9420 —, **weinige**, vinum rhei.
9421 **Ricinusöl**, n. 1. castor oil.
9422 **Rochellersalz**, n. 1. tartarated soda.
9423 **Rosmarinöl**, n. 1. oil of rosemary.
9424 **Safran**, m. 1. saffron.
9425 **Salbe**, f. salve, ointment.
9426 **Salbeiblätter**, pl. n. 1. garden sage.
9427 **Salep**, m. 1. salep or salop.
9428 **Salmiakgeist**, m. 1. spirits of hartshorn.
9429 **Salpetersäure**, f. nitric acid.
9430 **Salpeterweingeist**, m. 1. spirit of nitre.
9431 —, **versüszter**, sweet spirit of nitre.
9432 **Salz**, n. 1. salt;
9433 —, **englisches**, epsomsalts.
9434 **Sarsaparilla**, f. } sarsaparilla.
Sassaparilla, f. }
9435 **Sassafras**, n. 1. } sassafras, sassafras-wood.
Sassafrasholz, n. 1. }
9436 **Säure**, f. acid.
9437 **Scheidewasser**, n. 2. nitric acid.
9438 **Schlüsselblumenthee**, m. 1. primrose or longwort tea.
9439 **Schönheitswasser**, n. 2. cosmetic liquid.
9440 **Schwefeläther**, m. 2. sulphuric ether.
9441 **Schwefelwasser**, n. 2. sulphurated water.
9442 **Seidlitzpulver**, n. 2. Seidlitz powder.
9443 **Seifenspiritus**, m. 1. soap tincture.
9444 **Senföl**, n. 1. mustard oil.
9445 **Senfpflaster**, n. 2. mustard plaster.
9446 **Senna-or Senes-blätter**, n. 1. pl. (from Senes-baumblätter), senna-leaves.
9447 **Silbernitrat**, n. 1. nitrate of silver.
9448 **Spanishfliegenpflaster**, n. 2. Spanish fly blister.
9449 **Spirituosen**, m. 3. (from spiritus, m. 1. Hauch, Geist, Lebensgeist), alcoholic liquors.
9450 **Gebranntes Wasser**, n. 2. } spirits (beverage).
9451 **Geistige Getränke**, n. 1. pl. }
9452 **Stahlwein**, m. 1. steelwein.
9453 **Stärke**, f. starch.
9454 **Stimulant**, m. 1. } stimulant,
9455 **Reizmittel**, n. 1. } (from
9456 **stimulieren**, to stimulate).
9457 **Stinkasant**, m. 1. } assafœtida, devil's dung.
Teufelsdreck, m. 1. }
9458 **Süszholz**, n. 1. licorice root.
9459 **Taback**, m. 1. tobacco leaves.
9460 **Talg**, m. 1. sebum, tallow.
9461 **Teerwasser**, n. 2. tar-water.
9462 **Terpentinöl**, n. 1. } oil of turpentine.
Terpentinspiritus, m. 1. }
9463 **Terpentinölseife**, f. turpentine liniment.
9464 **Thymianöl**, n. 1. oil of thyme.
9465 **Tierkohle**, f. bone-charcoal, bone black.

9466 **Tollkirsche**, f. belladonna, deadly night shade.

9467 **Tollkirschenblätter**, n. 1. pl. belladonna leaves.

9468 **Tollkirschensalbe**, f. belladonna ointment.

9469 **Traganth**, m. 1. tragacanth.

9470 **Vanilla**, f. vanilla.

9471 **Vitriolöl**, n. 1. oil of vitriol.

9472 **Wachholderbeere**, f. juniperberry.

9473 **Wachholderbeerenwein**, m. 1. juniperberry wine.

9474 **Wachholderbeeröl**, n. 1. oleum juniperi.

9475 **Wachs**, n. 1. gelbes, grünes, weiszes, yellow, green, white wax.

9476 **Weinsteinsäure**, f. tartaric acid.

9477 **Wermut**, m. 1. wormwood.

9478 **Wundbalsam**, m. 1. vulnerary balsam.

9479 **Ziehpflaster**, n. 2. } drawing plaster, etc.
Zugpflaster, n. 2. }

9480 **Zittwerblütenextract**, m. & n. 1. extractum cinae.
Zittwersamen, m. 2. santonine seed.

9481 11. **GIFTE UND VERGIFTUNGEN**, Poisons and Poisoning in compounds:

9482 **Gift**, n. 1. poison, venom, virus, virulence.

9483 ——, **ätzendes**, corrosive poison.

9484 ——, **betäubendes**, narcotic poison.

9485 ——, **irritierendes**, irritating poison.

9486 ——, **narkotisches**, narcotic poison.

9487 ——, **septisches** or **zymotisches**, septic poison.

9488 **Alkoholvergiftung**, f. alcoholic poisoning.

9489 **Anilinvergiftung**, f. } poisoning by aniline.
9490 **Anilismus**, m. 1. }

9491 **Ansteckungsgift**, n. 1. } contagion, virus.
9492 **Ansteckungsstoff**, m. 1. }

9493 **Arsenik**, m. 1, arsenic

9494 **Blausäure**, f. hydrocyanic acid, prussic acid.

9495 **Bleivergiftung**, f. lead poisoning.

9496 **Blutvergiftung**, f. blood poisoning.

9497 **Bromvergiftung**, f. poisoning by the bromides.

9498 **Carbolvergiftung**, f. carbolic acid poisoning.

9499 **Chininvergiftung**, f. quinine poisoning.

9500 **Chloroformvergiftung**, f. poisoning by chloroform.

9501 **Cloakengasvergiftung**, f. poisoning from sewergas.

9502 **Contagionsgift**, n. 1. contagion, virus.

9503 **giftabtreibend**, adj. antidotal, antitoxic.

9504 **Giftarznei**, f. an antidote.

9505 **Giftfisch**, m. 1. poisonous fish.

9506 **Gifthahnenfusz**, m. 1. (plant) crawfoot, hemlock.

9507 **giftig**, adj. poisonous, infective, venomous.

9508 **giftige Mineralien**, n. 1. pl. poisonous minerals.

9509 **giftige Dämpfe**, m. 1. pl. poisonous vapors.

9510 **Giftigkeit**, f. virulence, the quality of being poisonous.

9511 **Giftkraut**, n. 1. venomous herb.

9512 **Giftkresse**, f. poisonous cress.

9513 **Giftlattich**, m. 1. poisonous lettuce, herba lactucae virosae.

9514 **Giftlattichextract**, m. & n. 1. extractum lactucae virosae (Germ. Pharm.)

9515 **giftlos**, adj. innocuous, nonpoisonous.

9516 **Giftmaterie**, f. poisonous matter or substance.

9517 **Giftmehl** n. 1. poisoned flour, white arsenic.

9518 **Giftmilbe**, f. argas persicus.

9519 **Giftmord**, m. 1. murder by poison.

9520 **Giftmittel**, n. 2. an antidote.

9521 **Giftpflanze**, f. poisonous plant.

9522 **Giftpilze**, f., } poisonous mushrooms, poisonous fungus.
9523 **Giftschwamm**, m. 1. }

9524 **Giftprüfung**, f. testing for poison.

9525 **Giftschein**, m. 1. warrant to buy poison.

9526 **Giftschlange**, f. venomous serpent.
9527 **Grünspan**, m. 1. acetate of copper, verdigris.
9528 **Gifttier**, n. 1. venomous animal.
9529 **Giftwurz**, m. 1. swallow wort, asclepias vincetoxicum.
9530 **Fingerhut**, m. 1. digitalis, foxglove.
9531 **Giftzahn**, m. 1. poison fang.
9532 **Jodvergiftung**, f. iodine poisoning.
9533 **Karbolvergiftung**, f. carbolic poisoning.
9534 **Klapperschlange**, f. rattlesnake.
9535 **Kohlendunstvergiftung**, f. poisoning by charcoal.
9536 **Kohlenoxidvergiftung**, f. } poisoning by carbonic acid.
9537 **Kohlensäurevergiftung**, f. } poisoning by carbonic acid.
9538 **Kröde**, f. toad.
9539 **Kupferschlange**, f. copper-snake.
9540 **Kupfervergiftung**, f. poisoning by copper.
9541 **Leichengift**, n. 1. cadaveric or septic poison.
9542 **Luftvergiftung**, f. air-poisoning.
9543 **Morphium**, n. 1. morphine.
9544 **Morphiumvergiftung**, f. poisoning by morphia.
9545 **Muschelvergiftung**, f. poisoning by shellfish.
9546 **Mutterkornvergiftung**, f. poisoning by ergot.
9547 **Nachtschatten**, m. 1. nightshade.
9548 **Natter**, f. adder.
9549 **Nikotin**, n. 1. nicotene.
9550 **Opium**, n. 1. opium.
9551 **Pestgift**, n. 1. pestilential poison.
9552 **Pyämie**, f. pyaemia, blood-poisoning.
9553 **pyämisch**, adj. pyaemic.
9554 **Quecksilbervergiftung**, f. mercurial poisoning.
9555 **Schierling**, m. 1. hemlock.
9556 **Schlangengift**, n. 1. poison of serpents or snakes.
9557 **Schleussenvergiftung**, f. poison by sewer gas.
9558 **Stechapfel**, m. 1. thorn-apple, stramonium (from v. ir.
9559 **stechen**, to sting, prick, pierce).
9560 **Strychnin**, n. 1. strychnine.
9561 **Tyrotoxikon**, n. 1. cheese poison.
9562 **Verpestung**, f. infection.
9563 **Viper**, f. viper.
9564 **Wurstvergiftung**, f. poisoning by sausage.
9565 **Wutgift**, n. 1. virus of hydrophobia, etc.
9566 §33. **ESSEN und TRINKEN**;
9567 **Lebens und Nahrungsmittel**, Eating and Drinking, and means of subsistence. (For compounds see also Appetite.)
9568 **Kost**, f. food, fare, diet, regimen.
9569 —, **schmale**, poor fare.
9570 **Lebensmittel**, n. 2. } means of subsistence, provisions, victuals. In compounds:
9571 **Nahrungsmittel**, n. 2. } means of subsistence, provisions, victuals. In compounds:
9572 1. **MAHLZEITEN**, f. pl. meals (lit. times of meals).
9573 **Fest**, n. 1. feast, banquet.
9574 **Festmahl**, n. 1. feast, banquet.
9575 **Frükstück**, n. 1. breakfast.
9576 **Gabelfrühstück**, n. 1. lunch.
9577 **Mahl**, n. 1. meal.
9578 **Mehlspeise**, f. farinaceous food.
9579 **Mittagessen**, n. 1. } dinner.
Mittagsmahl, n. 1. } dinner.
9580 **Abendbrot**, n. 1. } supper.
9581 **Abendessen**, n. 1. } supper.
9582 **Nachtmahl**, n. 1. } supper.
9583 (**Abendmahl und**
9584 **Nachtmahl** are used in the language of the church for the *Lord's Supper*.)
9585 2. **BROT**, n. 1. bread;
9586 —, **altbacken**, dry, stale bread;
9587 —, **belegtes** (from v. ir.
9588 —, **legen**, to lay, cover), e.g.
9589 —, **belegtes Butterbrot**,
9590 —, **frisches**, new bread;
9591 —, **geröstes**, toast-bread;
9592 —, **hausbacken**, home made bread.
9593 **Brotbrei**, m. 1. bread pap or pulp (for poultice.)
9594 **Brotkorb**, m. 1. bread basket.
9595 **Brotkümmel**, m. 2. caraway seed.
9596 **Brotkrumme**, f. crumb of bread.
9597 **Brotkruste**, f. } crust of bread.
9598 **Brotrinde**, f. } crust of bread.

9599 **Brotröster**, m. 2. bread-roaster.
9600 **Brotschnitte**, f. slice of bread.
9601 **Brotschrank**, m. 1. pantry, bread board.
9602 **Brotschnittchen**, n. 2. chip of bread, sipper.
9603 **Brotspende**, f. distribution of bread.
9604 **Brotumschlag**, m. 1. bread poultice.
9605 **Butterbrot**, n. 1. bread and butter.
9606 **Milchbrot**, n. 1. milkbread, French roll.
9607 **Roggenbrot**, n. 1. rye bread.
9608 **Schwarzbrot**, n. 1. brown bread.
9609 **Weiszbrot**, n. 1. white bread.
9610 **Weizen**, m. 2. wheat.
9611 **Weizenbrot**, n. 1. wheat bread.
9612 **Weizenmehl**, n. 1. wheat meal or flour.
9613 **Bäckerei**. f. bakery.
9614 **Backwerk**, n. 1. (from v. ir
9615 **backen**, to bake)
9616 **Gebäck**, n. 1. } pastry.
9617 **Biscuit**, n. 2. biscuit.
9618 **Kuchen**, m. 2. cake.
9619 **Pastete**, f. pastry, pie.
9620 **Semmel**, f. roll.
9621 **Torte**, f. tart.
9622 **Wassersuppe**, f. water porridge.
9623 **Zwieback**, m. 1. biscuit, etc.
9624 3. **EI**, n. 1. pl. *Eier*, eggs;
9625 ——, **auf** Butter, fried eggs;
9626 ——, **alte**, stale eggs;
9627 ——, **faule**, bad eggs;
9628 ——, **frische**, fresh or new eggs;
9629 ——, **gerührte**, buttered eggs;
9630 ——, **harte**, hard boiled eggs.
9631 ——, **weiche**, soft boiled eggs;
9632 **Eidotter**, m. 2. yolk of an egg.
9633 **Eikuchen**, m. 2. omelet, pancake.
9634 **Eiwein**, m. 1. eggwine.
9635 **Eiweisz**, n. 1. glaire, white of an egg.
9636 **Rühreier**, pl. (from rühren, to touch, strike, move), scrambled eggs.
9637 **Setzeier**, pl. (from v. a.
9638 **setzen**, to set), poached eggs.
9639 4. **FLEISCH**, n. 1. meat (flesh).
9640 ——, **gebratenes** (from braten, to roast), roasted meat;
9641 ——, **gekochtes**, boiled meat;
9642 ——, **gepöckelt**, pickled, salted meat.
9643 **Fleischbrühe**, f. broth, gravy.
9644 **Fleischkost**, f. meat diet, flesh diet.
9645 **Fleischkuchen**, m. 2. meat pie.
9646 **Fleischmahlzeit**, f. flesh meal.
9647 **Fleischnahrung**, f. animal food.
9648 **Fleischpastete**, f. meat pie, mince pie.
9649 **Fleischschnitte**, f. slice of meat.
9650 **Fleischspeise**, f. viands, flesh meals.
9651 **Fleischspiesz**. m. 1. meat spit.
9652 **Fleischsuppe**, f. broth.
9653 **Fleischtag**, m. 1. day on which meat is eaten; flesh day.
9654 **Fleischwage**, f. meat scales.
9657 **Hammelfleisch**. n. 1. mutton.
9658 **Hammelbraten**, m. 2. roast mutton.
9659 **Hammelcotelett**, n. 1.
9660 **Hammelrippchen**, n. 2. } mutton chops.
9661 **Hammelkeule**, f. leg of mutton.
9662 **Kalbfleisch**, n. 1. veal.
9663 **Kalbsbraten**, m. 2. roast veal.
9664 **Kalbscotelett**, n. 1. veal cutlet.
9665 **Kuhfleisch**, n. 1. cowflesh, } boeuf, beef.
9666 **Ochsenfleisch**, n. 1. oxmeat, } boeuf, beef.
9667 **Pöckelfleisch**, n. 1. corned beef.
9668 **Rauchfleisch**, n. 1. smoked beef (from
9669 **rauchen**, to smoke).
9670 **Rindfleisch**, n. 1. beef.
9671 **Rindfleischschnitt**, m. 1. beef steak.
9672 **Rinderbraten**, m. 2. **Rindsbraten**, m. 2. } roast beef.
9673 **Schinken**, m. 2. ham.
9674 **Schweinefleisch**, n. 1. pork.
9675 **Speck**, m. 1. bacon.
9676 **Suppenfleisch**, n. 1. soup meat, boiled meat.

9677 **Wildpret**, n. 1. game, venison.
9678 **Wurst**, f. sausage, etc.
9679 5. **FISCH**, m. 1. fish.
9680 **Aal**, m. 1. eel.
9681 **Auster**, f. oyster.
9682 **Barsch**, m. 1. perch;
9683 —, **amerikanish**, negro fish.
9684 **Forelle**, f. trout.
9685 **Hecht**, m. 1. pike.
9686 **Häring**, } m. 1. herring.
Hering, }
9687 **Hummer**, m. 2. lobster.
9688 **Karpfen**, m. 2. carp.
9689 **Krebs**, m. 1. crawfish.
9690 **Lachs**, m. 1. salmon.
9691 **Makrele**, f. mackerel.
9692 **Sardelle**, f. anchovy.
9693 **Schade**, f. shad; motherherring, mayfish.
9694 **Schildkröte**, f. tortoise, turtle.
9695 **Schleie**, f. tench.
9696 **Weiszling**, m. 1. whiting.
9697 6. **GEFLÜGEL**, n. 2. poultry.
9698 **Ente**, f. duck.
9699 **Entenbraten**, m. 2. roasted duck.
9700 **Fasan**, m. 1. pheasant.
9701 **Füllsel**, n. 2. stuffing.
9702 **Gans**, f. goose;
9703 **Gänsebraten**, m. 2. roasted goose;
9704 **Gänsebrust**, f. breast of a goose.
9705 **Spickgans**, f. smoked goose (from
9706 **spicken**, to lard.)
9707 **Henne**, f. } fowl,
9708 **Huhn**, n. 1. } chicken.
9709 **Rebhuhn**, n. 1. partridge.
9710 **Taube**, f. dove, pigeon.
9711 **Truthahn**, m. 1. turkey.
9712 7. **GEMÜSE**, n. 1. pl. } vegetables, greens, legumes, leguminous plants, lit. kitchenherbs.
9713 **Hülsenfrüchte**, f. pl. }
9714 **Küchenkräuter**, n. 1. pl. }
9715 **Blumenkohl**, m. 1. cauliflower.
9716 **Bohnen**, f. pl. beans.
9717 **Erbsen**, f. pl. peas.
9718 **Kartoffeln**, f. pl. potatoes.
9719 **Kohl**, m. 1. } cabbage.
9720 **Kraut**, n. 1. }
9721 **Korn**, n. 1. corn, grain, rye.
9722 **Linsen**, f. pl. lentils.
9723 **Möhren**, f. pl. carrots.
9724 **Reis**, m. 1. rice.
9725 **Rüben**, f. pl. gelbe (yellow) carrots.
9726 **Rüben**, f. pl. weisze (white) turnips.
9727 **Rüben**, f. pl. russische, Russian turnips.
9728 **Sauerkraut**, n. 1. (from sauer, acid), sourkrout.
9729 **Schoten**, f. pl. green peas.
9730 **Zwiebeln**, f. pl. onions.
9731 8. **FRUCHT**, f. pl. Früchte, fruit.
9732 **Obst**, n. 1. fruitage.
9733 **Ananas**, f. pine-apple.
9734 **Apfel**, m. 2. apple.
9735 **Aprikose**, f. apricot.
9736 **Beere**, f. berry.
9737 **Birne**, f. pear.
9738 **Chokolade**, f. chocolate.
9739 **Confect**, n. 1. confectionary.
9740 **Dattel**, f. date.
9741 **Eingemachtes**, n. 1. (fruit) in
9742 **Zucker** (sugar), *preserve.*
9743 **Eingemachtes**, n. 1. (fruit), e. g. such as
9744 **Gurken**, f. pl. cucumbers.
9745 **Pflaumen**, f. plums,
9746 **Zwiebeln**, f. pl. onions, etc., in salt, vinegar, etc., *picles.*
9747 **Eis**, n. 1. ice;
9748 **Eis-cream**, (ice-cream, Gefrorner Rahm, fr. v. ir.
9749 **frieren**, to freeze.)
9750 **Eisaufschlag**, m. 1. application of ice.
9751 **Eis-wasser**, n. 2. ice water.
9752 **Erdbeere**, f. strawberry.
9753 **Essig**, m. 1. vinegar.
9754 **Feige**, f. fig.
9755 **Gefrornes**, n. (from v. ir. frieren, to freeze.) } jelly.
9756 **Geronnenes**, n. (from v. ir. rinnen, to run.) }
9757 **Gallerte**, f. }
9758 **Gerste**, f. barley.
9759 **Hafer**, m. 2. oats.
9760 **Haferbrei**, m. 1. oatmeal, porridge.
9761 **Hafergrütze**, f. oatmeal groats.
9762 **Hafergrützschleim**, m. 1. } oatmeal water.
9763 **Haferschleim**, m. 1. }
9764 **Hafermehl**, n. 1. oatmeal.
9765 **Haferstärke**, f. oatstarch.

9766 **Hafertrank**, m. 1. oatmeal gruel.
9767 **Haselnusz**, f. hazel-nut.
9768 **Heidelbeere**, f. bilberry, fructus myrtilli.
9769 **Heidelbeerwein**, m. 1. myrtle wine.
9770 **Himbeere**, f. raspberry.
9771 **Himbeeressig**, m. 1. raspberry wine or vinegar.
9772 **Himbeersaft**, m. 1.) raspberry syrup.
9773 **Himbeersyrup**, m 1.) raspberry syrup.
9774 **Hollunderbeerenwein**, m. 1. elderberry wine.
9775 **Ingwer**, m. 2. ginger.
9776 **Kaffee**, m. 1. coffee.
9777 **Kirsche**, f. cherry.
9778 **Limonade**, f. lemonade.
9779 **Milch**, f. milk.
9780 **Muskatellertraube**, f. muscadine.
9781 **Muskatnusz**, f. nutmeg.
9782 **Nusz**, f. nut.
9783 **Pfirsich**, f. peach.
9784 **Pflaume**, f. plum.
9785 **Orange**, f. } orange.
9786 **Pomeranze**, f. } orange.
9787 **Pfahl**, m. 1. support (see Stütze).
9788 **Pfeffer**, m. 2. weiszer, white,
9789 ——, **roter**, red pepper.
9790 **Rahm**, m. 1. cream.
9791 **Rahmmesser**, n. 2. lactometer.
9792 **Rebe**, f. vine, branch on the vine,
9793 **Salz**, n. 1. salt.
9794 ——, **grobes**, coarse salt.
9795 **Kochsalz**, salt for cooking.
9796, **Salz. fein**, fine,
9797 **Tischsalz**, salt for the table.
9798 **Sodawasser**, n. 2. sodawasser (effervescent).
9799 **Stütze**, f. (from
9800 **stützen**, to support, uphold), support, prop.
9801 **Thee**, m. 1. tea.
9802 ——, **gemischter**, mixed tea.
9803 ——, **grüner**, green tea.
9804 ——, **schwarzer**, black tea.
9805 **Traube**, f. } grape.
9806 **Weintraube**, f. } grape.
9807 **Walnusz**, f. walnut.
9808 **Weinstock**, m. 1. vine.
9809 **Zimmt**, m. 1. cinnamon.
9810 **Zucker**, m. 2. sugar.
9811 **Zuckerwerk**, n. 1. sweetmeat.

9812 9. **WEIN**, m. 1. wine.
9813 **Apfelwein**, m. 1. cider.
9814 **Bordeaux**, m. 1. Bordeaux, claret.
9815 **Branntwein**, m. 1. brandy.
9816 **Burgunderwein**, m. 1. Burgundy.
9817 **Champagnewein**, m. 1. Champagne.
9818 **Doppelbier**, n. 1. ale.
9819 **Geistige Getränke**, n. 1. pl. } spirits (beverage), alcoholic liquors.
9820 **Spirituosen**, m. 3. pl. } spirits (beverage), alcoholic liquors.
9821 **Liqueur**, m. 1. liquor.
9822 **Mineralwasser**, n. 2. mineral water.
9823 **Moselwein**, m. 1. Moselle.
9824 **Muskateller**, m. 2. wine from muscadine grapes.
9825 **Portwein**, m. 1. port.
9826 **Punch**, m. 1. punch.
9827 **Rheinwein**, m. 1. Rhenish wine.
9828 **Rotwein**, m. 1. red wine.
9829 **Rum**, m. 1. rum.
9830 **Sherry**, m. 1. sherry.
9831 **Tokaier**, m. 2. Tokay.
9832 **Ungarwein**, m. 1. Hungarian wine.
9833 **Weiszwein**, m. 1. white wine, etc.
9834 10. **KLEIDUNG**, f. clothing.
9835 **Anzug**, m. 1, attire, dress, toilet.
9836 **Ärmel**, m. 2. sleeve.
9837 **Beinkleider**, n. 1. pl. } breeches, pantaloons.
9838 **Hosen**, f. pl. } breeches, pantaloons.
9839 **Corset**, n. 1. bodice, corsets.
9840 **Frauenhemd**, n. 1. chemise.
9841 **Frauenkleider**, n. 1. pl. female attire.
9842 **Futter**, n. 2. lining.
9843 **Gewand**, n, 1. dress, garment.
9844 **Gürtel**, m. 2. belt, sash, girdle.
9845 **Halbstiefel**, m. 2. half-boot.
9846 **Halsbinde**, f. necktie.
9847 **Halstuch**, n. 1. neckerchief.
9848 **Haube**, f. cap.
9849 **Hauskleid**, n. 1. morning dress.
9850 **Hemd**, n. 1. shirt.
9851 **Hosenträger**, m. 2. pl. suspenders.
9852 **Hut**, m. 1. hat.
9853 **Jacke**, f. jacket.

9854 **Kappe**, f.
9855 **Mütze**, f. } cap.
9856 **Kleid**, n. 1. dress.
9857 **Knopf**, m. 1. button.
9858 **Knopfloch**, n. 1. button-hole.
9859 **Kragen**, m. 2. collar.
9860 **Korsett**, n. 1. bodice, corsets.
9861 **Leib**, m. 1.
9862 **Leibchen**, n. 1. } bodice.
9863 **Mantel**, m. 2. cloak.
9864 **Mieder**, n. 2. bodice.
9865 **Morgenhaube**, f. morning cap.
9866 **Nachthaube**, f. night-cap.
9867 **Nachthemd**, m. 1. night-shirt.
9868 **Nachtjacke**, f.
9869 **Schlafjacke**, f. } night-jacket.
9870 **Nachtkappe**, f.
9871 **Nachtmütze**, f. } nightcap.
9872 **Nachtzeug**, n. 1. nightdress.
9873 **Pantoffel**, m. 2. slippers.
9874 **Pelz**, m. 1. fur.
9875 **Pelzkragen**, m. 2. fur collar.
9876 **Regenmantel**, m. 2. waterproof.
9877 **Rock**, m. 1. coat.
9878 **Schlafjacke**, f. skirt.
9879 **Schlafrock**, m. 1. dressing, night or study gown, chamber robe.
9880 **Schnürbrust**, f.
9881 **Schnürleib**, m. 1.
9882 **Schnürmieder**, n. 2. } (from schnüren, to lace, to tie), stays.
9883 **Schnürriemen**. m. 2. pl. laces.
9884 **Schuh**. m. 1. shoe.
9885 **Schuhband**, n. 1.
9886 **Schuhriemen**, m. 2. } shoelace, shoestring.
9887 **Schürze**, f. apron.
9888 **Socken**, m. 2. pl. socks.
9889 **Stecknadel**, f. pin.
9890 **Stiefel**, m. 2. boot.
9891 **Strumpf**, m. 1. stocking.
9892 **Strumpfbänder**, n. 1. pl. garters.
9893 **Tasche**, f. pocket.
9894 **Taschentuch**, n. 1. pocket-handkerchief.
9895 **Tracht**, f. costume, mode of dress.
9896 **Überrock**, m. 1. overcoat.
9897 **Überschuh**, m. 1. overshoe.
9898 **Unterhosen**, f. pl. drawers.
9899 **Unterrock**, m. 1. petticoat.
9900 **Wams**, m. 1. jacket.
9901 **Wäsche**, f. washing.
9902 **Weste**, f.
9903 **Chilet**, n. 1.
9904 **Kamisol**, n. 1. } waist coat, etc.
9905 11. **MÖBEL**, n. 2. pl. **Mobilien, movables**, movable goods, furniture, household-stuff (from
9906 **möblieren**, to fill with furniture).
9907 **Asche**, f. ashes.
9908 **Aschenkasten**, m. 2. ash-pan.
9909 **Backofen**, m. 2. oven (from v. ir.
9910 **backen**, to bake).
9911 **Bank**, f. bench.
9912 **Becher**, m. 2. cup, goblet, tumbler.
9913 **Becken**, n. 1.
9914 **Waschbecken**, n. 1. } basin, washbasin.
9915 **Besen**, m. 2. broom, besom.
9916 **Bett**, n. 1. bed.
9917 **Bettdecke**, f. blanket, cover, coverlet.
9918 **Bettlinen**, n. 2. sheeting, sheeting-linen.
9919 **Bettschieber**, m. 2.
9920 **Bettschüssel**, f. } bed-pan.
9921 **Bettstatt**, f.
9922 **Bettstelle**, f. } bedstead.
9923 **Betttuch**, n. 1. sheet.
9924 **Bettüberzug**, m. 1. bed-cover.
9925 **Bettvorhang**, m. 1.
9926 **Bettgardine**, f. } bedhanging, bed-curtain.
9927 **Bettwärmer**, m. 2.
9928 **Bettwärmflasche**, f.
9929 **Bettpfanne**, f. } bed-warmer, warming-pan, bed-pan.
9930 **Bettwäsche**, f. bed-linen, clothes.
9931 **Bettzeug**, n. 1. bedding, bed clothes.
9932 **Brennholz**, n. 1. firewood.
9933 **Bürste**, f. brush.
9934 **Dach**. n. 1. roof.
9935 **Dampf**, m. 1. steam, vapor.
9936 **Docht**, m. 1. wick.
9937 **Dunst**, m. 1. vapor.
9938 **Eimer**, m. 1. pail, bucket.
9939 **Fach**, n. 1. drawer.
9940 **Fasz**, n. 1. cask, barrel.
9941 **Federbett**, n. 1. featherbed.
9942 **Federmatratze**, f. spring-mattress.

9943 **Federmesser**, n. 2. penknife.
9944 **Fensterladen**, m. 2. window shutter.
9945 **Fensterscheibe**, f. pane of glass (in window).
9946 **Feuer**, n. 1. fire.
9947 **Feuerherd**, m. 1. fire place, hearth.
9948 **Fuszbank**, f. footstool.
9949 **Fuszbecken**, n. 2. foot basin.
9950 **Fuszboden**, m. 2. bottom, floor, ground.
9951 **Fuszdecke**, f. carpet, floor-cloth, foot-cloth.
9952 **Gabel**, f. fork.
9953 **Geheimfach**, n. 1. secret drawer.
9954 **Gaslampe**, f. gas-lamp.
9955 **Gaslicht**, n. 1. gas-light.
9956 **Haarbürste**, f. hairbrush.
9957 **Handtuch**, n. 1. towel.
9958 **Herd**, m. 1. hearth.
9959 **Holz**, n. 1. wood.
9960 **Hose**, f. gardenhose.
9961 **Kammer**, f. chamber, room.
9962 **Kamm**, m. 1. comb.
9963 **Keller**, m. 2. cellar.
9964 **Kerze**, f. candle.
9965 **Kessel**, m. 2. kettle.
9966 **Kissen**, n. 2. cushion, pillow.
9967 **Kleiderschrank**, m. 1. clothes press, wardrobe.
9968 **Klosett**, n. 1. } water-closet,
9969 **Abtritt**, m. 1. } privy.
9970 **Kochgerätschaften**, pl. (from
9971 **kochen**, to cook), cooking utensils.
9972 **Kohlen**, f. pl. coals.
9973 **Kölnisches Wasser**, n. 2. Eau de Cologne.
9974 **Kommode**, f. commode, chest of drawers.
9975 **Kopfkissen**, n. 2. pillow for the head.
9976 **Korb**, m. 1. basket.
9977 **Krankenstube**, f. } sick chamber,
9978 **Krankenzimmer**, n. 2. } sick room.
9979 **Krug**, m. 1. jug, pitcher.
9980 **Küche**, f. kitchen.
9981 **Küchengerät**, n. 1. } kitcken utensils,
9982 **Küchengeschirr**, n. 1. } furniture.
9983 **Küchenschrank**, m. 1. larder, kitchen closet.
9984 **Kutsche**, f. coach.
9985 **Lampe**, f. lamp.
9986 **Laterne**, f. lantern.
9987 **Lehnsessel**, m. 1. }
9988 **Lehnstuhl**, m. 1. } arm chair.
9989 **Armstuhl**, m. 1. }
9990 **Leuchter**, m. 2. candle-stick.
9991 **Licht**, n. 1. light.
9992 **Lichtputze**, f. } candle snuffer,
9993 **Lichtschere**, f. } a pair of snuffers.
9994 **Lichtschirm**, m. 1. light-screen, shade.
9995 **Löffel**, m. 2. spoon.
9996 **Eszlöffel**. m. 2. tablespoon.
9997 **Kaffeelöffel**, m. 2. } tea-
9998 **Theelöffel**, m. 2. } spoon.
9999 **Luftkissen**, n. 2. air-pillow.
10000 **Machwerk**, n. 1. (from
10001 **machen**, to make), bungling fabrications.
10002 **Matratze**, f. mattress.
10003 **Messer**, n. 2. knife.
10004 **Moskitonetz**, n. 1. } mosquito-bar,
10005 **Fliegennetz**, n. 1. } fly-net.
10006 **Nachtbecken**, n. 2. } cham-
10007 **Nachtgeschirr**, n. 1. } ber-
10008 **Nachttopf**, m. 1. } pot
10009 **Nachtlampe**, f. nightlamp.
10010 **Nachtstuhl**, m. 1. close-stool, chamber-stool.
10011 **Nagelbürste**, f. nail-brush.
10012 **Oberdecke**, f. cover, coverlet.
10013 **Ofen**, m. 2. stove, oven.
10014 **Ofenloch**, n. 1. mouth of a stove.
10015 **Ofenschirm**, m. 1. screen.
10016 **Ofenthüre**, f. stove door, vent door.
10017 **Officin**, f. drug store, apothecary shop.
10018 **Öl**, n. 1. oil.
10019 **Pfanne**, f. pan.
10020 **Pfropfen**, m. 2. cork.
10021 **Pfropfenzieher**, m. 2. cork-screw.
10022 **Polster**, n. 2. pillow.
10023 **Porcellan**, n. 1. porcelain.
10024 **Pult**, n. 1. desk, writing-desk.
10025 **Rauch**, m. 1. smoke.
10026 **Rost**, m. 1. grate.
10027 **Rouleau**, n. 1. blind.
10028 **Ruhekissen**, n. 2. pillow.
10029 **Schere**, f. scissors.
10030 **Regenschirm**, m. 1. umbrella.
10031 **Schirm**, m. 1. screen.
10032 **Schlafsessel**, m. 2. } easy
10033 **Schlafstuhl**, m. 1. } chair.

10034 **Schlafstube**, f. } bedroom,
10035 **Schlafzimmer**, n. 2. } bed-chamber.
10036 **Schlüssel**, m. 2. key.
10037 **Schlüsselloch**, n. 1, key-hole.
10038 **Schornstein**, m. 1. chimney.
10039 **Schrank**, m. 1. cupboard, press, shrine, wardrobe.
10040 **Schreibpult**, n. 1. } writing
10041 **Schreibtisch**, m. 1. } desk.
10042 **Schublade**, f. drawer.
10043 **Schüssel**, f. dish, platter, plate.
10044 **Serviette**, f. napkin.
10045 **Sopha**. n. 1. sofa.
10046 **Speiseschrank**, m. 1. pantry, safe.
10047 **Spuknapf**, m. 1. (from v. ir. speien, to spit), spittoon.
10048 **Stearinkerze**, f. stearin-candle.
10049 **Steinkohle**, f. coal.
10050 **Stiefelzieher**, m. 2. boot jack.
10051 **Steppdecke**, f. quilt.
10052 **Streichhölzchen**, n. 2. }
10053 **Schwefelholz**, n. 1. } match.
10054 **Zündhölzchen**, n. 2. }
10055 **Tasse**, f. cup.
10056 **Teller**, m. 2. plate.
10057 **Teppig**, m. 1. carpet.
10058 **Thür(e)**, f. door, portal.
Tischtuch, n. 1. (from } tablecloth,
10059 **Tisch**, m. 1. table), } tablecover.
10060 **Topf**, m. 1. pot.
10061 **Tragstuhl**, m. 1. carrying chair.
10062 **Trichter**, m. 2. funnel.
10063 **Unterbett**, n. 1. under-bed.
10064 **Untertasse**, f. saucer.
10065 **Wagen**, m. 2. waggon, carriage, coach.
10066 **Wäsche**, f. washing.
10067 **Waschnapf**, m. 1. } wash-top,
Waschbecken, n. 2. } wash-basin.
Waschtopf, m. 1. }
10068 **Waschtisch**, m. 1. } wash-
10069 **Waschtoilette**, f. } stand.
10070 **Waschschwamm**, m. 1. sponge.
10071 **Waschzuber**, m. 2. wash-tub with two handles.
10072 **Wasserhose**, f. waterspout, typhon.
10073 **Wasserklosett**, n. 2. } water-closet,
10074 **Abtritt**, m. 1. } privy.
10075 **Wohnung**, f. dwelling, residence.
10076 **Wollendecke**, f. woolen planket,
10077 **Zahnbürste**, f. toothbrush.
10078 **Zunder**, m. 2. tinder, etc.

PART THIRD.

DIALOGUES.

§ 34. 1. **Beim ersten Besuch** eines **Arztes.**	At the first visit of a physician.
Doktor. Guten Morgen--Tag--Nachmittag—Abend, mein Herr N., meine Dame (Frau) N., mein Fräulein N. Ich musz Sie um Entschuldigung bitten, dasz ich nicht sogleich kam, da ich nicht zu Hause war, als Sie für mich sandten (or schickten). Was fehlt Ihnen?	Good morning—day—afternoon—evening, Mr. N., Mrs. (Madam) N., Miss N. I must beg your pardon (I beg you to excuse me) for not coming directly, as I was not at home (being not at home), when you sent for me. Are you sick? What ails you? What's the matter?
Patient. Ich bin nicht gesund. Mir ist durchaus nicht wohl. Ich fühle sehr unwohl.	I am not well. I am not at all well. I feel very unwell—ill—sick.
Dok. Seit wann sind Sie unwohl?	How long have you been ill—sick—unwell?
Pat. Seit vorgestern Abend.	Since day before yesterday in the evening.
Dok. Was war der Anfang Ihres Unwohlseins—Ihrer Krankheit?	What was the beginning of your sickness?
Pat. Es begann mit Kopfweh and Frösteln (Fieberschauer).	It began with head-ache and shivering—a chill.
Dok. Wie fühlen Sie jetzt—gegenwärtig?	How are you feeling at present?
Pat. Ich bin, ich weisz nicht, wie ich's nennen soll, ungewöhnlich schwach, and kraftlos in allen meinen Gliedern.	I am, I know not how I shall call it, unusually weak and powerless in all my limbs.
Dok. Ist es Ihnen schwindelig, oder haben Sie nur Kopfweh?	Do you feel giddy (dizzy), or have you only head-ache.
Pat. Es ist mir nicht schwindelig, aber ich fühle zuweilen grosze Übelkeit, nahe zum Erbrechen.	I do not feel giddy, but I have sometimes a very disagreeable nauseating feeling.
Dok. Wie ist Ihr Appetit?	How is your appetite?
Pat. Mein Appetit ist sehr gering. Ich kann beinahe nichts essen, aber ich habe beständig groszen Durst.	I have but little appetite. I can scarcely eat anything, but I have always great thirst.
Dok. Lassen Sie mich Ihren Puls fühlen und Ihre Zunge besehen.—Ihr Puls ist etwas—ziemlich fieberhaft und Ihre belegte Zunge zeigt an, dasz Ihr Magen aus der Ordnung ist—nicht ist, wie er sein soll—verdorben ist.	Let me feel your pulse and look at your tongue. Your pulse is somewhat—tolerably—feverish, and your coated tongue indicates that your stomach is out of order—is not what it should be—is deranged.
Dok. Wie ist Ihr Schlaf?	How is your sleep?
Pat. Ich kann nur wenig schlafen, und meine Ruhe ist oftmals durch Träume gestört.	I can but little sleep, and my rest is often disturbed by dreams.

Dok. Gemäsz der Symptome (Merkmale) müssen Sie etwas Arznei gebrauchen, und am besten ist es, dasz Sie zu Bette gehen und sich ganz ruhig verhalten, wenigstens für eine kurze Zeit. Hier, lassen Sie diese Arznei bereiten, oder—nehmen Sie diese Arznei—und brauchen, oder—n e h m e n—S i e davon—jede Stunde—oder alle zwei Stunden—einen Eszlöffel voll, bis die Arznei wirkt, and dann, wann ich wieder komme, wollen wir weiter sehen, was zu thun ist.	According to the symptoms you must use some medicine, and it is the best that you go to bed and keep quiet, at least for a short time. Here, get this medicine prepared, and use—or take a tablespoonful of it every hour—or every two hours, until it operates, and then, when I come again, we will see what further is to be done.
Pat. Darf ich etwas essen, oder musz ich nüchtern bleiben.	May I eat something, or must I remain jejune—on an empty stomach?
Dok. Vorderhand essen Sie gar nichts, bleiben Sie ruhig im Bette liegen, and sehen Sie zu, dasz Sie sich nicht erkälten—Ich werde morgen früh wieder kommen, and in der Hoffnung, dasz Sie besser sein werden, verabschiede ich mich für heute.	At present do not eat anything, stay quietly in bed, and take care not to catch cold. I'll call again to-morrow morning, and in the hope that you will be better. I bid you good-bye for to-day.
2. Beim **zweiten Besuch** eines **Arztes.**	At the second visit of a physician.
Dok. Wie befinden Sie sich heute? Wie fühlen Sie heute? Ist Ihr Zustand schlimmer, schlechter, besser?	How are you to-day? How do you feel to-day? Is your condition worse or better?
Pat. Es scheint nicht besser—nicht viel besser zu gehen. Ich habe noch dasselbe Kopfweh, and obgleich die Arznei sehr gut gewirkt hat-ich muszte dreimal zu Stuhle gehen—so finde ich doch wenig Erleichterung, und meine Kräfte scheinen mich gänzlich zu verlassen.	I do not seem to be much better. I have still the same headache, and although the medicine has well operated, I was obliged to go to stool three times, I find not much relief, and my strength seems to leave me entirely.
Dok. Haben Sie einen Schmerz, Schmerzen, in Ihrer Seite, und wenn so, währt er, währen sie—lange, oder ist er—sind sie—nur von kurzer Dauer?	Have you pain, or pains in your side, and if so, does it, do they, continue long, or is it, are they, only of a short duration?
Pat. Ja, ich habe einen scharfen Schmerz in meiner Seite, besonders wann ich einen langen Atem ziehe.	Yes, sir, I have a sharp pain in my side, especially if I draw a long breath.
Dok. Haben Sie Schmerzen im Rücken?	Have you pains in your back?
Pat. Nicht besonders im Rücken, ich fühle Schmerzen beinahe überall.	Not especially in the back, I feel pains almost all over.
Dok. Warum sind Sie no niedergeschlagen?	Why are you so depressed?
Pat. Es scheint, Sie wissen nicht wie krank ich bin und wie viel ich leide.	It seems you do not know how sick I am and how much I suffer.

Dok. Allerdings, ich sehe wohl, dasz Sie sehr krank sind, und es ist mir nicht unbewuszt, dasz Sie auch Schmerzen haben, aber Sie sollten deshalb nicht so verstimmt sein, da Ihre Krankheit im jetzigen oder gegenwärtigen Zustande nicht gefährlich ist.	Certainly, I see indeed that you are very sick, and I am conscious—well aware—of the fact that you have also pains, but you should therefore not be so low-spirited, since your sickness in its present stage is not dangerous.
Pat. Denken Sie, dasz Aussicht vorhanden ist, dasz ich wieder gesund werde?	Do you think that there is a chance for my recovery.
Dok. Gewiszlich! Sie werden bald genesen, wenn Sie vorsichtig sind und Ihre Arznei pünktlich gebrauchen—einnehmen.	Assuredly! you will soon recover—convalesce, if you are careful and use—take your medicine regularly.
Pat. Was für eine Medizin werden Sie mir geben? Ich ziehe etwas Flüssiges den Pillen und Pulvern vor, da es mir schwer wird diese zu verschlucken.	What kind of medicine will you give me? I prefer some liquid medicine to pills and powders, which I find difficult to swallow.
Dok. Den Schmerz in der Seite zu lindern, und zur Erleichterung des Atems, gebrauchen Sie die Salbe, die ich Ihnen verschrieben habe, indem Sie die Seite und die Brust fleiszig damit einreiben.	To alleviate the pain in your side, and to ease your respiration, you must use the ointment (linament) I prescribed for you, rubbing diligently your side and breast therewith.
Pat. Was würden Sie mir raten zu essen, um wieder zu Kräften zu kommen-gelangen, da ich so sehr ermattet bin. Welche Diät musz—soll ich beobachten?	What would you advise me to eat in order to gain strength, as I am so very weak—What diet must I—should I observe?
Dok. Sie können zuerst irgend eine leicht verdauliche Speise genieszen, zum Beispiel: Fleisch-oder Hühnerbrühe, Grütze, geröstete Brotschnitte, erweicht in Milch, und dergleichen; and dann, ein wenig später, stärkere Nahrung, gänzlich gemäsz dem Verlangen eines gröszeren Appetits.	You can take at first any light food which is easily digested, e. g. skimmed beef or chicken-broth, gruel, milk-toast, and the like; and then, after a while, stronger food, wholly according to the demand of an increased appetite.
Pat. Kommen Sie morgen wieder, Herr Doktor; ich sehne mich sehr, so bald wie möglich wieder gesund zu werden.	Doctor, come again to-morrow; I am very anxious—or I long very much to become well again as soon as possible.
Dok. Es gibt nichts Ihre baldige Genesung zu verhindern, so viel ich nun sehen kann, vorausgesetzt, dasz nichts weiter geschieht, was jetzt nicht zu ersehen ist, und was ich nicht erwarte.	There is nothing to hinder your speedy recovery, so far as I can see now, provided nothing further happens—occurs—which at present cannot be forseen, and which I do not expect.
3. Beim **dritten Besuch** eines **Arztes.**	At the third visit of a physician.
Dok. Wie geht es? Wie befinden Sie sich heute?	How do you do to-day?
Pat. Ich befinde mich viel besser, bei weitem besser, als gestern.	I am much better, I thank you—by far better to-day than yesterday.
Dok. Wie steht's mit dem Kopfweh?	How is it with the head-ache?
Pat. Ich habe heute keine Kopfschmerzen, und ich fühle viel	I have no pain—pains—in my head to-day, and I feel much refreshed

frischer, indem ich letzte Nacht ziemlich gut geschlafen habe.

since I have slept pretty well last night.

Dok. Wie verhält es sich mit dem Schmerz—mit den Schmerzen—in der Seite? Sie scheinen viel freier--bei weitem besser—zu atmen. Haben Sie die Salbe angewandt? Ich kann sehen—sehr wohl wahrnehmen, d a s z d i e Medizin, welche ich Ihnen verschrieben habe, gute Wirkung gethan hat. und es freut mich sehr Sie bedeutend besser zu finden.

How is it with the pain—pains—in your side? You appear to breathe much easier—by far better—Did you use the ointment? I can see —I observe very well--that the medicine which I prescribed for you, has done good work, and I am very glad to find you so much better.

Pat. Der Schmerz in meiner Seite verliert sich allmählich—hat sich gänzlich verloren—und ich finde keine—gar keine Schwierigkeit zu atmen.

The pain in my side—gradually disappears—is entirely gone—and I have no difficulty in breathing.

Dok. Sie fühlen sich demnach sehr erleichtert. Ihre Kräfte werden sich, ohne Zweifel, bald vermehren, sobald das Fieber ganz—gänzlich gebrochen sein wird.

You feel therefore greatly relieved ; your strength, doubtless will become increased as soon as your fever shall be broken entirely.

Pat. Es scheint mir, dasz ich noch Fieber haben musz, indem ich immer noch Durst habe.

It seems to me that I must still have fever, since I am always thirsty.

Dok. Nehmen Sie von der Arznei, welche ich Ihnen jetzt verschreibe, alle zwei Stunden einen halben Thee-löffel voll, oder vier bis fünf von diesen Kügelchen, and wie ich hoffe, wird sich das Fieber bald legen, und den Durst wird etwas Limenade, oder etwas Himbeerenessig, gemischt mit ein wenig Wasser, stillen.

Take of the medicine, which I now prescribe for you, half a tea-spoon full every two hours, or from four to five of these lozenges, and I hope the fever will soon be reduced, and your thirst will be relieved by lemonade or by raspberry syrup, mixed with some water.

Pat. Wie lange musz ich noch im Bette bleiben? Ich möchte das Bett gar zu gern verlassen.

How long must I still remain in bed? I would like very much to leave the bed.

Dok. Bleiben Sie nur noch heute ruhig im Bett. Sie sind noch zu schwach zum Aufstehen. Wenn Sie morgen stärker fühlen, so mögen Sie das Bett verlassen, wenigstens für eine kurze Zeit.

Remain only still to-day quietly in bed; you are yet too weak to leave your bed. If you are stronger to-morrow, you may get up, at least for a short time.

Pat. Der üble Geschmack in meinem Munde hat sich verloren, und es scheint, dasz mein Appetit sich vermehrt hat. Erlauben Sie mir, Herr Doktor, zu essen, was ich liebe, oder musz ich immer noch eine besondere Diät beobachten?

The bitter taste in my mouth has left me and it seems that my appetite is increasing ; do you allow me, doctor, to eat what I like, or must I still restrict myself to a special diet?

Dok. Sie müssen noch nicht essen, was Sie wollen, and namentlich müssen Sie alle fetten und sauren Speisen vermeiden, and soviel als möglich sich allein auf Mehlspeisen beschränken, and nur wenig Gemüse essen.

You must not yet eat what you like, but avoid in particular all fatty and sour food, and confine yourself, as much as possible, to farinaceous substances and eat but few vegetables.

Pat. Darf ich gar kein Fleisch auch kein kaltes Fleisch essen? — Must I eat no meat at all, not even cold meat?

Dok. Sie können Fleisch-und Hühnerbrühe and dergleichen öfters genieszen, und auch etwas Hammelfleisch—oder Hammelsrippchen, and etwas Huhn,und gebratene Kartoffeln, and dürres, gekochtes Obst und Reis, etc. — You can often take as food meat or chicken-broth and the like, and some boiled or roasted chicken or mutton, or mutton-chops and roasted potatoes, and cooked dried fruit and rice, etc.

Pat. Darf ich Kaffee und Thee bei den Mahlzeiten und sonst auch während des Tages Wasser mit Eis trinken? — May I drink at meals coffee and tea and also ice-water during the day?

Dok. Trinken Sie Ihren Kaffee und Thee nur mäszig stark, und trinken Sie nur wenig Eiswasser auf ein mal. Ihre Genesung is sicher, aber es wird einige Zeit nehmen, bis Sie wieder ganz gesund werden sein. Eine Luftveränderung—oder Aufenthalt im Lande für einige Wochen—Monate, würde Ihrer Gesundheit ungemein zuträglich sein, etc. — Drink your coffee and tea only moderately strong and drink but little ice-water at one time. Your convalescence is sure, but it will take some time, till you will be entirely well. A change of air—or a stay in the country for several weeks or months, would be uncommonly beneficial for your health, or would be a great benefit to your health, etc.

§ 35. Idiomatische Phrasen und Sprichwörter. — Idiomatic Phrases and Proverbs.

Abschied nehmen. e. g. Ich nehme Abschied. — To take leave, to bid adieu; e. g. I take leave. (To shake hands with.)

Acht geben, sich in Acht nehmen, Vorsicht haben. — To take care or precaution,

Aufmerksamkeit schenken or widmen. — To pay attention.

Auf baldiges Wiedersehen. — Till I see you again. I hope to see you again.

Auf der Stadtuhr ist es ein Uhr. — 'Tis one o'clock by the town clock.

Aufgeschoben ist nicht aufgehoben (prov.). — A reprieve is no acquittance.

Auf jeden Fall. — At all events, at any rate.

Auf Regen folgt Sonnenschein. — After rain comes sunshine.

Aller Anfang ist schwer (prov.). — Every beginning is hard (difficult).

Alles zum besten kehren. — To turn everything to the best advantage.

Am Kopfe, am Fusze, an den Füszen leiden. — To feel pain in one's head, foot, feet, etc.

Am Morgen, Mittag, Abend, etc. — In the morning, at noon, in the evening, etc.

Anstatt zu gehen, hören, gehorchen, etc. — Instead of going, of listening, of obeying, etc.

Armut ist keine Schande (prov.). — Poverty is no disgrace.

Armut thut weh (prov.). — Poverty is a sharp weapon.

Aus dem Regen in the Traufe kommen (prov.). — To fall out of the frying pan into the fire.

Aus der Not eine Tugend machen. — To make a virtue of necessity.

Aus Dankbarkeit. — From or out of gratitude.

Aus Pflicht, aus Freude. — From or out of duty, from or for joy.

Aus freien Stücken. — Of one's own accord.

Aus Mitleiden or Barmherzigkeit. — For pity's sake.

Aus Scham, aus Verdrusz.	From or out of shame, from or out of vexation.
Befinden Sie sich wohl?	Are you well!
Bei wem?	At whose house?
Beim Anbruche des Tages.	At the breaking of day.
Beim or gegen Einbruch der Nacht.	At or about the close of the evening.
Bleibet nicht zu lang aus.	Do not stay beyond your time.
Da mögen Sie zusehen.	That is your lookout.
Da steckt etwas dahinter.	There is some mystery about it.
Damit hat es gute Zeit.	There is no hurry with that.
Danke! Danke Ihnen!	Thank you.
Das Essen, Frühstück, Mittagessen, Abendessen, ist fertig.	Breakfast, dinner, supper, is ready.
Das freut mich sehr.	I am very glad of it.
Das glaube ich.	I believe so, that I believe.
Das geht ihn nichts an.	That does not concern him.
Das geht Sie nichts an.	That does not concern you, etc.
Das geht nicht mit rechten Dingen zu.	'Tis not at all right about this.
Das hat nichts zu sagen.	No matter about it.
Das hat nichts zu bedeuten.	It means nothing.
Das thut nichts.	That does not matter, etc.
Das ist etwas Anderes.	That is a different thing.
Das ist gleichviel.	That is all the same.
Das ist seine Sache.	That concerns him.
Das kann ihm niemand verdenken.	No one can blame him for that.
Das Licht, die Sonne scheint mir ins Gesicht.	The light—the sun is in my eyes.
Das Werk lobt den Meister (prov.).	The master is known by his work.
Das wird dir nach Hause kommen (prov.).	That will come upon thy head.
Der Arzt besucht meine Mutter täglich.	The doctor attends my mother every day.
Dem sei wie ihm wolle.	Be that as it may.
DerMensch denkt,Gott lenkt(prov.).	Man proposes, God disposes.
Der Wievielste ist heute?	What day of the month is this?
Den Gelehrten ist gut prediger. (prov.).	A word is enough to the wise.
Dieser Hut steht Ihnen gut.	This hat fits or becomes you well.
Die Mühe ist gering.	No trouble at all.
Die Zeit mit etwas zubringen.	To spend the time in something.
Darf ich Sie um eine Gefälligkeit bitten oder ersuchen?	May I ask a favor of you? May I trouble you?
Ehrlich währt am längsten (prov.).	Honesty is the best policy.
Eigner Herd is Goldes wert (prov.)	Nothing is like home.
Eile mit Weile (prov.). Eile thut kein gut (prov.).	The more haste, the worse speed.
Ein für allemal.	Once for all.
Ein gutes Wort findet eine gute Stelle.	A good word always tells.
Einen auf die Achsel klopfen.	To tap one on the shoulder.
Einem das Wort reden.	To intercede or plead for one or in one's favor.
Einen Gott glauben.	To believe in a God.
Eine Gelegenheit vom Zaune brechen (prov.).	To seek a pretext.
Er geht auf Reisen.	He goes abroad.
Er hat sich aus dem Staube gemacht.	He has taken himself off.

(175)

Er ist der deutschen Sprache mächtig.	He is master of the German language.
Er ist von Geburt ein Franzose.	He is a Frenchman by birth.
Er ist zu Allem zu gebrauchen.	He is fit for anything.
Er ist zu arm um eine solche Ausgabe zu machen.	He cannot afford to spend so much.
Er macht sich Gedanken darüber.	He troubles his head about it.
Er trinkt lieber Kaffee als Thee.	He likes coffee better than tea.
Er verdient sein Brot.	He makes his living.
Er weisz sich in alles zu finden oder zu schicken.	Nothing comes amiss to him.
Er, sie, es hat sich erkältet.	He, she, it has taken cold.
Er, sie, es hat allen Glauben verloren.	He, she, it has lost all credit.
Ende gut, Alles good (prov.).	All's well that ends well. The evening crowns the day.
Es fehlt mir, ihm, ihr, nichts.	Nothing ails me, him, her. Nothing is the matter with me, him, her.
Es freut mich sehr.	I am very glad (of it.)
Es friert mich sehr.	I am very cold.
Es geht mir durchs Herz.	That strikes me to the very heart.
Es geht mir zu Herzen.	It grieves me.
Es geht nichts über das Reisen.	There is nothing like traveling.
Es geschieht ihr, ihm, ihnen recht.	It serves her, him, them right.
Es hat viel or nicht viel, wenig or nichts or gar nichts zu bedeuten.	It is of *much* or of *not much*, of no consequence, or of no consequence whatever.
Es hat Not, es hat keine Not.	There is need, there is no need.
Es ist der Mühe wert.	It is worth while.
Es ist nicht der Mühe wert.	It is not worth while.
Es ist ewiger Schade	It is a great pity.
Es ist mir lieb.	I am glad of it.
Es ist mir um so lieber.	I like it all the better.
Es ist schon gut.	It is enough.
Es ist an dem, dasz sie geht.	Her time of going is near.
Es steckt im Blut.	It runs in the blood.
Es thut mir leid.	I am very sorry for it.
Etwas los werden.	To get rid of something.
Frisch und gesund.	Healthful and gay ; safe and sound.
Frisch gewagt ist halb gewonnen (prov.).	Well begun is half done.
Ganz der Ihrige.	I am yours with all my heart.
Geh hin im Frieden !	Depart in peace !
Geh ! Go along ! Geht !	Get you gone !
Geh doch !	Pray, be gone ! Go !
Gewalt geht über Recht.	Might is more than right.
Glauben Sie so leicht davon zu kommen ?	Do you think to escape thus ?
Gleich und Gleich gesellt sich gern (prov.).	Birds of a feather flock together.
Gott befohlen !	Farewell ! Adieu !
Gott sei Dank !	Thank God ! God be praised !
Grüszen Sie mir Ihre Fräulein Nichte vielmal !	Remember me most kindly to your niece.
Grüszen Sie mir Ihren Herrn Oheim.	My compliments to your uncle.
Guten Morgen—Nachmittag—Abend—Nacht.	Good morning, day, afternoon, evening, night.

Guter Hoffnung ; Mutes ; Laune sein.	To be with child ; to have courage, to be in good humor, to be in good spirits.
Hast du Geld bei dir?	Have you any money about you?
Hat Ihre Frau Mutter einen Arzt?	Does any one, any doctor attend your mother?
Haben Sie Ihre Meinung—Gesinnung geändert?	Have you changed your mind?
Heute über acht Tage—vierzehn Tage—ein Jahr.	A week—a fortnight—a year from to-day.
Hunger ist der beste Koch (prov.)	Hunger is the best cook—sauce.
Ich befinde mich sehr wohl.	I am very well.
Ich bin es, du bist es, etc.	It is I—it is thou, etc.
Ich bitte, Pray. Ich bekümmere mich nicht darum.	I do not care, etc.
Ich gehe meinem Vater entgegen.	I go to meet my father.
Ich glaube wohl.	I dare say—
Ich habe mir den Arm—das Bein, etc.—gebrochen.	I have broken my arm—my leg, etc.
Ich habe nichts daran auszusetzen.	I find no fault with it.
Ich kann ihn nicht los werden.	I cannot get rid of him.
Ich konnte nichts dabei gewinnen.	It was of no advantage to me.
Ich kann nichts dafür.	It is not my fault. I cannot help it.
Ich kann ihn nicht ausstehen, wegen seines Leichtsinns.	I cannot bear him on account of his levity.
Ich konnte mich des Lachens kaum enthalten.	I could scarcely keep from laughing.
Ich möchte wissen was das ist.	I would like to know what it is.
Ich nehme Sie beim Wort.	I take you at your word.
Ich war im Begriffë fortzugehen.	I was about to start.
Ich werde Sie nach Hause begleiten.	I shall see you home.
Ich wünsche Ihnen viel Glück.	I wish you much happiness.
Ich würde es gern thun.	I would like to do it.
Ich will ihm zeigen, was das heiszt.	I will show him, what it is.
Ich suche meinen Bruder.	I am looking for my brother.
In die Hände klopfen.	To clap one's hands.
Ist der Tisch gedeckt?	Is the cloth laid?
Ich werde es nicht versäumen Ihrem Wunsche nachzukommen.	I shall not fail to fulfill your desire.
Ist das Ihr wahrer Ernst?	Are you very serious.
Jahr aus, Jahr ein.	Every year. All the year round.
Jedem Narren gefällt seine Kappe.	Every one has his hobby.
Jeder is sich selbst der Nächste (prov.).	Charity begins at home.
Ich habe Sie seit letztes Frühjahr nicht gesehen.	I have not seen you since last spring.
Kauf ist Kauf, geschehen ist geschehen (prov.).	A bargain is a bargain.
Kehren Sie sich nicht daran!	Never mind that!
Kommt Zeit, kommt Rat (prov.).	Let time shape.
Lassen Sie sich von ihm raten!	Be advised by him!
Lassen Sie mich nicht im Stich!	Do not disappoint me!
Lassen Sie uns spazieren gehen!	Let us take a walk!
Machen Sie Ihrer Frau Mutter meine Empfehlungen.	Give my regards to your mother.
Man glaubt von ihm dasz—	He is suspected of—
Meinen besten Dank.	I thank you very much.
Mir ist alles einerlei.	It is all the same to me.

12

Mit jemand ehrlich zu Werke zu gehen.	To deal honestly with one.
Mit Ihrer Erlaubnis.	By your leave.
Müsziggang ist aller Laster Anfang.	Idleness is the beginning or parent of vice.
Nehmen Sie sich in Acht!	Take care of yourself!
Nehmen Sie etwas ein?	Do you take anything?
Neue Besen kehren gut (prov.).	New brooms sweep clean.
Not bricht Eisen (prov.). Not kennt kein Gebot.	Necessity has no law.
Not lehrt beten (prov.).	Necessity teaches to pray. Necessity teaches many things.
Nun, was soll alles dieses bedeuten!	Well, and what of all this?
Recht gebetet, ist halb studiert.	Praying right, is studied half.
Recht gern.	Willingly.
Seit wann sind Sie krank?	How long have you been unwell?
Sie hat ihre Zeit.	She has her courses.
Sie ist ihrer Zeit nahe.	She is near her time—reckoning.
Sie mögen—können thun, was Sie wollen.	Do as you please—anything you please.
Soll ich Sie rufen lassen?	Shall I send for you?
Soll ich Sie es wissen lassen?	Shall I send you word about it?
So viel ich kann,—so viel ich weisz.	As far as I can—as far as I know.
So viel ich mich erinnere.	To the best of my knowledge—or remembrance.
So viel Köpfe, so viel Sinne (prov.).	So many men, so many minds.
So viel ich weisz.	For aught I know.
Sprechen Sie nicht davon.	Do not mention it.
Übung macht den Meister (prov.).	Practice makes perfect.
Um so besser.	So much the better.
Unkraut verdirbt nicht.	Ill-weeds grow apace.
Unrecht Gut gedeiht nicht (prov.).	Ill-gotten goods do not prosper.
Vergessen Sie mich nicht bei Ihrem Herrn Schwager.	Give my kind regards to your brother-in-law.
Versichern Sie Ihre Frau Schwester meiner Hochachtung.	Present my respect to your sister.
Was fehlt Ihnen?	What ails you? What is the matter with you?
Was haben Sie am Backen?—am Halse, etc.	What ails your cheek?—your neck? etc.
Was halten Sie davon?	What think you of it?
Was ist zu thun?	What is to be done?
Was liegt mir daran?	What do I care?
Was soll das heiszen?	What is the meaning of this? What does it signify?
Wann die Not am grözsten, is Gott (Gottes Hülfe) am nächsten (prov.).	When times are at the worst they will certainly mend.
Wenn es Ihnen gefällt, so nehmen Sie es.	If you like it—if you are pleased with it, take it.
Wer zuerst kommt, malt zuerst (prov.).	First come, first served.
Wer alles will, bekommt nichts (prov.).	All grasp, all lose.
Wer nichts wagt, gewinnt nichts (prov.).	Nothing venture, nothing have.
Wer hat nach mir gefragt.	Who has asked for me?
Wesz das Herz voll ist, (desz) geht der Mund über (prov.).	What the heart thinketh, the mouth speaketh.

Wie befinden Sie sich?	How do you do?
Wie der Herr, so der Knecht (prov.).	Like master, like men.
Wie befindet man sich in Ihrem Hause?	How do they all do at home?
Wie die Arbeit, so der Lohn (prov.).	As the work, so the pay
Wie Einige glauben mögen.	As some may suppose.
Wie heiszen Sie? Wie ist Ihr Name?	What is your name?
Wie es der Gebrauch mit sich bringt.	According to custom.
Willens sein.	To have the intention.
Zeit bringt Rosen (prov.).	Time brings everything to pass, lit. Time brings roses, etc.

§ 36. Schedule of the Terminations of Each Declension.

	STRONG OR OLD DECLENSION.							WEAK OR NEW DECLENSION.		
	CLASS I. Masc. and Neuter.				CLASS II. Masc.and Neut.		CLASS III. Masc.	CLASS IV. Feminine.		
					SINGULAR.					
N.	—		—		—	—	—e	—	—	—
G.	—es or s		—es or s		—s	—s	—en	—	—	—
D.	—e		—e		—	—	—en	—	—	—
A.	—		—		—	—	—en	—	—	—
					PLURAL.					
N.	—e	¨[1]—e	—e	¨[1]—er[2]	¨[1]—	¨[1]—	—en	¨[1]—e	—en	—n
G.	—e	¨—e	—e	¨—er	¨—	¨—	—en	¨—e	—en	—n
D.	—en	¨—en	—en	¨—ern	¨—n	¨—n	—en	¨—en	—en	—n
A.	—e	¨—e	—e	¨—er	¨—	¨—	—en	¨—e	—en	—n
					SINGULAR.					
	Masc.		Neut.		Masc.	Neut.				
N.	Berg.	Ball,	Beil,	Buch,	Vater,	Kloster,	Knabe,	Hand,	Art,	Gabe.
G.	Berges	Balles.	Beiles,	Buches	Vaters,	Klosters,	Knaben,	Hand,	Art,	Gabe.
D.	Berge,	Balle,	Beile.	Buche,	Vater,	Kloster.	Knaben,	Hand,	Art,	Gabe.
A.	Berg,	Ball,	Beil,	Buch,	Vater,	Kloster,	Knaben,	Hand,	Art,	Gabe.
					PLURAL.					
	Masc.		Neut.		Masc.	Neut.				
N.	Berge,	Bälle,	Beile,	Bücher,	Väter,	Klöster,	Knaben,	Hände,	Arten,	Gaben.
G.	Berge,	Bälle,	Beile,	Bücher,	Väter,	Klöster,	Knaben,	Hände.	Arten,	Gaben.
D.	Bergen	Bällen	Beilen	Büchern	Vätern,	Klöstern	Knaben.	Händen,	Arten.	Gaben.
A.	Berge,	Bälle,	Beile,	Bücher,	Väter,	Klöster,	Knaben,	Hände,	Arten,	Gaben.

[1] These dots show the plural modified.

[2] This plural ending *er* is a deviation, occurring mostly in *neuter monosyllabic* nouns, though, xceptionally, it is also transferred upon some *masculine* nouns (see § 27, II, B. b. 2, note) of my Grammar.

§37. Complete List of Irregular Verbs, with the Changes in the Various Tenses, Etc.

Infinitive.	Present Indicative.	Imperfect.		Imperative.	Past Participle.
		Indicative.	Subjunctive.		
Backen, to bake,	bäckst, bäckt	buk (backte)	bücke (backte)	backe	gebacken
Bedingen, to contract,	. . . . . .	bedung	bedünge	bedinge	bedungen
Bedürfen, to need,	bedarf, bedarfst, bedarf	bedurfte	bedürfte	none	bedurft
Befehlen, to command,	befiehlst, befiehlt	befahl	befähle	befiehl	befohlen
Befleiszen, to apply one's self.	. . . . . .	beflisz	beflisse	befleisz(e)	beflissen
Beginnen, to begin,	. . . . . .	begann	begänne	beginne	begonnen
Beiszen, to bite,	. . . . . .	bisz	bisse	beisz(e)	gebissen
Bergen, to conceal,	birgst, birgt	barg	bärge or börge	birg	geborgen
Bersten, to burst.	berstest or (i)	borst or barst	bürste	berste or birste	geborsten
Besinnen, to meditate,	. . . . . .	besann or besonn	besänne or besönne	besinne	besonnen
Besitzen, to possess,	. . . . . .	besasz	besäsze	besitze	besessen
Betrügen, to deceive,	. . . . . .	betrog	betröge	betrüge	betrogen
Bewegen, to induce (when it means move it is regular),	. . . . . .	bewog	bewöge	bewege	bewogen
Biegen, to bend,	. . . . . .	bog	böge	biege	gebogen
Bieten, to offer,	. . . . . .	bot	böte	biete	geboten
Binden, to bind,	. . . . . .	band	bände	binde	gebunden
Bitten, to beg,	. . . . . .	bat	bäte	bitte	gebeten
Blasen, to blow,	bläsest, bläset or bläst,	bliesz	bliese	blase	geblasen
Bleiben, to remain,	. . . . . .	blieb	bliebe	bleibe	geblieben
Bleichen, to lose color (when it means whiten it is regular,	. . . . . .	blich	bliche	bleiche	geblichen
Braten, to roast,	bratest or brätst, bratet or brät,	bratete or briet	brate or (briete)	brat(e)	gebraten
Brechen, to break,	brichst, bricht	brach	bräche	brich	gebrochen
Brennen, to burn,	. . . . . .	brannte	brennete	brenne	gebrannt
Bringen, to bring,	. . . . . .	brachte	brächte	bringe	gebracht
Denken, to think,	. . . . . .	dachte	dächte	denke	gedacht
Dingen, to hire,	. . . . . .	dung	dünge	dinge	gedungen
Dreschen, to thrash,	drischest, drischet or drischt,	drosch or (a)	drösche or (ä)	drisch	gedroschen
Dringen, to press,	. . . . . .	drang	dränge	dringe	gedrungen
Dürfen, to be permitted,	(see bedürfen)	. . . .	. . . . . .	. . . .	gedurft
Einschlafen, to fall asleep,	(see schlafen)	. . . .	. . . . . .	. . . .	eingeschlafen

INFINITIVE.	Present Indicative.	IMPERFECT.		Imperative.	Past Participle.
		Indicative.	Subjunctive.		
Empfangen, to receive,	empfängst, empfängt,	empfing	empfinge	empfang (e)	empfangen
Empfehlen, to recommend,	empfiehlst, empfiehlt	empfahl	empfähle	empfiehl	empfohlen
Empfinden, to feel,	. . . .	empfand	empfände	empfinde	empfunden
Entsprechen, to answer,	entsprichst, entspricht	entsprach	entspräche	entsprich	entsprochen
Erbleichen, to lose color,	(see bleichen)	. . . .	. . . . . .	. . . .	erblichen
Erfrieren, to freeze,	(see frieren)	erfror	. . . . .	. . . .	erfroren
Er, { kiesen, küren, } to choose,	. . . . . .	erkor	erköre	erküre	erkoren
Erlöschen, to become extinct,	erlischest, erlischt	erlosch	erlösche	erlösche (lisch)	erloschen
Ersaufen, to get drowned,	(see saufen)	. . . .	. . . . . .	. . . .	ersoffen
Erschallen, to resound,	. . . .	erscholl	erschölle	erschall (e)	erschollen
Erscheinen, to appear,	(see scheinen)	. . . .	. . . . . .	. . . .	erschienen
Erschrecken, to get frightened,	erschrickst, erschrickt	erschrack	erschräcke	erschrick	erschrocken
Ertrinken, to be drowned,	(see trinken)	. . . .	. . . . . .	. . . .	ertrunken
Erwägen, to consider,	(see wägen)	. . . .	. . . . . .	. . . .	erwogen
Essen, to eat,	issest, isset or iszt	asz	äsze	isz	gegessen
Fahren, to drive,	fährst, fährt	fuhr	führe	fahre	gefahren
Fallen, to fall,	fällst, fällt	fiel	fiele	fall(e)	gefallen
Fangen, to catch,	fängst, fängt	fing	finge	fange	gefangen
Fechten, to fight,	fichst, ficht	focht	föchte	fechte or (i)	gefochten
Finden, to find,	. . . . . .	fand	fände	finde	gefunden
Flechten, to twine,	flichst (flechtest), flicht	flocht	flöchte	flicht	geflochten
Fliegen, to fly,	(fleugst, fleugt, poetical)	flog	flöge	fliege (fleuch)	geflogen
Fliehen, to flee,	(fleuchst, fleucht, poetical)	floh	flöhe	fliehe (fleuch)	geflohen
Flieszen, to flow,	(fleuszest, fleuszt, poetical)	flosz	flösse	fliesze (fleusz)	geflossen
Fragen, to question,	. . . . . .	frug or fragte	früge	frage	gefragt
Fressen, to devour,	frissest, frisset (friszt)	frasz	fräsze	frisz	gefressen
Frieren, to freeze,	. . . . . .	fror	fröre	friere	gefroren
Gähren, to ferment,	. . . .	gohr	göhre	gähre	gegohren
Gebären, to bring forth,	(gebierst, gebiert)	gebar	gebäre	gebäre (gebier)	geboren

INFINITINE.	Present Indicative.	IMPERFECT.		Imperative.	Past Participle.
		Indicative.	Subjunctive.		
Geben, to give,	gibst, gibt	gab	gäbe	gib	gegeben
Gebieten, to command,	(see bieten)	. . . .	. . . . . .	. . .	geboten
Gedeihen, to thrive,	. . . .	gedieh	gediehe	gedeihe	gediehen
Gefallen, to please,	(see fallen)	. .	. . . . . .	. . . .	gefallen
Gehen, to go,	. . . .	ging	ginge	geh(e)	gegangen
Gelingen, to succeed,	. . . .	gelang	gelänge	gelinge	gelungen
Gelten, to be worth,	gilst, gilt	galt	gälte or gölte	gilt	gegolten
Genesen, to recover,	. . . .	genasz	genäsze	genese	genesen
Genieszen, to enjoy,	. . . .	genosz	genösse	geniesz(e)	genossen
Geraten, to fall into,	(see raten)	. . . .	. . . . . .	. . . .	geraten
Geschehen, to happen,	es geschiehet or geschieht	geschah	geschähe	geschehe	geschehen
Gewinnen, to win,	. . . .	gewann	gewänne	gewinne	gewonnen
Gieszen, to pour,	(geuszest, geuszt, poetical)	gosz	gösse	giesz(e)	gegossen
Gleichen, to resemble,	. . . .	glich	gliche	gleiche	geglichen
Gleiszen, to shine, to glisten,	. . . .	glisz	glisse	gliesze	geglissen
Gleiten, to glide,	. . . .	glitt	glitte	gleite	geglitten
Glimmen, to gleam,	. . . .	glomm	glömme	glimme	geglommen
Graben, to dig,	gräbst, gräbt	grub	grübe	grabe	gegraben
Greifen, to gripe,	. . . .	griff	griffe	greif(e)	gegriffen
Haben, to have,	hast, hat	hatte	hätte	habe	gehabt
Halten, to hold,	hältst, hält	hielt	hielte	halt(e)	gehalten
Hangen, to hang,	hängst, hängt	hing	hinge	hange	gehangen
Hauen, to hew,	. . . .	hieb	hiebe	hau(e)	gehauen
Heben, to raise,	. . . .	hob	höbe, or hübe	hebe	gehoben
Heiszen, to call,	. . . .	hiesz	hiesze	heisze	geheiszen
Helfen, to help,	hilfst, hilft	half	hälfe or hülfe	hilf	geholfen
Keifen, to chide,	. . . .	kiff	kiffe	keif(e)	gekiffen
Kennen, to know,	. . . .	kannte	kennete	kenne	gekannt
Klieben, to cleave,	. . . .	klob	klöbe	kliebe	gekloben
Klimmen, to climb,	. . . .	klomm	klömme	klimme	geklommen
Klingen, to sound,	. . . .	klang	klänge	klinge	geklungen
Kneifen, to pinch,	. . . .	kniff	kniffe	kneif(e)	gekniffen
Kommen, to come,	. . . .	kam	käme	komm	gekommen
Können, to be able, can,	kannst, kann	konnte	könnte	none	gekonnt
Kriechen, to creep,	(kreuchst, kreucht,—poetical)	kroch	kröche	krieche	gekrochen
Küren, to choose,	(see erküren)	. . . .	. . . . . .	. . . .	gekoren

INFINITIVE.	Present Indicative.	IMPERFECT. Indicative.	Subjunctive.	Imperative.	Past Participle.
Laden, to load,	(lädst, lädt)	lud	lüde	lade	geladen
Lassen, to let,	lässest, lässet or läszt,	liesz	liesz	lasse or lasz	gelassen
Laufen, to run,	läufst, läuft	lief	liefe	lauf(e)	gelaufen
Leiden, to suffer,	. . . .	litt	litte	leide	gelitten
Leihen, to lend,	. . . .	lieh	liehe	leihe	geliehen
Lesen, to read,	liesest, lieset, liest	las	läse	lies	gelesen
Liegen, to lie,	. . . .	lag	läge	liege	gelegen
Lügen, to lie,	. . . .	log	löge	lüge	gelogen
Mahlen, to grind,	(mählst, mählt)	mahlte	mahlete	mahl(e)	gemahlen
Meiden, to shun,	. . . .	mied	miede	meide	gemieden
Melken, to milk,	(milkst, milkt)	molk	mölke	melke or milk	gemolken
Messen, to measure,	missest, misset, miszt	masz	mäsze	misz	gemessen
Miszfallen, to displease,	(see fallen)	. . . .	. . . . . .	. . . .	miszfallen
Mögen, —may,	mag, magst, mag, subj. möge	mochte	möchte	none	gemocht
Müssen, must,	musz, muszt, musz, subj. müsse	muszte	muszte	none	gemuszt
Nehmen, to take,	nimmst, nimmt	nahm	nähme	nimm	genommen
Nennen, to name,	. . . .	nannte	nennete	nenn(e)	genannt
Pfeifen, to whistle,	. . . .	pfiff	pfiffe	pfeif(e)	gepfiffen
Pflegen, to cherish,	. . . .	pflog	pflöge	pflege	gepflogen
Preisen, to praise,	. . . .	pries	priese	preise	gepriesen
Quellen, to gush,	quillst, quillt	quoll	quölle	quelle or quill	gequollen
Rächen, to avench,	. . . .	räche, roch	rächete or röchete	räche	gerächt or gerochen
Raten, to advise,	rätst, rät	riet	riete	rat(e)	geraten
Reiben, to rub,	. . . .	rieb	riebe	reibe	gerieben
Reiszen, to tear,	. . . .	risz	risse	reisz(e)	gerissen
Reiten, to ride,	. . . .	ritt	ritte	reite	geritten
Rennen, to run,	. . . .	rannte	rennete	renne	gerannt
Riechen, to smell,	. . . .	roch	röche	riech(e)	gerochen
Ringen, to wring,	. . . .	rang	ränge	ringe	gerungen
Rinnen, to run,	. . . .	rann	ränne or rönne	rinne	geronnen
Rufen, to call,	. . . .	rief	riefe	rufe	gerufen
Salzen, to salt,	. . . .	salzte	salzete	salze	gesalzet or gesalzen
Saufen, to drink,	säufst, säuft	soff	söffe	sauf(e)	gesoffen
Saugen, to suck,	. . . .	sog	söge	sauge	gesogen
Schaffen, to create,	. . . .	schuf	schüfe	schaffe	geschaffen
Scheiden, to part,	. . . .	schied	schiede	scheide	geschieden
Scheinen, to appear,	. . . .	schien	schiene	scheine	geschienen

Complete List of Irregular Verbs—*Continued.*

Infinitive.	Present Indicative.	Imperfect.		Imperative.	Past Participle.
		Indicative.	Subjunctive.		
Schelten, to scold,	schiltst, schilt	schalt	schälte or schölt	schilt	gescholten
Scheren, to shear,	schierst, schiert	schor	schöre	schier	geschoren
Schieben, to shove,	. . . . .	schob	schöbe	schieb(e)	geschoben
Schieszen, to shoot,	. . . . . .	schosz	schösse	schiesz(e)	geschossen
Schinden, to flay,	. . . . . .	schund	schünde	schinde	geschunden
Schlafen, to sleep,	schläfst, schläft	schlief	schliefe	schlaf(e)	geschlafen
Schlagen, to strike,	schlägst, schlägt	schlug	schlüge	schlage	geschlagen
Schleichen, to sneak,	. . . . . .	schlich	schliche	schleiche	geschlichen
Schleifen, to whet,	. . . . . .	schliff	schliffe	schleife	geschliffen
Schleiszen, to slit,	. . . . . .	schlisz	schlisse	schleisz(e)	geschlissen
Schliefen, to slip,	(schleufst, schleuft)	schloff	schlöffe	schliefe (schleuf)	geschliffen
Schlieszen, to shut,	. . . . . .	schlosz	schlösse	schliesz(e)	geschlossen
Schlingen, to sling,	. . . . . .	schlang	schlänge	schlinge	geschlungen
Schmeiszen, to smite,	. . . . . .	schmisz	schmisse	schmeisz (e)	geschmissen
Schmelzen, to melt,	(schmilzest, schmilzt)	schmolz	schmölze	schmelze or schmilz	geschmolzen
Schneiden, to cut,	. . . . . .	schnitt	schnitte	schneide	geschnitten
Schnieben, to snuff, to breathe, blow,	. . . . . .	schnob	schnöbe	schniebe	geschnoben
Schrauben, to screw,	. . . . . .	schrob	schröbe	schraube	geschroben
Schreiben, to write,	. . . . . .	schrieb	schriebe	schreibe	geschrieben
Schreien, to cry,	. . . . . .	shrie	shrie	schrei(e)	geschrieen
Schreiten, to stride,	. . . . . .	schritt	schritte	schreite	geschritten
Schwären, to fester,	schwierst, schwiert	schwor	schwöre	schwäre	geschworen
Schweigen, to be silent,	. . . . . .	schwieg	schwiege	schweig (e)	geschwiegen
Schwellen, to swell,	schwillst, schwillt	schwoll	schwölle	schwelle or schwille	geschwollen
Schwimmen, to swim,	. . . . . .	schwamm	schwämme	schwimm (e)	geschwommen
Schwinden, to vanish,	. . . . . .	schwand	schwände	schwinde	geschwunden
Schwingen, to swing,	. . . . . .	schwang	schwänge	schwinge	geschwungen
Schwören, to swear,	. . . . . .	schwor or schwur	schwöre or schwüre	schwör(e)	geschworen
Sehen, to see,	siehst, sieht	sah	sähe	sieh(e)	gesehen
Sein, to be,	bin, bist, ist, sind, seid, sind, subj, sei, seiest, sei	war	wäre	sei	gewesen
Senden, to send,	. . . . . .	sandte	sendete	sende	gesandt or gesendet

INFINITIVE.	Present Indicative.	IMPERFECT.		Imperative.	Past Participle.
		Indicative.	Subjunctive.		
Sieden, to boil,	. . . .	sott	sötte	siede	gesotten
Singen, to sing,	. . . .	sang	sänge	singe	gesungen
Sinken, to sink,	. . . .	sank	sänke	sinke	gesunken
Sinnen, to think,	. . . .	sann	sänne or sönne	sinne	gesonnen
Sitzen, to sit,	. . . .	sasz	säsze	sitze	gesessen
Sollen, shall,	. . . .	sollte	sollte	none	gesollt
Spalten, to split,	. . . .	spaltete	spaltete	spalte	gespalten or gespaltet
Speien, to spit,	. . . .	spie	spie	spei(e)	gespieen
Spinnen, to spin,	. . . .	spönne	späune or spönne	spinne	gesponnen
Spleiszen, to split,	. . . .	spleiszte	splisse	spleisze	gesplissen
Sprechen, to speak,	sprichst, spricht	sprach	spräche	sprich	gesprochen
Sprieszen, to sprout,	. . . .	sprosz	sprösse	spriesz(e)	gesprossen
Springen, to spring,	. . . .	sprang	spränge	springe	gesprungen
Stechen, to prick,	stichst, sticht	stach	stäche	stich	gestochen
Stecken, to stick,	. . . .	stak	stäke	stecke	gesteckt
Stehen, to stand,	. . . .	stand or stund	stände or stünde	steh	gestanden
Stehlen, to steal,	stiehlst, stiehlt	stahl	stähle or stöhle	stiehl	gestohlen
Steigen, to ascend,	. . . .	stieg	stiege	steig(e)	gestiegen
Sterben, to die,	stirbst, stirbt	starb	stärbe or störbe	stirb	gestorben
Stieben, to disperse,	. . . .	stob	stöbe	stieb(e)	gestoben
Stinken, to stink,	. . . .	stank	stänke	stinke	gestunken
Stoszen, to push,	stöszest, stöszt	stiesz	stiesze	stosz(e)	gestoszen
Streichen, to stroke,	. . . .	strich	striche	streich(e)	gestrichen
Streiten, to strive,	. . . .	stritt	stritte	streite	gestritten
Thun, to do,	thue, thust, thut	that	thäte	thu(e)	gethan
Tragen, to carry,	trägst, trägt	trug	trüge	trage	getragen
Treffen, to hit,	triffst, trifft	traf	träfe	triff	getroffen
Treiben, to drive,	. . . .	trieb	triebe	treibe	getrieben
Treten, to tread,	trittst, tritt	trat	träte	tritt	getreten
Triefen, to drip,	. . . .	troff	tröff	triefe	getroffen
Trügen, to deceive,	. . . .	trog	tröge	trüge	getrogen
Trinken, to drink,	. . . .	trank	tränke	trink(e)	getrunken
Verbergen, to conceal,	(see bergen)	. . . .	. . . . . .	. . . .	verborgen
Verbieten, to forbid	(see bieten)	. . . .	. . . . . .	. . . .	verboten
Verbleiben, to remain,	(see bleiben)	. . . .	. . . . . .	. . . .	verblieben
Verbleichen, to lose color,	(see bleichen)	. . . .	. . . . . .	. . . .	verblichen
Verderben, to ruin,	verdirbst, verdirbt	verdarb	verdärbe or verdürbe	verdirb	verdorben

Complete List of Irregular Verbs—*Continued.*

Infinitive.	Present Indicative.	Imperfect.		Imperative.	Past Participle.
		Indicative.	Subjunctive.		
Verdrieszen, to vex,	. . . . . .	es verdrosz	verdrösse	none	verdrossen
Vergessen, to forget,	vergissest, vergiszt	vergasz	vergäsze	vergisz	vergessen
Verhehlen, to hide,	. . . . . .	verhehlte	verhehlete	verhehle	verhehlet, verhohlen
Verlieren, to lose,	. . . . . .	verlor	verlöre	verliere	verloren
Verlischen, Verlöschen, } to become extinct,	(see erlöschen)	. . . .	. . . . .	. . . .	verloschen
Verschwinden, to disappear,	(see schwinden)	. . . .	. . . . .	. . . .	verschwunden
Verwirren, to entangle,	. . . . . .	verworr	verwörre	verwirr	verworren
Verzeihen, to pardon,	. . . . . .	verzieh	verziehe	verzeih	verziehen
Wachsen, to grow,	wächsest, wächst	wuchs	wüchse	wachse	gewachsen
Waschen, to wash,	wäschest, wäscht	wusch	wüsche	wasche	gewaschen
Wägen, Wiegen, } to weigh,	. . . . . .	wog	wöge	wäge or wiege	gewogen
Weben, to weave (to move is regular,	. . . . . .	wob	. . . . .	. . . .	gewoben
Weichen, to yield,	. . . . . .	wich	wiche	weiche	gewichen
Weisen, to show,	. . . . . .	wies	wiese	weise	gewiesen
Wenden, to turn,	. . . . . .	wandte or wandt or wendete	wendete	wende	gewandt or gewendet
Werben, to sue, to recruit,	wirbst, wirbt	warb	wärbe	wirb	geworben
Werden, to become,	wirst, wird	ward or wurde	würde	werde	geworden
Werfen, to throw,	wirfst, wirft	warf	wärfe or würfe	wirf	geworfen
Winden, to wind,	. . . . . .	wand	wände	winde	gewunden
Wissen, to know,	weisz, weiszt, weisz	wuszte	wüszte	wisse	gewuszt
Wollen, to will,	will, willst, will	wollte	wollte	none	gewollt
Zeihen, to accuse,	. . . . . .	zieh	ziehe	ziehe	geziehen
Ziehen, to draw,	(zeuchst, zeucht, — poetical)	zog	zöge	zieh(e) or (zeuch)	gezogen
Zwingen, to force,	. . . . . .	zwang	zwänge	zwinge	gezwungen

INDEX

OF

GERMAN WORDS AND MEDICAL TERMS.

(197)

I.

J.

K.

(221)

L.

M.

N.

Qu.

R.

S.

T.

W.

Z.

INDEX

OF

ENGLISH WORDS AND MEDICAL TERMS.

17

B.

E.

G.

H.

I.

19

N.

O.

P.

QU.

R.

S.

U.

V.

W.

X

Y

Z

In its issue of August 3d, 1893, the *Independent, New York*, speaks of the *second* edition thus: "This is a second edition revised and enlarged generally. The chief change is the introduction throughout the work of the new *Official Orthography* adopted by the German governments and now in general use in Germany. The *excellent practical* features noticed by us in the first edition are preserved in this, while it has gained both in fullness and systematic arrangement. The rules and tabulations are worked out in a clean and simple manner. Needless matter is cut away and nothing retained which will in any way retard the student's progress or confuse his mind. The success of the first edition has been sufficient to show the practical usefulness of the work."

The *Public Ledger* of Philadelphia, in one of its recent issues, in regard to the second edition, says: "This book comprises a grammar, reader and dictionary in one volume. Dr. Losch is a distinguished and successful teacher here in Philadelphia of his native language, and has applied his scientific training to developing a good manual for the rich and flexible *Deutsche Sprache*. As all doctors now who wish to keep up with the sciences must be able to read German, it is not surprising that many of the numerous testimonials to the ease and pleasure derived from Losch's system come from medical practitioners. German students, however, of merely literary or linguistic ambitions, will find in Losch's book a competent and comprehensive guide. His methods are without confusion, and his declensions and conjugations lead directly to the insight of structural German. The chief change to be noted in this edition is the use throughout the book of the new official orthography adopted by the German governments and in general use throughout Germany."

Rev. Dr. John S. Stahr, President of Franklin and Marshall College, Lancaster, Pa., says: "I have examined Dr. Henry Losch's 'Improved Method and Complete Manual for the Study of the German Language' with some care, and I am ready to say that I am well pleased with it. The arrangement of the matter, the copious exercises and selections, and the skillful exhibition of the principles of Syntax make it a valuable aid to the study of this noble language. This single volume, well mastered, will serve to give the learner a very fair knowledge of the language, not only in theory, but also in practice."

Rev. P. F. Fogarty, of Tamaqua, Pa., says: "I regard this Grammar as a most excellent treatise on the subject."

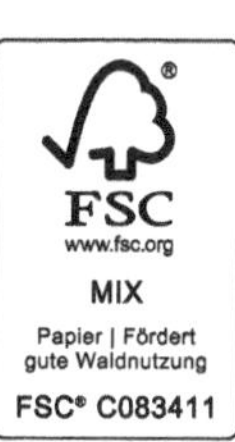

Zeitfracht Medien GmbH
Ferdinand-Jühlke-Straße 7
99095 Erfurt, Deutschland
produktsicherheit@kolibri360.de